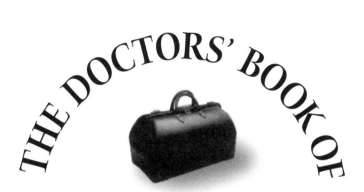

THE DOCTORS' BOOK OF
SYMPTOMS
and
TREATMENTS

YOUR GUIDE TO ACHES, PAINS, AND OTHER PHYSICAL PROBLEMS; ILLNESSES; MEDICAL TESTS; AND SURGERIES

THE EDITORS OF CONSUMER GUIDE™
with Northwestern University Medical School
& Gary J. Martin, M.D.

PUBLICATIONS INTERNATIONAL, LTD.

Louis Weber, CEO
Publications International, Ltd.
7373 North Cicero Avenue
Lincolnwood, Illinois 60712

Permission is never granted for commercial purposes.

Manufactured in U.S.A.

8 7 6 5 4 3 2 1

ISBN: 0-7853-2594-8

Note: Neither the Editors of Consumer Guide® and Publications International, Ltd., nor the authors, consultants, editors, or publisher take responsibility for any possible consequences from any treatment, procedure, exercise, dietary modification, action, or application of medication or preparation by any person reading or following the information in this book. The publication of this book does not constitute the practice of medicine, and this book does not attempt to replace your physician or your pharmacist. Before undertaking any course of treatment, the authors, consultants, editors, and publisher advise the reader to check with a physician or other health care provider.

CONSULTANTS

Northwestern University Medical School is located in Chicago, Illinois. The missions of the Northwestern University Medical School are education, research, and professional services, a major component of the latter being the delivery of high-quality patient care. The Medical School supports the overall mission of the University to achieve excellence in its scholarly and service programs and to participate in its framework for distinction. The provision of excellent medical education that builds on the foundation provided by the core academic disciplines is of the highest priority. The Medical School seeks to provide leadership in scientific discovery, intellectual inquiry and creativity, and innovative performance. Through its teaching, research, and professional service, the Medical School strives to achieve a leadership position in shaping health and research policy by encouraging faculty, staff, and student involvement at local and national levels.

Northwestern Medical Faculty Foundation is a premier multispecialty medical group consisting of health care professionals who are full-time faculty in the clinical departments of Northwestern University Medical School. The faculty members, jointly with a professional staff of administrative and clinical support personnel, are committed to providing exemplary medical care to patients in a sensitive and service-oriented environment. It is the Foundation's mission to support the teaching and research functions of the Northwestern University Medical School through a commitment to the Medical School's goals and objectives. Further, it is the Foundation's mission to create a health care delivery system in which innovation in patient care services, sound practice management techniques, and responsible allocation of resources are used to create an environment in which health care professionals can be educated and prepared for a changing health care environment and society's future medical needs. Within this environment, it is the Foundation's mission to support and facilitate the evolution of scientific endeavors from the laboratory to the direct delivery of patient care.

Gary J. Martin M.D., is Chief of the Division of General Internal Medicine at Northwestern University Medical School. He is an associate professor and is board certified in Internal Medicine and Cardiovascular Disease. He has provided primary care since 1984 as a member of the Northwestern Medical Faculty Foundation and as an attending physician at Northwestern Memorial Hospital of Chicago.

CONTRIBUTORS

Martin J. Arron, M.D.
General Internal Medicine

Mark K. Bowen, M.D.
Orthopedics

Michelle Baer, M.D.
Obstetrics and Gynecology

Steven Brem, M.D.
Neurosurgery

Jennifer A. Bierman, M.D.
General Internal Medicine

Wade Bushman, M.D., Ph.D.
Urology

CONTRIBUTORS *continued*

David Conley, M.D.
Otolaryngology

Thomas Corbridge, M.D.
Pulmonary Medicine

Therese A. Denecke, M.S., R.N.,
C.S., F.N.P.
Primary Care Nursing

Albert L. Ehle, M.D.
Neurology

Robert S. Feder, M.D.
Ophthalmology

David Fishman, M.D.
Gynecologic Oncology

Marilynn C. Frederiksen, M.D.
Obstetrics and Gynecology

William Friedrich, D.D.S.
Dentistry

Luther Gaston, M.D.
Obstetrics and Gynecology

Darren R. Gitelman, M.D.
Neurology

William J. Gradishar, M.D.
Medical Oncology

Zoran M. Grujic, M.D.
Neurology

Michael Haak, M.D.
Orthopedics

Nanci Fink Levine, M.D.
Obstetrics and Gynecology

John R. Lurain III, M.D.
Gynecologic Oncology

Michael T. Margolis, M.D.
Gynecology

Helen Gartner Martin, M.D.
Sleep Disorders and Pulmonary Medicine

Tacoma McKnight, M.D.
Obstetrics and Gynecology

Patricia Naughton, M.D.
Obstetrics and Gynecology

Gary A. Noskin, M.D.
Infectious Diseases

Harold J. Pelzer, M.D., D.D.S.
Otolaryngology

Robert V. Rege, M.D.
Surgery and Surgical Critical Care

Douglas Reifler, M.D.
General Internal Medicine

Jack M. Rozental, M.D., Ph.D.
Neurology

Frank R. Schmid, M.D.
Rheumatology

Arvydas D. Vanagunas, M.D.
Gastroenterology

Sybilann Williams, M.D.
Gynecologic Oncology

David T. Woodley, M.D.
Dermatology

CONTENTS

INTRODUCTION · 6

You can make the most effective use of this book when you understand how it is organized. Take a moment to read about our cross-referencing method.

SYMPTOMS · 7

This section discusses, in alphabetical order, a variety of physical problems, such as cough and headache, and their possible causes and treatments. Whether your symptoms are mild or severe, these profiles will help you understand why you may have them and what you can do about them.

ILLNESSES · 74

From AIDS to varicose veins, this section covers dozens of conditions and illnesses. Organized alphabetically, the profiles include possible causes, symptoms, and treatments.

TESTS AND SURGERIES · 279

When you're faced with taking a medical test or having a surgical procedure, you want to know what to expect. This section covers the most common tests and surgeries, with detailed explanations of the procedures, pre- and post-procedure care, complications and risks, and recovery. Profiles are arranged alphabetically.

INDEX · 386

INTRODUCTION

Everyone suffers from headaches, bellyaches, and an assortment of aches, pains, and other physical problems from time to time. Most of them are minor, transient problems of no great significance. Nevertheless, questions inevitably arise. Should you call the doctor? Could the symptom mean something serious? Is an over-the-counter medication appropriate?

Symptoms and Treatments will give you quick answers to many of your questions. Whether the problem is as innocent as a stuffy nose or as serious as colon cancer, in the following pages you'll get the facts about causes, symptoms, treatment options, complications, tests, surgical procedures, and even prevention tips. Armed with this information, you'll be able to take better care of yourself and to ask more precise questions at the doctor's office.

This book is divided into three sections: Symptoms, Illnesses, and Tests and Surgeries. The profiles are arranged alphabetically in each section and contain cross references to other profiles of related interest. You can easily identify the cross references because they are printed in SMALL CAPITAL LETTERS. For instance, when reading the profile on chest pain, you will find ANGINA mentioned under the section on possible causes. Since ANGINA is printed in small capital letters, you know that you can find a profile on it in the Illnesses section of the book. The profile on chest pain also mentions ANGIOPLASTY as a possible treatment. Since it is printed in small capital letters, you'll know that you can find a profile on that procedure in the Tests and Surgeries section of the book.

These days, it's more important than ever to be an informed health care consumer. *Symptoms and Treatments* can help you understand your symptoms and illnesses and assess the benefits and risks of treatments. This knowledge is the first step toward obtaining the highest quality health care.

SYMPTOMS

ABDOMINAL PAIN

There are many causes of abdominal pain, and it is one of the most frequent reasons patients seek medical attention or advice.

Most causes of abdominal pain are not dangerous and need little, if any, investigation. Some features, however, that point to more serious causes include abdominal pain

- That is constant and prolonged (over two hours)
- Associated with persistent VOMITING
- Associated with a high FEVER (over 101°F)
- That is sudden and awakens the patient
- Made worse by movement, coughing, or sneezing

CAUSES

The causes of abdominal pain range from the very common (GASTROENTERITIS, IRRITABLE BOWEL SYNDROME, and indigestion) to the less frequent (appendicitis, GALLSTONES, ULCER, PANCREATITIS, and DIVERTICULAR DISEASE) to the uncommon (aortic ANEURYSM and INTESTINAL OBSTRUCTION).

APPROACH

The patient's MEDICAL HISTORY provides the clue to the cause of abdominal pain in many instances. Pain made better or worse by eating may point to ULCER or PANCREATITIS. Pain that diminishes with bowel movements suggests IRRITABLE BOWEL SYNDROME or narrowing of the large intestine. Pain associated with VOMITING may suggest an INTESTINAL OBSTRUCTION. Women are prone to gynecologic causes of abdominal pain, and a menstrual history may be helpful.

The location of the pain and the way it radiates are important features. For example, ULCER pain is typically pinpointed just below the end of the breast bone, while pain caused by PANCREATITIS or GALLSTONES frequently starts above the belly button and travels straight into the back.

Laboratory tests may include evaluation of the BLOOD COUNT or other BLOOD TESTS. If the MEDICAL HISTORY or PHYSICAL EXAMINATION indicates serious problems, X rays (RADIOGRAPHY) of the stomach and intestine, COMPUTED TOMOGRAPHY, ULTRASOUND, or ENDOSCOPY may be in order.

TREATMENT OPTIONS

If the pain is severe, prolonged, or associated with the dangerous symptoms listed above, it is best to avoid solid food. The patient may take clear liquids, if tolerated, and should seek medical attention.

ABDOMINAL SWELLING

Although usually an insignificant symptom, many illnesses can be signaled by abdominal swelling. If the abdominal swelling is prolonged and visibly obvious to others, this symptom could represent serious medical problems.

CAUSES

The intestine itself lacks typical pain receptors, and when the wall of the intestine is minimally stimulated or stretched, patients may experience the subjective symptom of distension without any objective evidence of it. This is very common in patients with IRRITABLE BOWEL SYNDROME whose intestinal nerve receptors may have a lower threshold for sensing intestinal action.

Fluid accumulation within the abdomen can also cause abdominal swelling. Fluid accumulation can result from various causes such as

- CONGESTIVE HEART FAILURE
- Cirrhosis of the liver
- Nephrotic syndrome of the kidney including KIDNEY FAILURE
- Intra-abdominal cancer (especially OVARIAN CANCER in women)

INTESTINAL OBSTRUCTION from many causes may also result in this symptom, but is typically accompanied by ABDOMINAL PAIN and VOMITING.

APPROACH

The PHYSICAL EXAMINATION will frequently detect any serious cause for abdominal swelling. At times, ULTRASOUND probing or COMPUTED TOMOGRAPHY of the abdomen may be done to rule out the more potentially dangerous causes of abdominal swelling.

TREATMENT OPTIONS

Minor dietary modifications such as restricting dairy products and reducing fat content may help some patients with benign abdominal swelling (see IRRITABLE BOWEL SYNDROME).

More serious underlying conditions such as various forms of cancer or cirrhosis of the liver must be treated by a physician immediately.

Many people feel some abdominal swelling, or distension, after a meal. In this situation, however, the symptom does not have a serious medical cause or consequence.

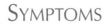

ANKLE SWELLING

> Ankle swelling is an example of a symptom that directly affects only one area of the body but indicates possible systemic problems.

The term *swollen ankles* includes any visibly apparent increase in size or puffiness in the lower legs. It is a sign of excess fluid pooling in the lower legs, called *edema*.

CAUSES

The most common cause of ankle swelling is V<small>ARICOSE VEINS</small>. Less commonly, ankle swelling can be caused by an injury such as a sprain or bone damage.

Less common but more serious causes include

- Thrombophlebitis
- C<small>ONGESTIVE HEART FAILURE</small>
- Nephrotic syndrome—damage to the filtering function of the kidneys (see K<small>IDNEY FAILURE</small>)
- Liver damage that causes decreased protein production and fluid retention

APPROACH

Clues from an individual's M<small>EDICAL HISTORY</small> include any known heart, kidney, or liver disease or any symptoms related to those organs, especially if swelling is associated with B<small>REATHING DIFFICULTY</small>. Without shortness of breath and with fluid retention limited to the leg, V<small>ARICOSE VEINS</small> would be the most common explanation.

A P<small>HYSICAL EXAMINATION</small> might focus on the neck veins and signs of fluid retention in other parts of the body, with close attention to any bone tenderness.

Diagnostic tests might include blood flow studies of the leg to look for blood clots (U<small>LTRASOUND</small>), X rays of the bones (R<small>ADIOGRAPHY</small>) if an injury is suspected, or B<small>LOOD TESTS</small> to assess kidney and liver function. Tests of cardiac function include echocardiography (U<small>LTRASOUND</small>).

TREATMENT OPTIONS

Treatment of the underlying condition should, in general, alleviate ankle swelling; however, general measures to treat the symptom include

- Elevation of the leg above the level of the heart
- Elastic stockings that prevent blood and fluid from pooling in the lower leg
- Diuretics such as hydrochlorothizaide or furosemide to control severe edema, although their use is rare

APPETITE, LOSS OF

The symptom of appetite loss, or anorexia, by itself has limited diagnostic significance. The degree of anorexia, however, does provide a useful index of the severity of many diseases.

CAUSES

Loss of appetite is quite common to a large number of debilitating diseases, but if it is the only symptom, it has very limited diagnostic value. Many people with chronic diseases such as MULTIPLE SCLEROSIS, CROHN DISEASE, RHEUMATOID ARTHRITIS, and AIDS can lose their appetite. Stress, anxiety, and DEPRESSION are certainly frequent contributors to a loss of appetite. If the anorexia persists and is *not* accompanied by WEIGHT LOSS, it is less likely to be related to an illness.

Anorexia can be the first sign of infectious HEPATITIS, even preceding yellowing of the skin. Cancers of various types, including STOMACH CANCER and PANCREATIC CANCER, can cause loss of appetite and progressive WEIGHT LOSS.

Anorexia nervosa is a psychophysiologic condition usually occurring in women and girls; it is characterized by refusal of food, fear of becoming obese, distorted sense of body image, and MENSTRUAL IRREGULARITIES.

APPROACH

Loss of appetite deserves investigation if it is protracted and is accompanied by WEIGHT LOSS. Stress, anxiety, and DEPRESSION are very common causes, and their presence may be explanation enough for the symptom. A general PHYSICAL EXAMINATION will help determine whether diagnostic testing is necessary. BLOOD TESTS, including a BLOOD COUNT, test of thyroid function, and screening chemistries, provide a good picture of general health and can be an effective screen for any serious illness responsible for the anorexia.

TREATMENT OPTIONS

Treatment should be directed at the underlying cause of the loss of appetite. Pharmacologic appetite stimulants, as a general rule, are not very effective and carry some risk, although agents such as megestrol acetate are useful in some patients with chronic debilitating illnesses such as AIDS and cancer.

> The medical term for loss of appetite is *anorexia*. This symptom can be caused by a number of illnesses or may result from a psychological problem.

BACKACHE

Backache is a common symptom that may affect as many as 20 percent of all Americans at any given time. There is a 90 percent lifetime chance that one will have an episode of back pain at some time.

Although back pain frequently strikes after lifting or straining, it may also occur without an obvious cause. Most back pain episodes improve or resolve within about six weeks.

CAUSES

The vast majority of backaches occur because of overuse. Heavy lifting or repetitive twisting and turning activities may contribute to backache.

Inflammatory conditions such as RHEUMATOID ARTHRITIS, systemic LUPUS ERYTHEMATOSUS, and others may also cause backache. And backache is a primary symptom of ankylosing spondylitis—a condition that affects a very small population, mostly men.

OSTEOPOROSIS may cause a localized compression fracture in the spine, causing pain.

Tumors and infections of the spine, all of which can cause back pain, are very rare.

Kidney infection can also cause back pain.

In rare instances, sudden severe back pain may be caused by the rupture of an aortic ANEURYSM.

APPROACH

The course of the backache is an important feature; for example, if it started with an injury or overuse episode, other causes can be ruled out. The PHYSICAL EXAMINATION will be directed toward the muscles, range of motion, and response to stresses on the spine. The doctor will also be interested in any sensation or reflex changes in the lower extremities.

More involved diagnostic studies, such as RADIOGRAPHY, COMPUTED TOMOGRAPHY, and MAGNETIC RESONANCE IMAGING are useful in only a small number of cases.

TREATMENT OPTIONS

The initial treatment for backache usually can be self-directed. Rest and over-the-counter analgesics such as aspirin, acetaminophen, or ibuprofen are usually all that is required. Persistent pain may benefit from treatment with prescription medicines and some exercises or physical therapy. In rare cases, LUMBAR DISK REMOVAL surgery may be needed for a persistently problematic HERNIATED DISK.

BOWEL CONTROL, LOSS OF

An isolated episode of fecal incontinence is not an uncommon experience and should not be a source of major concern. Recurrent episodes of fecal incontinence, however, are abnormal and require medical evaluation.

Bowel control involves five aspects; they are
- The ability to sense stool filling the rectum
- The ability to distinguish the nature of rectal contents (gas, liquid, or solid)
- The ability of the rectum and large bowel to store feces for variable periods of time
- The ability of valves (rectal sphincters) to open and close in a controlled fashion
- The ability of the pelvic muscles to maintain the rectum at a sharp angle in the abdomen, retarding the passage of stool by mechanical means

Disruption of any of these mechanisms can cause fecal incontinence.

CAUSES

An isolated instance of fecal incontinence can usually be attributed to stress, sensitivity to food, or an acute episode of DIARRHEA. Prolonged or recurrent fecal incontinence, however, may have multiple causes that are related to several general categories, including
- Functional impairment or decreased mental capacity, including any severe, chronic, debilitating illness in which a patient is bedridden
- Decreased capacity of the rectum as a result of a tumor (COLORECTAL CANCER), surgical resection of part of the intestine, or aging
- Decreased rectal sensation because of DIABETES or stool impaction (see INTESTINAL OBSTRUCTION)
- Damaged rectal sphincters or damage to the nerves that control their function such as unrecognized trauma from vaginal delivery in women, spinal cord problems, or laxity of pelvic muscles with aging

APPROACH

Isolated episodes of fecal incontinence, although obviously distressing to the patient, may not require extensive evaluation. A PHYSICAL EXAMINATION would involve a digital examination of the rectal sphincter and a test of the sensation

Fecal incontinence is rare in young people; it occurs more often in older patients.

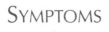
around the rectum to determine if stool impaction (see INTESTINAL OBSTRUCTION), local inflammation, or nerve damage is the cause.

Repeated episodes of fecal incontinence would be evaluated by several measures, including

- Sigmoidoscopy or colonoscopy (see ENDOSCOPY) to assess the capacity of the rectum and reveal any obstruction or inflammation
- A barium X ray (RADIOGRAPHY) of the colon
- In complicated cases, tests of rectal sphincter and nerve function or tests of anorectal motility, which involve placing a small balloon in the rectum

At times, X-ray studies (RADIOGRAPHY) of rectal function called *defecography* or *proctography* may be done by placing small amounts of barium within the rectum and recording the process of defecation.

TREATMENT OPTIONS

If fecal incontinence is related to stool impaction (see INTESTINAL OBSTRUCTION), the impaction needs to be evacuated with cleansing enemas, and the physician may implement a treatment program for chronic CONSTIPATION. In other circumstances, a variety of therapeutic options may be employed depending on the underlying cause of fecal incontinence.

Other options that may help with a fecal incontinence problem include

- Bowel training programs
- Biofeedback techniques
- Pharmacologic agents (such as psyllium to increase the bulk of the stool)
- Surgical procedures

Except for incontinence related to obvious prolapse of the rectum, in which the rectum drops out through the anus, surgery should be employed only after nonsurgical methods have failed.

BREAST PAIN OR LUMPS

Women of all ages can have breast pain or lumps. About one in ten women will get BREAST CANCER at some time in their life, usually between the ages of 50 and 70. Ninety percent of women, therefore, will never get BREAST CANCER. It is important to remember that there are many other causes of breast symptoms, and most are not serious.

CAUSES

Breast pain and tenderness can be caused by
- FIBROCYSTIC BREAST DISEASE
- Benign tumors
- BREAST CANCER
- Infection such as mastitis or an abscess
- Tenderness from hormones related to pregnancy, estrogen replacement therapy, birth control pills, or premenstrual syndrome

APPROACH

The MEDICAL HISTORY and PHYSICAL EXAMINATION will focus on caffeine intake, risk factors for BREAST CANCER, signs of infection such as FEVER, cellulitis near the nipple, and any recent use of medication. The examination will help distinguish a cyst from a more suspicious lump. A follow-up examination in one month or at a different time in the woman's cycle may also be useful.

Persistent or suspicious lumps generally need to undergo a BIOPSY. Mammogram (RADIOGRAPHY) and ULTRASOUND may be helpful, but mammography misses about ten percent of BREAST CANCER, so BIOPSY remains necessary.

TREATMENT OPTIONS

Decreasing caffeine and increasing vitamin E intake to 400 to 800 IU per day seems to help many women with pain from FIBROCYSTIC BREAST DISEASE.

Most women immediately think of cancer when they find a lump in the breast or have breast pain. But usually something else is the cause. It is still very important, however, to investigate these symptoms.

BREATHING DIFFICULTY

A majority of people with breathing difficulties adopt an increasingly inactive lifestyle which can, in many cases, aggravate their condition.

Breathing is normally not a conscious activity, except during exercise. A number of medical conditions alter this state, so that breathing is noticeable with minimal or no activity. Such conscious or labored breathing is often described as air hunger or shortness of breath. The medical term is *dyspnea*.

CAUSES

The most obvious and most common causes of breathing difficulties are lung conditions such as

- ASTHMA
- Chronic bronchitis (BRONCHITIS, CHRONIC)
- EMPHYSEMA
- PNEUMONIA

When lung conditions are the cause, other respiratory symptoms such as wheeze, COUGH, sputum production, and chest pain may be present.

A number of nonlung conditions cause dyspnea as well, but they are usually accompanied by other symptoms. For example:

- CONGESTIVE HEART FAILURE results in episodes of shortness of breath that cause sleep problems and ANKLE SWELLING.
- Severe ANEMIA is often accompanied by pale-colored nail beds and conjunctiva (the lining of the eyelids).
- Neuromuscular weakness may cause generalized weakness or specific coordination problems such as difficulty rising from a chair or SWALLOWING DIFFICULTIES.
- Anxiety and hyperventilation are suspected in patients with certain personality traits and no other evidence of disease.

It should be noted that most dyspneic patients minimize their sense of breathlessness by adopting an increasingly sedentary lifestyle. This lack of any regular physical exercise results in general deconditioning and possibly overweight or sore throat, all of which can further aggravate the sense of shortness of breath.

APPROACH

A physician will first take a careful MEDICAL HISTORY and perform a PHYSICAL EXAMINATION. However, more extensive testing is often needed to confirm the cause of dyspnea. Testing can include

- Chest X ray (RADIOGRAPHY)
- PULMONARY FUNCTION TESTING
- Arterial blood gas analysis (BLOOD TESTS)
- Complete BLOOD COUNT

If the diagnosis is not apparent after these tests, further information may be gathered with a formal exercise test, which is useful to distinguish between lung and nonlung causes of breathlessness, and echocardiography (ULTRASOUND) to assess cardiac function.

TREATMENT OPTIONS

Dyspnea is most effectively treated by addressing the underlying medical condition. For example:

- In patients with lung disease, such as EMPHYSEMA, treatment should be aimed at improving lung function.
- In patients with CONGESTIVE HEART FAILURE, drugs such as digoxin, furosemide, or enalapril should be prescribed to improve heart function, thus decreasing breathing problems.
- In patients with ANEMIA, the red BLOOD COUNT should be restored by nutritional supplementation after the underlying cause of the ANEMIA is determined.

BRUISING, UNEXPLAINED

Unexplained bruising of the skin can be insignificant, or it can be a sign of a blood or bone marrow disorder. A sudden onset of unexplained bruising should be evaluated to determine the cause.

A bruise is nothing more than blood under the skin. If blood leaks out of a blood vessel for any reason, a bruise forms. It may be red, yellow, orange, or blue. Blue usually indicates a deeper bruise. The color is caused by the blood pigment, hemoglobin, reflected through skin tissue.

CAUSES

The most common cause of a bruise is blunt trauma to the skin, causing an opening in one of the skin blood vessels. Even after an insect bite, the injured vessel may leak into the skin and cause a bruise. People who have accumulated a lot of sunlight over a lifetime tend to have fragile skin blood vessels. They will notice very easy bruising in sunlight-exposed areas, such as the forearms. In these individuals, bruises often form just from normal pressure on the skin, without any injury or trauma.

A severe vitamin C deficiency can cause easy bruising. The classic sign of this deficiency, called *scurvy*, is a little bruise with a corkscrew-shaped hair rising from the bruise. Scurvy is very rare today.

When injured, the blood vessels should clot. If a problem exists with the elements in the blood that clot the vessels, the result may be thin blood that does not clot well and readily seeps out of the skin blood vessels, causing a bruise with even minor trauma. Possible causes include

- LEUKEMIA
- A defect in one of the clotting elements of the blood, particularly the platelets (thrombocytopenia)
- A problem with the bone marrow (which makes blood elements and cells) such as that caused by chemotherapy, alcohol, or insecticides.

If a person takes a lot of aspirin or another nonsteroidal anti-inflammatory drug such as ibuprofen, the platelets in the blood do not clot properly and the person may bruise easily. In addition, patients who take systemic corticosteroid medications such as prednisone often have thin skin and bruise easily.

The sudden onset of small red bruises on the lower legs and feet or on the forearms and wrists in conjunction with FEVER and general illness must be taken very seriously. These symptoms may indicate an acute life-threatening infection such as Rocky Mountain spotted fever or spinal meningitis. Viral illness, drug allergies, and connective tissue diseases such as systemic LUPUS ERYTHEMATOSUS are other serious conditions in which the skin blood vessels become inflamed and leak blood, causing small bruises.

APPROACH

Often, a MEDICAL HISTORY combined with a PHYSICAL EXAMINATION can indicate the cause of the bruising problem. For example, sun-induced bruising is very common in middle-aged and elderly people, particularly those with fair complexions. The appearance of bruises on sun-exposed areas of the body usually makes this diagnosis self-evident. The physician may inquire about any medications the patient is taking, such as aspirin, ibuprofen, or prednisone.

The sudden onset of generalized bruising or bruising after an activity in which such bruising usually does not occur (such as water skiing, light exercise, rowing, jumping, and so on) dictates a careful examination by a physician. In addition, laboratory tests should be done to evaluate the clotting elements in the blood and to make sure that the bone marrow is producing the right amounts of blood cells and platelets (see BLOOD TESTS; BLOOD COUNT).

The sudden onset of small bruises over the arms, hands, lower legs, and feet in association with FEVER and generalized illness must be considered a serious infection or vasculitis until proved otherwise. BLOOD TESTS (white BLOOD COUNT, bacterial CULTURE) may be taken to evaluate whether the patient has an infection. To determine the possibility of vasculitis, the physician will ask about any recent illnesses and medications. To diagnose vasculitis, BLOOD TESTS and a BIOPSY of the skin are often necessary.

TREATMENT OPTIONS

When bruising stems from a serious condition such as LEUKEMIA, bone marrow disorders, systemic infection, or vasculitis, the treatment depends upon the cause. For simple, benign causes of bruising (use of aspirin, ibuprofen, corticosteroids, or other medications), the treatment is stopping the medication if possible. Sometimes use of these medications is necessary, and the patient must learn to live with some easy bruising of the skin. For easy bruising due to the accumulation of sunlight and perhaps other types of light over a lifetime, the only effective treatment is keeping the skin covered.

CHEST PAIN

Although many people associate chest pain with heart attack, this symptom is not always a sign of life-threatening illness. Many conditions—some very mild—can cause discomfort in the chest.

Sudden severe chest discomfort is a potentially ominous symptom; it should be considered an emergency that requires rapid evaluation by a medical professional. Milder, recurrent, episodic chest discomfort, however, can be evaluated more leisurely in the setting of an office visit.

CAUSES

Common causes of chest pain include
- Muscle or ligament strain in the chest wall
- Gastrointestinal problems such as inflammation of the esophagus, peptic ulcer disease (see ULCER), upper colon problems, and heartburn
- Psychological problems such as anxiety, DEPRESSION, or panic attacks
- Heart and lung problems such as pleurisy, pericarditis, and ANGINA (the most common cardiac cause)

HEART ATTACK (called *myocardial infarction*), tears in the aorta sometimes associated with ANEURYSM, and PULMONARY EMBOLISM are among the life-threatening causes.

APPROACH

Severe sudden chest pain needs to be evaluated rapidly with a careful MEDICAL HISTORY, PHYSICAL EXAMINATION, ELECTROCARDIOGRAPHY, and often a chest X ray (RADIOGRAPHY) to ascertain whether the symptom is being caused by a life-threatening condition. Characteristics of the pain can be important clues. Some questions might include
- What brings on the pain—effort, cold wind, swallowing, changes in position?
- What makes the pain go away—antacids, rest, changes in position?
- What is associated with the pain—BREATHING DIFFICULTY, nausea?
- What is the nature of the pain—burning, pressure, or sharp pain?

Tests that may be useful include
- ELECTROCARDIOGRAPHY
- BLOOD PRESSURE TESTING
- X ray (RADIOGRAPHY) of the chest and stomach
- Treadmill tests (CARDIAC STRESS TEST)
- Exploration of psychosocial stressors and other clues to anxiety or DEPRESSION

COUGH

In general, cough protects the lung by forcefully eliminating harmful elements from the tracheobronchial tree. It is a vital mechanism to clear foreign material (as when food "goes down the wrong pipe"), pus (as in PNEUMONIA), and excess mucus (as in ASTHMA and chronic bronchitis [BRONCHITIS, CHRONIC]). On the other hand, cough that does not produce mucus—a dry cough—may not be of obvious benefit.

All of us experience cough during upper respiratory tract infections such as the common cold. Cough in this setting may last for several weeks, but it invariably goes away on its own. Cough that is present for more than a month is distinctly unusual and suggests another medical condition.

> Coughing is a common symptom that rarely signifies a serious problem, but a cough that continues for months or years invariably disrupts life, resulting in fatigue, sleep problems, and isolation.

CAUSES

The most common causes of cough include
- Cigarette smoking (chronic smoker's cough)
- Air pollution
- Postnasal drip (see NOSE, STUFFY OR RUNNY)
- ASTHMA
- Gastroesophageal reflux (heartburn)
- EMPHYSEMA
- Chronic bronchitis (BRONCHITIS, CHRONIC)
- Cystic fibrosis
- Upper respiratory tract infections such as the common cold or INFLUENZA
- Head and neck cancer, such as LARYNGEAL CANCER
- LUNG CANCER
- Bronchiectasis (abnormal dilation of the bronchial tree leading to collection of mucus)
- CONGESTIVE HEART FAILURE
- Anxiety
- Pulmonary fibrosis or scarring
- PNEUMONIA
- Tuberculosis
- Some medications such as ACE inhibitors (enalapril or captopril) commonly used in HYPERTENSION

APPROACH

The single most important factor in patients with chronic cough is whether or not they smoke. The cough can be eliminated about 50 percent of the time if a smoker completely stops smoking.

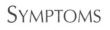

Another significant factor is whether the cough is productive of mucus or whether it is dry. Productive cough is seen in conditions such as chronic bronchitis (BRONCHITIS, CHRONIC) and bronchiectasis, whereas chronic dry cough or minimally productive cough may be seen in chronic postnasal drip, ASTHMA, heartburn, or drug-induced cough.

Routine tests to establish the cause of cough include

- Chest or sinus X rays (RADIOGRAPHY)
- PULMONARY FUNCTION TESTING
- A provocative test when ASTHMA is suspected (but not proved by routine PULMONARY FUNCTION TESTING)
- Monitoring of esophageal acidity or radiographic studies (RADIOGRAPHY) when heartburn is suspected

TREATMENT OPTIONS

The most effective treatment for cough is treatment of the underlying condition. For example:

- For cough associated with the common cold, expectorants are useful to loosen thick sputum that is difficult to clear.
- For dry cough, cough suppressants may be tried; increasing water intake decreases the sense of throat tickle in many cases.
- For cough associated with smoking, complete cessation of smoking is the only effective treatment.
- For chronic productive cough related to chronic bronchitis (BRONCHITIS, CHRONIC) and EMPHYSEMA, smoking cessation combined with bronchodilator medications such as theophylline or albuterol improves cough.
- For productive cough, cough suppressants and antihistamines are best avoided as these medications will interfere with mucus clearance.
- For a dry or minimally productive cough in non-smokers with a normal chest X ray (RADIOGRAPHY), speech therapy techniques and specific breathing techniques are extremely helpful to decrease unnecessary throat clearing and cough. Such techniques are preferable to cough suppressant medications, which are generally quite disappointing for these patients

DIARRHEA

Diarrhea is the passage of large volumes of unformed or liquid stool. It is not just the frequency of the stool, but the volume passed that determines whether a patient has diarrhea. Physicians define diarrhea as a volume of stool greater than 200 grams (approximately six ounces) in a 24-hour period. Some patients may have the urge to defecate frequently, but unless the stool is unformed and the volume large enough, it does not constitute diarrhea.

> Diarrhea is a very common symptom and is usually not a sign of serious illness; it most commonly resolves after a few days.

CAUSES

Diarrhea is most frequently a self-limited illness of three or four days and is usually caused by an infection. The most common infection is caused by a virus such as rotavirus or Norwalk agent virus, but bacteria such as *Salmonella*, *Shigella*, *Campylobacter*, and toxigenic *Escherichia coli* (the cause of "traveler's diarrhea") are also culprits.

Dietary causes of diarrhea are also very common but tend to last 24 hours or less and include overindulgence in rich food, lactose intolerance, and food poisoning. Overuse of artificially sweetened foods, candies, or soft drinks may also induce diarrhea.

Various medications (prescription and over-the-counter) such as antacids and antibiotics are also very common causes of diarrhea.

Diarrhea that lasts more than three or four weeks may be caused by a large variety of diseases, including chronic PAN-CREATITIS, sprue (a rare sensitivity to wheat protein), and bacterial overgrowth that causes diarrhea by interfering with intestinal absorption of nutrients.

Recurrent diarrhea can also be a sign of IRRITABLE BOWEL SYNDROME.

APPROACH

Most diarrhea is self-limited, runs its course in several days, and does not need evaluation. However, investigation by a physician is warranted if the patient experiences
- Diarrhea that lasts more than four weeks
- High FEVER (higher than 101°F)
- ABDOMINAL PAIN
- Diarrhea that awakens one from a good sleep
- RECTAL BLEEDING

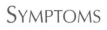
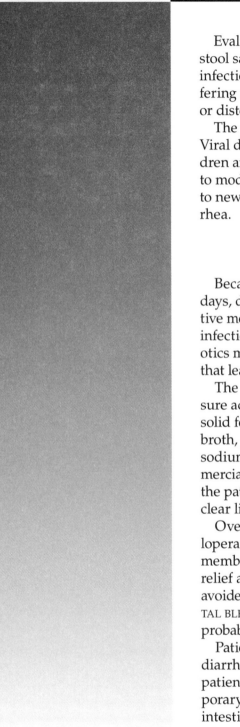

Evaluation includes a PHYSICAL EXAMINATION and possibly a stool sample to determine if the patient has a serious bacterial infection. The physician focuses on whether the patient is suffering from DEHYDRATION and whether the abdomen is tender or distended (see ABDOMINAL PAIN; ABDOMINAL SWELLING).

The patient's recent history may provide important clues. Viral diarrhea, for example, may start in infants or young children and then spread through the family. Travel (even travel to modern and industrialized areas) may expose the patient to new bacteria or viruses, and certain foods may induce diarrhea.

TREATMENT OPTIONS

Because most cases of diarrhea run their course in several days, direct treatment is often not needed. There is no effective medication for the most common cause of diarrhea—viral infection—and it remains quite controversial whether antibiotics make any major difference even in bacterial infections that lead to diarrhea.

The most important way to prevent complications is to insure adequate hydration. This can be achieved by limiting solid food and maintaining a diet of clear liquids (soft drinks, broth, juices, and water) supplemented by some source of sodium such as crackers. Liquid supplements are also commercially available but are not always needed, especially if the patient can maintain hydration through the liberal use of clear liquids (two quarts or more in a 24-hour period).

Over-the-counter medications to slow diarrhea such as loperamide can be used with discretion, but it must be remembered that these agents provide only some symptomatic relief and do not cure diarrhea. These agents should be avoided if there is substantial ABDOMINAL PAIN, FEVER, or RECTAL BLEEDING. Agents such as pectin that absorb water are probably safe, but their benefits are questionable.

Patients can resume their normal diets once the volume of diarrhea has decreased and their appetite returns. In some patients, consumption of dairy products may produce a temporary relapse because the diarrheal illness has depleted the intestine of the enzyme (lactase) that helps with the digestion of milk.

DIZZINESS

Doctors find it useful to divide dizziness into four categories:

- *Light-headedness* is a mild sensation that represents about one-third of all people who see the doctor for dizziness.
- *Vertigo* is a more intense spinning sensation; it represents another one-third of cases.
- *Dysequilibrium* involves unsteadiness, balance problems, or stumbling; it represents about one-fifth of cases.
- *Presyncope* is an episode of near FAINTING OR FAINTNESS; it represents only a few percent of cases.

CAUSES

As a general rule, light-headedness is associated with anxiety, DEPRESSION, panic attacks, or stress-related problems.

Vertigo is usually caused by an inner-ear problem or a problem in a related portion of the brain. The body uses minute changes in position in the inner ear as a balancing device, hence these structures are suspect in cases of vertigo.

Dysequilibrium, or unsteadiness, can be caused by a number of problems with the body's sensory systems. These include problems with the nerves in the legs that help tell the brain the exact position of the ground. Vision problems (for example, CATARACTS) can also cause unsteadiness as can problems with the balance centers of the brain and inner ear.

Presyncope, or near-fainting spells, are usually caused by low blood pressure. Most commonly, low blood pressure is related to problems with the tone of the blood vessels and the nervous system reflexes responsible for maintaining adequate blood pressure when standing up. Less often, presyncope is related to heart rhythm irregularities (ARRHYTHMIAS). Actual FAINTING OR FAINTNESS and its causes are discussed elsewhere.

APPROACH

Other symptoms associated with dizziness can be a clue to the underlying cause.

- Changes in hearing or a ringing in the ears (EAR, RINGING OR BUZZING) when combined with vertigo-like dizziness suggest the inner ear or the nerves in that area might be involved.

People use the word dizziness to describe a number of different feelings. These feelings can range from brief light-headedness to a near fainting spell. Dizziness is not usually serious, but on rare occasion it can be caused by problems that should not be ignored.

- Vomiting and headache combined with dizziness can be signs of serious problems with the nervous system.
- Dizziness associated with certain types of head movements may be clues to inner-ear problems or problems with the circulation to the brain.
- Dizziness associated with arm or leg weakness; numbness in the arm, leg, or face; difficulty talking; vision disturbances; or clumsiness may all be clues to a circulation problem in the brain such as a transient ischemic attack (see stroke).

Besides asking questions about related symptoms such as the ones mentioned above, the doctor may perform standing blood pressure tests and some blood tests and may also listen to the heartbeat.

To examine the nervous system, the doctor may want to observe walking and certain head motions. A hearing test may also be needed. Depending on the initial results, more involved tests of the nervous system may be required, including magnetic resonance imaging, computed tomography, and electroencephalography.

Treatment Options

Treatment of dizziness involves treating the underlying cause. The two most common types of vertigolike dizziness are benign positional vertigo and labyrinthitis (an inflammation of the inner ear). These problems are usually treated with the drug meclizine. Problems associated with low blood pressure can be treated with certain drugs to raise the blood pressure, such as fludrocortisone, or drugs to treat the arrhythmia causing the problem, such as procainamide, atenolol, and digoxin. For patients with dysequilibrium, correcting vision problems is sometimes the answer.

If the problem is persistent and has no apparent cause, certain exercises are sometimes useful in suppressing the feeling of vertigo. Using assisted walking devices such as canes or walkers can also be helpful. Stress reduction techniques and treatment for anxiety or depression help many patients with light-headedness.

In rare cases, surgery could be required for some of the inner-ear and brain-stem problems that cause dizziness.

EAR, RINGING OR BUZZING

Tinnitus is the name for a noise that is heard in one or both ears without any obvious external stimulus. It may be described as a ringing, buzzing, or even hissing. The pitch and intensity vary among individuals. Tinnitus can be present without any obvious cause, but is usually a symptom of another illness. Therefore, all patients with tinnitus should be evaluated by a physician.

CAUSES

It is thought that the source of tinnitus is the hair cells that conduct hearing. The damaged hair cells in the inner ear send an abnormal signal to the brain that is interpreted as tinnitus.

Tinnitus is frequently caused by medications, including over-the-counter drugs. The most common medications that can cause tinnitus are aspirin, ibuprofen, and medications for RHEUMATOID ARTHRITIS such as hydroxychloroquine.

A variety of ear-related problems can cause tinnitus. Frequently, processes involving the middle ear can cause ringing. These include fluid or infections in the middle ear, eustachian tube dysfunction (inability to clear or pop one's ear), or disorders of the middle-ear bones.

Tinnitus can also be caused by inner ear disorders. One of the more common is Meniere disease. This disease usually has a triad of symptoms including tinnitus, fluctuating hearing loss, and vertigo (DIZZINESS). Some systemic illnesses may affect the inner ear, too. These include inflammatory or infectious illnesses such as labyrinthitis.

Unfortunately, tinnitus can be associated with more severe illnesses. Patients whose tinnitus can be heard by others may have a vascular tumor affecting the ear. This type of tinnitus is usually pulsatile in nature and is heard with every heartbeat. It is frequently accompanied by a hearing loss. Tinnitus that affects only one ear that also has a hearing loss can be a sign of a problem involving the hearing nerve or the brain stem. There are tumors known as acoustic neuromas that can cause this scenario. Fortunately, these tumors are uncommon and benign.

If the tinnitus is associated with weakness, VISION DISTURBANCES, and incoordination, the possibility of a transient ischemic attack should be considered (see STROKE).

Trauma that causes a concussion or damage to the ear drum can also provoke tinnitus.

A ringing or buzzing in the ear is a symptom frequently associated with hearing loss. All patients who experience it should have a hearing test.

APPROACH

The evaluation of this symptom would start with a MEDICAL HISTORY focusing especially on recent medication use, past illnesses, and possibly any acoustically traumatic events. Other associated symptoms, such as DIZZINESS or hearing loss, may help narrow the possibilities. A hearing test and an examination of the ear in question with an otoscope (a device for looking in the ear canal) are also usually performed. A general PHYSICAL EXAMINATION, particularly a neurologic examination of the head, is helpful.

More extensive tests may be necessary depending on the suspected diagnosis. MAGNETIC RESONANCE IMAGING of the head may be done to locate structural problems in the ear or tumors that affect hearing. A BLOOD COUNT to rule out ANEMIA and blood flow studies (ULTRASOUND) to test the circulation to the brain may also be appropriate.

TREATMENT OPTIONS

There are a number of medications that may be of some benefit. They include several antidepressant medications such as amitriptyline, anti-anxiety medications such as diazepam, diuretics such as hydrochlorothiazide, and steroids such as prednisone.

For people with moderate to severe hearing loss, a hearing aid can sometimes help. The increased sound delivered to the ear through the hearing aid can help make the tinnitus less noticeable.

There are also devices that produce white noise to help mask the tinnitus. Such a device can be worn in the ear, or a larger one can be placed in the patient's environment. The results with these devices, however, have not been encouraging.

Many patients join support groups usually sponsored through the American Tinnitus Association. This association provides continuing education through seminars and newsletters. In some severe cases, patients are referred for psychiatric counseling. There are many individuals who have stressors in life that can make the tinnitus worse, and counseling may be an option for them. Biofeedback has also been used with some success.

EARACHE

Although commonly thought of as a problem that affects children, earaches can and do occur in people of all ages. In an effort to identify the cause of and best treatment for this symptom, careful evaluation of the ear and its anatomy is essential.

CAUSES

Common causes of earache include
- Middle-ear infections
- Ear-canal infections (swimmer's ear)
- Swelling of the lymph glands in the area
- External ear infections
- Disturbances of the joint of the jaw (temporo-mandibular disorder)

Less common causes of ear pain include
- Infections of the mastoid bone behind the ear (mastoiditis)
- Foreign bodies in the external ear canal
- Tonsillitis
- Herpes zoster infections (SHINGLES) of the nerve pathway around the ear
- Pressure-related injury (called *barotrauma*) to the eardrum
- Wax impactions

APPROACH

The history of the symptom, including the onset, duration, character, specific location, and intensity of the earache, is very important in identifying the cause.

Intense pain in the ear followed by rapid resolution and purulent discharge from the ear suggests a middle-ear infection with subsequent perforation of the eardrum. Viral infections of the middle ear usually accompany or immediately follow an upper respiratory tract infection such as the common cold or INFLUENZA.

Earache associated with chewing suggests temporomandibular disorder or an infection of the external areas of the ear.

Earache is a common complaint that prompts many visits to doctors' offices and emergency departments.

Pain behind the ear in an individual who has experienced recurrent ear infections for a long time suggests infection of the mastoid bone (mastoiditis). This type of radiating pain can also be a sign that the pain is being referred from another area such as infected tonsils (tonsillitis). A vague or intense pain around the ear can herald the eruption of a herpes zoster rash (SHINGLES).

People who swim regularly may develop an infection of the external ear canal, so a history of recent swimming can be a diagnostic clue. Recent airline travel may also be a clue; airline travel is associated with pressure injuries. An acute onset of pain and a diminished sense of hearing after swimming, showering, or attempting to clean one's ears could be evidence of an earwax blockage in the external canal.

Most of the above conditions can be quickly diagnosed by a physician who takes the relevant MEDICAL HISTORY and inspects the ear. During an examination of the ear, the physician will probably look in the ear canal with a special device called an *otoscope* and may feel the surrounding structures for clues as to the exact location of the pain.

Occasionally, a specialist in ear, nose, and throat medicine (an otolaryngologist) may be needed to perform more thorough or complex diagnostic evaluations.

TREATMENT OPTIONS

Treatment of earache involves addressing the underlying cause:

- Bacterial infections of the middle and external ear necessitate antibiotic therapy with amoxicillin, trimethoprim, or sulfamethoxazole.
- Viral infections may require antiviral therapy (acyclovir for herpes zoster infection) and therapy, such as decongestant medication, aimed at relieving specific aspects of the symptom.
- Wax impactions or the presence of foreign matter in the ear canal requires removal of the offending material.

EYE PAIN

Eye pain can be characterized in three ways. A patient may complain of
- A foreign body sensation—irritation, scratchiness, a sandy sensation, or a stinging feeling—like something is in the eye
- Aching or deep discomfort, like a toothache or dull pressure
- ITCHING

CAUSES

A foreign body sensation nearly always feels like something is indeed in the eye. More often than not, there is no foreign body. However, some activities, such as standing or walking out in the wind, working under a car, or grinding metal, can increase the likelihood that a foreign body is responsible for the sensation.

This type of discomfort can also be the first symptom of an eye infection, conjunctivitis, or corneal ulcers. Contact lens wearers at risk for infections involving the front tissue of the eye should immediately remove the contact lens from the affected eye.

Chronic dry eye or corneal abrasion are examples of noninfectious causes of foreign body sensation.

Aching discomfort is often a symptom of deeper inflammation of the eye. However, this symptom may occur in patients who need glasses but choose not to wear them. It can also occur in patients prone to crossed or wall eyes.

Eye pain can also be caused by head or neck problems away from the eye such as
- Tooth decay
- Abnormal jaw function (temporomandibular disorder)
- Sinus disease
- RHEUMATOID ARTHRITIS of the neck.

Pain that occurs away from the true source is called *referred pain*. Infections or inflammations within the eye or the eye socket (such as blepharitis) and sudden elevations in the inner fluid pressure of the eye (GLAUCOMA) can cause this type of discomfort.

ITCHING is usually associated with allergy. This can be a drug allergy, hay fever, a reaction to makeup, or a reaction to some other environmental stimulus.

Eye pain ranges from minor irritation to achiness to stinging. Although it usually indicates a problem with the eye itself, it can also be associated with conditions elsewhere in the body.

APPROACH

Persistent pain, especially in the presence of redness or VISION DISTURBANCES, should prompt a call to the ophthalmologist. The eye doctor will ask several questions, such as

- What was happening when the pain began?
- Was the onset of pain sudden or gradual, and how long has it lasted?
- Has it ever occurred before?
- Is the pain constant or intermittent?
- Is it severe or mild, and is the intensity changing?
- Are there associated eye problems such as redness, light sensitivity, VISION DISTURBANCES, or eye discharge?
- Was the eye injured in any way?
- Are there any significant past medical or eye problems?

A foreign body sensation must be carefully evaluated by a doctor. The affected eye needs to be inspected for the presence of a foreign particle; this includes flipping the upper lid to look for a hidden foreign body.

TREATMENT OPTIONS

Avoiding the allergen or causal substance will prevent the release of the chemicals in the eye responsible for the symptoms. Cold compresses made by soaking a wash cloth in cold tap water should be held over the closed eyes for a few minutes several times each day for symptomatic relief.

Unless the symptom is quite mild, a physician and possibly an ophthalmologist should be consulted. An eye examination may be necessary to determine the best course of action. While aspirin or acetaminophen may help reduce pain from any cause, the best solution is to uncover the source of the problem and address it.

FAINTING OR FAINTNESS

Fainting or faintness (known medically as *syncope*) is not usually the sign of a major problem. Most people will feel faintness from simply standing up too quickly after squatting or lying down. Less often, fainting or faintness is a sign of a serious disease.

CAUSES

Fainting is generally caused by the body's inability to maintain adequate blood pressure in the brain, thus depriving the brain of oxygen and leading to a loss of consciousness. This inadequate blood pressure can be caused by something as simple as standing for extended periods.

Less common causes include
- Seizures
- Heart rhythm abnormalities (ARRHYTHMIAS) or pumping problems
- Low blood sugar levels
- Low blood oxygen levels
- Specific physical situations that interfere with brain circulation (for example, coughing)

In approximately one-fourth of all cases, no exact cause is ever determined despite reasonable efforts.

APPROACH

Clues that may indicate the underlying cause of fainting or faintness include
- The position of the individual at the time of the episode (for example, getting up from bed)
- The activity the individual was engaged in (for example, straining physical work)
- The general situation (for example, standing in a hot, stuffy, crowded room)
- Any specific provocation (for example, the sight of blood or a large needle)

A further investigation into an episode of fainting would include consideration of any associated symptoms such as
- Weakness in the arm
- BREATHING DIFFICULTY
- Nausea
- CHEST PAIN
- Seizures

The feeling of almost passing out is a common experience. About one third of healthy young people report having had at least one episode of faintness.

A MEDICAL HISTORY of underlying heart disease and the use of medications that commonly affect blood pressure or heart rhythm may also help with the diagnosis. Certain drugs used to treat hypertension that may be pertinent include

- Hydrochlorothiazide
- Captopril
- Atenolol
- Nifedipine

Psychotropic drugs may also be of interest. These include

- Amitriptyline
- Chlorpromazine

A PHYSICAL EXAMINATION would focus on BLOOD PRESSURE TESTING while lying down and then while standing for at least two minutes. The physician may also check neurologic function and the arteries in the neck and heart, depending on what the underlying cause is suspected to be.

Additional tests are usually not necessary, but may include

- ELECTROCARDIOGRAPHY
- Various BLOOD TESTS
- Tilt-table testing

TREATMENT OPTIONS

Most fainting spells are isolated events, but they do warrant the review of a physician. Recurrent episodes are treated based on the underlying cause. For example, fainting caused by inadequate blood pressure when standing may be treated with elastic stockings that keep blood from pooling in the legs, a high-salt diet to increase blood pressure, or drugs such as fludrocortisone.

FATIGUE

Fatigue is discomfort or loss of efficiency experienced after physical or mental activity. It is distinct from weakness, which is a loss of power or strength, and from sleepiness, which is a difficulty or inability to stay awake.

When fatigue lasts for more than a few months, it is classified as chronic. Chronic fatigue is an exceedingly common symptom. It is one of the top ten reasons adults seek medical attention.

CAUSES

A wide range of illnesses and circumstances can cause chronic fatigue, including

- Psychological conditions such as DEPRESSION, anxiety, bereavement, and stress
- Excessive use of caffeine, alcohol, sedatives, or illicit drugs
- Some prescription drugs such as atenolol and methyldopa used to treat HYPERTENSION
- Disorders that interfere with sleep such as irregular nighttime breathing, called *sleep apnea* and restless leg syndrome, called *nocturnal myoclonus*
- Illnesses that affect the major body systems or organs such as the heart, lungs, kidneys, liver, blood, and nervous system
- Chronic infections, particularly viral HEPATITIS and certain forms of tuberculosis

The chronic fatigue syndrome is a well-publicized, rare cause of unremitting fatigue. It is 50 to 100 times less common than any other cause of chronic fatigue. In a significant minority of patients, a cause of the fatigue is never identified despite an extensive medical and psychological evaluation.

APPROACH

In some cases, the illness inducing the fatigue is readily apparent, but if not, the investigation into the symptom usually begins with a discussion of possible related symptoms. For example, if the fatigue is accompanied by BREATHING DIFFICULTY during exertion, heart and lung problems may be sus-

As many as one-quarter of the people seeing their primary care physician have fatigue of sufficient severity that it significantly compromises their ability to meet their daily responsibilities and to enjoy life.

pected; sleepiness, loud snoring, and HEADACHE may indicate a sleep disorder.

Given that psychological disorders are exceedingly common causes of fatigue, an inquiry into an individual's mood, intellectual functioning, and stress level is important. Referral to a mental health professional may be helpful.

A complete MEDICAL HISTORY may uncover clues from the health of other family members or from recent use of prescription or nonprescription drugs. Although the results of a PHYSICAL EXAMINATION are usually normal, in some cases it can reveal an underlying illness.

More sophisticated diagnostic tests are usually reserved until a specific cause is suspected. However, if no illness or cause can be suspected from the MEDICAL HISTORY and PHYSICAL EXAMINATION, further investigation may include BLOOD TESTS to assess the patient's

- BLOOD COUNT
- Liver function
- Kidney function
- Pancreas function
- Thyroid function

TREATMENT OPTIONS

Therapy is, of course, aimed at treating the underlying disease. However, even when a specific cause is not identified, symptoms can usually be minimized by therapies that are designed to

- Enhance sleep
- Improve physical fitness
- Maintain mental health

FEVER

Fever is usually a sign of infection and is most often self-limited. Low-grade fever (that is, a fever less than 100.5°F) is commonplace with upper respiratory infections such as the COMMON COLD. Higher temperatures (10l°F to 104°F) are seen with flulike illness (INFLUENZA). The associated symptoms are the main determining factor in deciding about further diagnostic tests or specific treatment.

CAUSES

Viral illnesses are a common cause of fever. Examples include
- Common cold
- INFLUENZA
- HEPATITIS
- Viral meningitis
- AIDS
- Mononucleosis

Bacterial illnesses that can cause a fever include
- PNEUMONIA
- Bacterial meningitis
- Otitis (ear infection)
- Sinusitis
- Urinary tract infection (BLADDER INFECTION)
- PELVIC INFLAMMATORY DISEASE
- Appendicitis
- Lyme disease
- Toxic shock syndrome
- Tuberculosis
- BLOOD POISONING
- Endocarditis

Fever can be a symptom of some forms of cancer, including
- HODGKIN DISEASE
- LEUKEMIA
- Lymphoma (LYMPHOMA, NON-HODGKIN)

Autoimmune diseases that can cause fever include
- LUPUS ERYTHEMATOSUS
- Sarcoidosis
- CROHN DISEASE
- Scleroderma

Parasitic diseases such as malaria and amebiasis also cause fever.

Fever that persists for days, is very high (104°F or higher), or is associated with other worrisome symptoms requires medical evaluation.

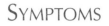
APPROACH

A MEDICAL HISTORY and PHYSICAL EXAMINATION will usually provide sufficient clues to make a diagnosis. CULTURES of the blood, urine, sputum, or spinal fluid (see LUMBAR PUNCTURE) may be necessary in some cases.

The most useful clues leading to a diagnosis include

- Any RASH or bruising (BRUISING, UNEXPLAINED) on the skin or mucous membranes of the mouth
- COUGH or BREATHING DIFFICULTY
- HEADACHE
- Nausea, VOMITING, or DIARRHEA
- Swollen glands
- Any localized pain
- Night sweats (SWEATING, EXCESSIVE)
- Bladder or pelvic symptoms such as pain during urination (URINATION, PAINFUL) and urethral or VAGINAL DISCHARGE;
- Painful testes (TESTICLES, PAINFUL OR SWOLLEN)

TREATMENT OPTIONS

For self-limited viral infections, treatments may include

- Acetaminophen or ibuprofen (aspirin is to be avoided in children and young adults)
- Antibiotics for specific bacterial or parasitic infections
- Adequate fluids to replace the loss from perspiration

For any persistent fever, a diagnosis should be sought so that specific treatment can be given for the underlying cause.

HALLUCINATIONS

Hallucinations are false sensory perceptions. They can involve vision, hearing, or, occasionally, touch and feeling. In some instances, the hallucinating individual is aware that the perceptions are not real, but in other cases, the hallucinations are perceived as being real. When hallucinations occur as part of mental illness, there are usually other behavioral and thought disturbances that accompany them, and the hallucinations are typically voices.

CAUSES

Drugs and psychiatric illness are the most common causes of hallucinations. Drugs—including alcohol, prescription drugs, and especially illicit psychedelic drugs (LSD, psilocybin, and mescaline)—can produce all types of hallucinations.

Less commonly, the symptom can be produced by brain diseases such as
- STROKE
- Transient ischemic attack
- Tumor
- Seizures such as those in epilepsy

APPROACH

Evaluation of the patient with hallucinations includes
- A MEDICAL HISTORY, in which the onset and nature of the hallucinations are determined, as are any other problems that preceded or appear to be related to their onset, such as drug and alcohol use
- A PHYSICAL EXAMINATION, which usually focuses on mental and neurologic function as well as any evidence of systemic illness
- Laboratory tests, the nature and extent of which are determined by the initial clinical examination and commonly include BLOOD TESTS and URINALYSIS
- Psychiatric evaluation for patients who appear to have no physical cause for their hallucinations

TREATMENT OPTIONS

Treatment is determined by the cause. Drugs such as haloperidol, risperidone, and thioridazine can be very effective in psychiatric causes and can also counteract hallucinations produced by other drugs.

Hallucinations can be symptoms of serious disease, but more often, they have a simple cause.

HEADACHE

There are many different types of headaches, but they can roughly be divided into two categories: 1) those that are not dangerous or not associated with a dangerous disease or condition; and 2) those that require immediate medical attention. Fortunately, the vast majority of headaches are trivial and fall into the former category.

CAUSES

Benign headaches have a variety of causes, and although they can be very unpleasant, they are usually self-limiting to some degree. The most common causes are
- Muscle tension
- Eye strain
- Mild viral infection such as the common cold or INFLUENZA
- Stress, anxiety, or mild DEPRESSION
- Dental pain such as a toothache
- MIGRAINE HEADACHE
- Caffeine withdrawal
- HYPERTENSION
- Side effects of some medications such as fluoxetine, nitroglycerin, antihypertensive drugs such as nifedipine, and bronchodilator drugs such as theophylline
- Minor trauma to the head

Less common are headaches that are caused by very serious problems:
- The "thunderclap" headache—the sudden onset of intense head pain—could be caused by a ruptured ANEURYSM.
- Headache associated with FEVER, malaise (general feeling of being unwell), confusion, and NECK PAIN could be caused by meningitis (inflammation of the membrane surrounding the brain and spinal cord).
- Headache after a head cold associated with FEVER, malaise, and purulent nasal discharge could be caused by acute sinusitis.
- Headache associated with low-grade FEVER, malaise, muscle pain, and a loss of appetite (APPETITE, LOSS OF) in patients older than 50 could be caused by an inflammation of the arteries called *temporal arteritis.*
- Headache associated with nausea and VOMITING, weakness on one side of the body, NUMBNESS,

seizures, speech difficulty, SWALLOWING DIFFICULTIES, VISION DISTURBANCES, HALLUCINATIONS, or personality changes could be caused by a brain tumor or a clot in the brain (hematoma).

APPROACH

The physician will probably begin with a detailed medical history focusing on medication use, previous illness, and family medical history. The nature of and symptoms associated with the headache are also crucial. Important aspects include

- How long they have been occurring
- Whether they have changed over time
- Their frequency
- Their duration
- Whether they have a distinct location
- Whether they are preceded by specific symptoms such as vision disturbances or nausea (see MIGRAINE HEADACHE)
- Their character
- What makes them worse or better

A complete PHYSICAL EXAMINATION is usually performed with special attention paid to the cranial nerves, which give function and sensation to the head, and the blood vessels in the head and neck. BLOOD TESTS and an eye examination (visual acuity test) may provide more clues. More complex diagnostic tests may include

- MAGNETIC RESONANCE IMAGING of the head and neck
- Angiography (a form of RADIOGRAPHY used to image blood vessels)
- ELECTROENCEPHALOGRAPHY

TREATMENT OPTIONS

Treatment, of course, depends on the underlying cause of the headaches. Most benign headaches respond to pain killers, either over-the-counter varieties (such as aspirin, acetaminophen, and ibuprofen) or prescription (for example, mild narcotics such as codeine). Stress headaches can sometimes be treated by removing the stressor or by learning stress-reduction techniques. MIGRAINE HEADACHES can sometimes be prevented with medical treatment.

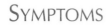

ITCHING

> Itching is common and most often due to a benign condition.

Itching is a symptom that is related to a mild pain but is perceived differently. Scratching probably helps relieve itching by overstimulating the area to the point where the nerve impulses from the skin to the brain are no longer felt. People tend to itch and scratch more in the evenings and around bedtime when other external stimuli are lessened and the itching is more noticeable.

CAUSES

There are many internal and external causes of this symptom, including

- Any common skin disease, such as PSORIASIS or DERMATITIS
- A topical agent that irritates the skin or to which a person is allergic, such as poison ivy resin, a perfume, a type of clothing, or a cosmetic
- A product that a person has used for many years without a problem, which suddenly becomes a source of itching
- Dry skin, very common in the middle-aged and elderly, which can result from the use of hot water, frequent bathing, and the generous use of soaps and detergents
- A complex of conditions consisting of easily irritable skin, hay fever, ASTHMA, and frank periods of skin DERMATITIS
- A number of diseases of the internal organs such as chronic KIDNEY FAILURE or primary biliary cirrhosis
- A high red blood-cell count (see BLOOD COUNT) due either to genetics or to chronic lung diseases, which causes itching especially when one is getting out of a hot shower
- Reaction to certain medications such as hydrochlorothiazide
- An underlying malignancy, especially lymphoma (see LYMPHOMA, NON-HODGKIN), although this is rare

APPROACH

A MEDICAL HISTORY of childhood or other skin diseases, ASTHMA or hay fever, and systemic diseases is taken. A list of current medications is compiled along with a critical evaluation of the need for these medications. Then a determination is made as to whether the onset of the itching corresponded to the onset of the use of one or more of the current medications. The types of personal soaps, fragrances, moisturizing creams, fabric softeners, laundry powders, and bathing habits may give clues to the cause of itching. The habit of frequently bathing with harsh soaps and hot water suggests that dry skin is the culprit.

PHYSICAL EXAMINATION of the skin is necessary, and skin conditions such as DERMATITIS are directly viewed. When skin dries out, it may exhibit a patchy DERMATITIS (redness with scale). A localized scaly red patch on the feet, soles, groin, or flank may suggest a fungal infection that often itches. In this case, the scale must be scraped and examined for fungi.

When no obvious cause for the itching can be ascertained and when it is persistent, the physician will search for an underlying cause. This evaluation will include a chest X ray (RADIOGRAPHY), evaluation of the BLOOD COUNT, and examination of certain biochemical elements associated with blood, kidney, and liver disease (see BLOOD TESTS). When lymphoma (LYMPHOMA, NON-HODGKIN) limited to the skin is considered, a skin BIOPSY must be obtained for microscopic examination. If possible, medication should be discontinued to see if the itching improves or abates.

TREATMENT OPTIONS

- Avoiding frequent bathing, hot water, and harsh soaps
- Using topical agents that bring moisture back to the skin
- Soaking in a tub without soap and then applying these topical agents immediately after soaking
- The use of antihistamines such as diphenhydramine or hydroxyzine
- Avoiding wool or polyester fabrics and potentially irritating topical preparations such as fragrances, harsh body soaps, cosmetics, and astringents
- Treating any underlying skin disease or systemic disease
- Specific therapy for itching due to certain internal diseases (Patients with severe kidney disease may need to have their itching treated with ultraviolet light treatments.)

MEMORY PROBLEMS

Nearly everyone notices changes in memory as they get older, but not all components of memory are affected by the aging process.

Mild changes in memory function do occur as people age, but these changes should not substantially interfere with performance. Some changes, though, are signs of other problems.

From a practical point of view, what people notice as they age is particular difficulty remembering names, the need for additional repetitions to learn new items, and some degree of randomness to the memory errors they make (that is, items are not consistently forgotten). When the memory system is affected by actual disease, there is a more consistent inability to recall items, and repetition of material is less and less effective in improving memory performance. Progressive decline in memory eventually attacks old knowledge—which is usually minimally affected by the aging process—and performance deteriorates in most, if not all, daily activities.

CAUSES

There are many factors that affect memory processes. Even in healthy people, the decreased attentiveness that can accompany lack of sleep or moderate illness may be enough to cause apparent difficulties in memory performance. However, performance usually returns to normal when the offending factor resolves.

Drug intoxicants can cause varying degrees of memory problems. Prescription drugs that can cause subtle deficits in attention or metabolic processes involved in memory include

- Sedatives such as lorazepam and triazolam
- Psychoactive drugs such as antidepressants or major tranquilizers
- Diuretics such as hydrochlorothiazide and furosemide
- Steroid hormones such as prednisone

Chemical intoxicants other than medications can also affect memory and attention functions. These substances include

- Alcohol
- Volatile agents or gases such as toluene and carbon monoxide
- Illicit drugs
- Heavy metals such as lead, arsenic, and mercury

Systemic disorders affecting the body in general can interfere with memory. These disorders include

- Cardiovascular disorders such as CONGESTIVE HEART FAILURE

- Pulmonary disorders such as EMPHYSEMA
- Renal (kidney) disorders such as KIDNEY FAILURE
- Hepatic (liver) disorders such as cirrhosis
- Endocrine (glandular) disorders such as Cushing syndrome, HYPOTHYROIDISM, and HYPERTHYROIDISM
- Certain cancers such as small-cell LUNG CANCER
- Deficiencies of vitamin B_{12} or thiamin
- Infections that cause FEVER, particularly in the elderly

Environmental agents or situations can cause disorientation and apparent memory problems. These include

- Hospitalization
- Isolation
- Absence of day and night cues

Finally, brain disorders can directly affect memory areas. These disorders include

- Degenerative disorders such as ALZHEIMER DISEASE and PARKINSON DISEASE
- Vascular diseases of the brain such as ATHEROSCLEROSIS, ANEURYSM, and STROKE
- Trauma such as concussion
- Brain infections such as meningitis, encephalitis, and syphilis
- Brain tumors
- Severe epilepsy

APPROACH

Diagnosis of memory disorders almost always begins with a detailed MEDICAL HISTORY and a PHYSICAL EXAMINATION, including a complete neurologic and mental status assessment. Mental status examination is a detailed review of various cognitive functions to check performance of attention, memory, language, visual-spatial function, abstract reasoning, insight, behavior, and judgment.

BLOOD TESTS can be useful to check for metabolic disturbances, systemic infections, and nutrient deficiencies.

Further tests, performed only when unusual features have been detected on earlier examination, can include

- ELECTROENCEPHALOGRAPHY
- COMPUTED TOMOGRAPHY
- MAGNETIC RESONANCE IMAGING
- LUMBAR PUNCTURE

MENSTRUAL IRREGULARITIES

Menstruation is not always a perfectly predictable process, and many irregularities in the cycle are not cause for concern.

Some variation in regularity and length of menses is normal, but persistent changes may be related to an underlying problem. Common menstrual irregularities include
- Mid-cycle spotting
- Missed period
- Heavier or lighter menstrual flow

(See VAGINAL BLEEDING for related problems.)

CAUSES

Of course, pregnancy may be the cause of a missed period, but stress, both emotional and physical, can also cause a missed or delayed period. Birth control pills often help regulate menses, but any variation in type of pill or time of day the pill is taken, as well as missed pills, may throw off the cycle.

Other common causes of menstrual irregularity are
- FIBROID TUMORS
- Systemic bleeding disorders such as decreased number of platelets or other clotting protein disorders
- ENDOMETRIOSIS
- Thyroid imbalance (HYPERTHYROIDISM or HYPOTHYROIDISM)

APPROACH

The common diagnostic approach includes
- A MEDICAL HISTORY, focusing especially on past menstrual history and any clues to systemic illness (hormone imbalances, bleeding disorders)
- A PHYSICAL EXAMINATION, including pelvic examination and PAP SMEAR
- A pregnancy test, either by BLOOD TEST or URINALYSIS
- BLOOD TESTS to check the level of thyroid hormone
- Other diagnostic tests (see VAGINAL BLEEDING)

TREATMENT OPTIONS

- Different preparations of birth control pills are frequently tried.
- Special causes of VAGINAL BLEEDING may require other therapies.
- Progressively bothersome FIBROID TUMORS may require surgical FIBROID TUMOR REMOVAL.

NECK PAIN

Most people experience some neck pain or neck ache for a limited time after an overuse episode or injury. Neck pain after an automobile crash or a severe fall or injury should be evaluated to exclude a bone fracture or ligament injury.

CAUSES

The most common cause of neck ache or neck pain is overuse of the neck muscle; this may be due to a positioning problem (as may occur when working on a computer) or because of repetitive motions. Injuries involving falls or automobile crashes are also common; these injuries should be carefully evaluated and may require some time to resolve.

Rarely, meningitis and inflammatory conditions such as RHEUMATOID ARTHRITIS can be the cause of neck pain. Pain from the heart may also radiate into the neck (see ANGINA).

APPROACH

A MEDICAL HISTORY will be taken, including how the neck pain started. If the injury was traumatic, the way in which the neck was stressed may be helpful in deciding which part of the neck (disk, ligaments, muscles) has been injured. Radiating pains into the arms or shoulders may be associated with nerve root problems; the doctor will also ask about any sensation or muscle strength changes.

The PHYSICAL EXAMINATION will be focused on the neck; range of motion testing, as well as direct examination of the muscles, may point toward the diagnosis. Upper extremity strength and sensation testing for those patients with radiating pain complaints may pinpoint where the nerve roots are irritated. X rays (RADIOGRAPHY) are especially useful to eliminate the chance that a bone fracture is present in cases in which the neck pain has a traumatic cause.

TREATMENT OPTIONS

Most neck pain will respond to
- Rest and over-the-counter analgesics such as ibuprofen or acetaminophen
- A change in sleeping position to let the neck rest in the neutral position
- Prescription medicines such as etodolac and exercises or physical therapy

A large percentage of the population will experience neck pain at some time. Most often, the symptom is the result of overuse of the neck muscle.

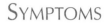

NOSE, STUFFY OR RUNNY

Stuffy nose is perhaps the most commonly experienced symptom. Its causes run the gamut from minor irritations to major illnesses.

When the lining of the mucous membranes in the nasal passages become inflamed, one experiences a stuffy nose; when they produce excess mucus, one has a runny nose. Although a stuffy or runny nose is not usually a sign of serious illness, any nasal congestion lasting longer than a week should be investigated by a physician.

CAUSES

Stuffy or runny nose can be the result of
- Allergies, usually to pollen, dust, or molds
- Infections, either viral (the common cold or INFLUENZA), bacterial, or fungal
- Anatomic abnormalities such as a deviated septum
- Nasal polyps or enlarged adenoids
- Systemic disease such as granulomatosis—a rare disorder affecting the sinuses, lungs, and kidneys
- Tumors, either benign or malignant

APPROACH

The investigation into the cause of a stuffy nose usually begins with a PHYSICAL EXAMINATION, in which the nose may be inspected visually. More extensive evaluation might include ENDOSCOPY of the nasal passages. To examine the internal structures, plain X rays (RADIOGRAPHY) may be useful, but COMPUTED TOMOGRAPHY is often preferred.

If specific causes are suspected, more targeted diagnostic testing may be performed, including
- ALLERGY TESTING
- Nasal air-flow measurements
- BIOPSY of suspicious areas

TREATMENT OPTIONS

Obstructions can sometimes be treated surgically, sometimes with lasers or cryosurgery. Septoplasty is a procedure to correct a deviated septum. Adenoidectomy is a procedure to remove enlarged adenoids.

Treatments aimed at alleviating the symptom include
- Topical steroid nasal sprays
- Decongestants such as pseudoephedrine
- Antihistamines such as chlorpheniramine
- Allergy shots

NUMBNESS

Numbness is a sensory disturbance that consists of loss of sensation, the occurrence of abnormal sensations, or pain. When a sensory disturbance takes the form of an abnormal spontaneous sensation, such as burning, tingling, or "pins and needles," it is called a *paresthesia*. A *dysesthesia* is a disturbance in which an unpleasant and painful sensation is produced by a stimulus that is usually painless.

CAUSES

There are many causes of numbness. The location of the symptoms, the mode of onset, and the accompanying symptoms help to determine what part of the nervous system is causing the numbness. In general, sensory impairment can happen as a result of brain, spinal cord, or peripheral nerve involvement.

Some characteristics that suggest a serious cause of numbness are
- A sudden onset
- Involvement on one side of the body only
- Association with other symptoms such as VISION DISTURBANCES, slurred speech, weakness, and disequilibrium (see DIZZINESS)

Common types of sensory loss and their causes include
- Sciatica, characterized by shooting pain and sensory loss in the back of the leg, most often caused by a HERNIATED DISK or RHEUMATIOID ARTHRITIS of the lower back
- Peripheral neuropathy, characterized by a gradual onset of numbness and tingling in both feet, caused by such diseases as DIABETES and alcoholism, which damage the ends of long nerves
- Benign forms of sensory loss, in which a person may, for example, hyperventilate and experience tingling of all the extremities and of the mouth, caused by anxiety
- The combination of numbness of one part of the body and slurred speech, possibly caused by a STROKE
- Sensory loss involving only a part of a limb and associated with sharp pain, suggesting a pinched nerve

> Numbness itself is difficult to treat without knowledge of the underlying cause.

APPROACH

Testing for numbness includes
- A complete MEDICAL HISTORY to assess possible drug-related or injury-related problems
- A PHYSICAL EXAMINATION, including a full neurologic examination, to determine what parts of the body are involved, how the numbness started, how it has progressed, and if there are any associated symptoms such as weakness, VISION DISTURBANCES, DIZZINESS, or difficulties with walking or any other specific tasks
- Depending on the patient's MEDICAL HISTORY and PHYSICAL EXAMINATION results, electromyography and nerve conduction studies to evaluate the peripheral nerves and help determine whether numbness is caused by a "pinched nerve" or a peripheral neuropathy
- BLOOD TESTS to determine whether a peripheral neuropathy is the cause of numbness and to exclude DIABETES, vitamin deficiencies, and other possible causes related to systemic illness
- MAGNETIC RESONANCE IMAGING or COMPUTED TOMOGRAPHY of the brain and spinal cord, if abnormalities in these structures are believed to be the origin of the numbness

TREATMENT OPTIONS

The treatment of a sensory disturbance is directed at the underlying cause.

RASH

Rashes appear in various forms: small, clear, fluid-filled bumps (vesicles); red raised bumps (papules); flat red spots (macules); and raised red bumps with pus inside that may drain (pustules).

CAUSES

- Infections such as SHINGLES, Lyme disease, syphilis, ringworm, and scabies; childhood infections such as measles, rubella, and chicken pox; rare infections such as Rocky Mountain spotted fever and toxic shock syndrome
- Allergic or autoimmune diseases such as systemic LUPUS ERYTHEMATOSUS, hives (allergic drug reactions, some types of DERMATITIS), and sarcoidosis
- PSORIASIS
- Forms of SKIN CANCER (rare)

APPROACH

A MEDICAL HISTORY can be helpful in identifying irritants such as detergents, oils, and heavy metals such as nickel or mercury found in leather products. Clues to a more systemic illness include mouth ulcers and swollen joints or lymph glands. Any new drug ingestion, including over-the-counter or health food store products, or viral infection should be reported to the doctor. Family history of PSORIASIS or DERMATITIS may be suggestive—ITCHING may be a useful clue.

The PHYSICAL EXAMINATION may include looking at the entire body's skin, the lymph nodes, and the abdomen. Characterizing the rash by location and type of rash helps to limit the possibilities of causes.

FEVER is an important clue. Scrapings, CULTURE, or even BIOPSY may be needed as well as certain BLOOD TESTS. ALLERGY TESTING for contact DERMATITIS may occasionally be necessary.

TREATMENT OPTIONS

Antihistamines such as diphenhydramine may be used for ITCHING. Steroid creams such as triamcinolone, anti-fungal drugs such as griseofulvin and fluconazole, or even systemic treatment with antibiotics or prednisone may be needed depending on the underlying disease.

Rashes are very common and have a variety of causes ranging from infections to irritants to serious internal problems.

RECTAL BLEEDING

Most frequently, rectal bleeding is not dangerous or life threatening even if it is recurrent.

Rectal bleeding is the passage of visible red blood through the rectum, usually with a bowel movement. It is a very common occurrence. Blood is seen primarily on the toilet paper or streaking the stool; on rare occasion, it is large in volume with clots. Most often the amount of blood passed is quite small and not immediately dangerous, although it should ultimately be discussed with a health care professional.

CAUSES

The most common causes of rectal bleeding are HEMORRHOIDS and anal fissures. Nearly all of us have HEMORRHOIDS, which are cushions of vascular tissue that line the rectal opening. Since HEMORRHOIDS are rich in blood vessels, they can bleed easily. Anal fissures are small cuts or scrapes in the anus that occur with straining during bowel movements. Anal fissures will frequently cause pain with defecation or burning after a bowel movement and at times can squirt blood into the toilet. Other causes of rectal bleeding occur less often but are more serious, including COLON POLYPS, COLORECTAL CANCER, and vascular malformations.

APPROACH

It is always appropriate to consult with a health professional about rectal bleeding. The physician will examine the rectum digitally. If the bleeding is recurrent or the source is not obvious, the physician may use anoscopy, sigmoidoscopy, or colonoscopy (all forms of ENDOSCOPY).

TREATMENT OPTIONS

Bleeding from HEMORRHOIDS or anal fissures can be alleviated by
- Adding stool softeners or fiber to the diet
- Sitting in a warm bath or tub
- Cleansing the anus with mild soap and water after bowel movements
- Tissues medicated with nonallergenic lotions
- Multiple local surgical techniques (HEMORRHOID BANDING, HEMORRHOID REMOVAL, application of cautery or heat, topical injection), especially in severe or repeatedly bothersome cases

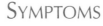

SKIN CHANGES

Moles are cells related to pigment-producing cells called *melanocytes* and can have a tan, brown, or black color. When a mole changes, this may be cause for some concern. A mole that bleeds, becomes elevated, becomes larger, changes color, or changes shape should be evaluated by a professional.

CAUSES

Benign causes of moles becoming darker or appearing larger occur
- During pregnancy
- While taking hormones such as oral contraceptives or estrogen replacement therapy
- With increased exposure to sunlight
- After injury to the mole and during the natural healing process

However, the main significant concern is when a mole changes because the cells within the mole become cancerous (SKIN CANCER). Melanoma is a pigmented SKIN CANCER that is of great concern, and this is the most dangerous cause of skin changes.

APPROACH

Melanoma can be cured when it is caught early and the pigmented tumor has not invaded the skin too deeply (see MALIGNANT MELANOMA REMOVAL). Therefore, the most conservative approach is to have any changing mole evaluated as soon as possible.

The doctor will evaluate the mole visually, perhaps with the aid of an optivisor or dermatoscope, which helps bring out the detailed features of the mole. During the evaluation, the clinician will record the mole's characteristics, making credit and debit columns out of its features.

On the credit side, the physician would like to see a symmetric mole that
- Is flat and nonpalpable
- Has even, homogeneous color
- Has a regular, clear border
- Does not have notching of the perimeter or fingers of pigment extending from the border

> Moles are sometimes present at birth, but they more often appear during childhood and adolescence. Skin changes are likely during pregnancy as well.

All of these features suggest that the mole is benign. Some moles may have one or more hairs growing from them, and this also is usually considered a benign feature.

Features that suggest a mole has atypical cells and may be a melanoma include: asymmetry, irregular border, and variegated hues of tan, yellow, brown, red, and black.

Treatment options

Benign moles, or *nevi*, do not need to be treated. Moreover, if the patient desires to have the mole removed for cosmetic purposes, the clinician needs to inform the patient that he or she will be trading the mole for a scar.

One approach is to remove the mole by performing a shave BIOPSY. This type of wound does not require sutures, but the patient is inconvenienced by the necessity of tending to the wound on a daily basis for 10 to 16 days. There is also a recurrence rate of about 5 to 7 percent.

Alternatively, the mole can be excised with an elliptical incision and the margins of the ellipse sutured closed. The patient can have the sutures removed in 7 to 14 days, depending upon the site.

If the lesion is suspected to be a melanoma (SKIN CANCER), the physician will excise it (MALIGNANT MELANOMA REMOVAL) to provide enough material for the pathologist to determine its depth. This is important because the thickness and depth of the melanoma have implications for prognosis and treatment options.

If there is only slight suspicion that the lesion is a melanoma, but it has features that are atypical or are of concern, the physician may elect to remove it or at least obtain a BIOPSY of the specimen for viewing under the microscope by a trained dermatopathologist.

STOOL, ABNORMAL APPEARANCE

Many things influence the color and consistency of stool. Variations in size and color most frequently relate to changes in the diet and transit through the digestive tract. It is not unusual to see vegetable material (corn kernels, tomato skin) in stool. Bile from the liver and gallbladder interacts with dietary substances to give stool its color, which may normally vary from brown to green or even yellow. The amount of fiber in the diet dramatically influences the volume and consistency of stool.

CAUSES

Only several abnormalities in stool appearance should give rise to some concern. Stools that are pitch black and loose in consistency may represent bleeding in the stomach or upper intestinal system. Bacteria degrading small amounts of blood will cause the stool to turn black. However, the use of iron, bismuth subsalicylate, and occasionally beets or spinach may also cause stool to turn black.

The shape of stools is quite variable and rarely an indicator of underlying disease. Although physicians have worried that narrowing of stools may represent the development of cancer, it is rare that this symptom is of any dangerous significance.

Stools frequently float in the toilet and this is not a marker of illness but relates to the volume of air trapped within the stool. Stools that are greasy or have visible oil droplets may represent problems with adequate intestinal digestion or absorption of food.

Visible red blood with stools, although most frequently related to minor RECTAL BLEEDING from HEMORRHOIDS, should raise some concern and deserves discussion with a health professional.

APPROACH

A dietary and MEDICAL HISTORY are usually the beginning of an inquiry into this symptom. The physician will digitally examine the rectum to be sure there are no abnormalities. OCCULT BLOOD TESTING can detect any tiny amounts of blood hidden in the stool. At times, sigmoidoscopy (a form of ENDOSCOPY) may be performed through the rectum. If there is concern that there is internal bleeding or that digestive organs are not functioning properly, barium X rays (RADIOGRAPHY) of the stomach, small intestine, or colon may be done.

Only a few abnormalities in stool appearance, such as blackened stool or red blood with stools, may be cause for concern; other problems are usually not significant.

SWALLOWING DIFFICULTIES

Swallowing difficulties may result from problems within the esophagus itself or with the muscles in the throat that initiate swallowing.

The esophagus is a long muscular tube that runs from the throat into the stomach. It has no function in digesting food but serves as a conduit for food to pass into the stomach. Although gravity does most of the work, the esophagus has a muscular coat that aids in propelling food forward. The patient may experience food getting caught in the back of the throat, behind the breast bone, or in the "pit" of the stomach. Swallowing may also be painful.

CAUSES

Swallowing difficulties should be attended to, as their causes can be serious. Causes include
- Narrowing of the esophagus due to scarring from acid reflux (peptic stricture)
- Development of a tumor
- Muscular weakness of the esophagus due to neurologic illness (myasthenia gravis) or STROKE
- Excessive muscular contraction of the esophagus
- Lower esophageal sphincter's lack of contraction
- Acid reflux and infections of the esophagus

APPROACH

Most swallowing problems require careful investigation. Barium X rays (RADIOGRAPHY) of the esophagus or gastrointestinal ENDOSCOPY are frequently the initial studies. More sophisticated tests of swallowing function, such as motility testing and video fluoroscopy (RADIOGRAPHY) of the throat and larynx, performed while a patient swallows a small amount of barium paste, may also be required.

TREATMENT OPTIONS

Treatment should be specifically directed toward the underlying cause of the problem. Empiric treatment with acid-blocking drugs (cimetidine) or motility agents (metoclopramide) before diagnostic testing is rarely done and only when gastroesophageal reflux is the cause. Retraining of swallowing by a speech pathologist may be helpful in those patients with a neurologic illness.

SWEATING, EXCESSIVE

Excessive sweating, particularly of the palms, soles, and underarms, is a common problem. Excessive sweating, called *essential hyperhidrosis*, is rarely an indicator of a medical problem, but there are very rare causes of excessive sweating that stem from significant underlying disorders.

CAUSES

Excessive sweating can be caused by
- Rare neurologic diseases in which there is a genetic imbalance in the autonomic nervous system
- A disturbance in the hypothalamus of the brain
- A metabolic condition, such as DIABETES, HYPERTHYROIDISM, obesity, or pregnancy
- Spinal cord disorders
- Chronic infection, such as tuberculosis or malaria
- Medications, such as INSULIN
- Genetic skin disorders
- Lymphoma (LYMPHOMA, NON-HODGKIN)

APPROACH

An underlying neurologic disease can usually be detected during a careful MEDICAL HISTORY and a PHYSICAL EXAMINATION including neurologic examination. Most of the time, an extensive search for the cause of the excessive sweating is not done. However, if other clues are suggestive of possible metabolic disorders, BLOOD TESTS to assess factors such as thyroid function may be performed.

TREATMENT OPTIONS

Treatment can be difficult. The topical application of aluminum chloride, either alone or under clear plastic cling wrap, to the area of excessive sweating can control (not cure) the problem. The use of medicated powders such as Zeasorb applied to the skin after a bath or shower and after drying well may be helpful. If excessive sweating of the feet is associated with severe odor, the additional application of an antibiotic solution such as clindamycin or erythromycin to decrease the bacterial flora of the skin may help.

Another approach to excessive sweating of the palms, soles, or underarms is iontophoresis. This procedure involves placing the skin in a solution with a mild electric current.

Although inconvenient to the patient, excessive sweating usually does not indicate a medical problem.

TESTICLE, PAINFUL OR SWOLLEN

Regular testicular self-examination should be a part of every man's hygiene routine, and abnormalities should be reported to a physician.

At times, men may develop a severe pain or a swelling in the scrotum. Not all causes of testicular pain and swelling have serious repercussions, but scrotal swelling should always be evaluated by a physician.

CAUSES

Acute pain in the scrotum may occur as a result of
- Viral infections, such as mumps, in young men
- Bacterial infections, such as epididymitis
- Torsion or twisting of the testicle that compromises the blood supply to the testicle

Nontender swellings of the scrotum may represent
- Benign cysts in the epididymis
- A collection of fluid around the testicle (hydrocele)
- Malignant tumors of the testicle (TESTICULAR CANCER)

APPROACH

The most important clues to scrotal pain and swelling are found in the patient's MEDICAL HISTORY. Information about the onset of the symptoms, the duration of the mass or swelling, and the degree of tenderness in various positions is very helpful. The PHYSICAL EXAMINATION by the doctor can often reveal the source of the problem. When necessary, an ULTRASOUND of the scrotum may be very useful to image the mass.

TREATMENT OPTIONS

In general, many scrotal swellings or other benign conditions need not be treated unless they cause symptoms because of their large size. Viral inflammation of the testicles, such as that in mumps, often resolves spontaneously. Bacterial infections respond well to antibiotics.

Testicular torsion represents a surgical emergency because of possible damage to the testicle from impaired blood supply; in this case, a simple surgical procedure to untwist the testicle is performed immediately.

Solid masses in the scrotum may represent a malignancy (TESTICULAR CANCER) and require surgical exploration and removal.

TONGUE PAIN

Tongue pain is a symptom that must never be ignored. Unless there is a history of recent trauma (such as biting or burning the tongue) the complaint requires a medical or dental examination.

CAUSES

The most obvious cause of tongue pain would be trauma. Biting one's tongue or eating scalding hot food can leave acute as well as residual pain.

Infections of the tongue are another possible explanation. Bacterial, fungal, and viral infections can lead to generalized tongue pain. These are usually accompanied by other symptoms associated with infection, such as swelling and redness.

Sore tongue is a symptom seen in several vitamin deficiency syndromes. Sore tongue associated with ANEMIA and neurologic weakness may be a sign of vitamin B_{12} deficiency. Folate deficiency can also lead to a red, sore tongue with ANEMIA and weakness.

Among the more serious conditions heralded by a sore tongue are ORAL CANCER and DIABETES.

APPROACH

A PHYSICAL EXAMINATION would involve visual examination and palpation (directly feeling the area) of the tongue. A MEDICAL HISTORY might focus on eating habits, alcohol use, tobacco use, and surgical history to explore the possibility of a vitamin deficiency. Diagnostic tests include
- CULTURE to test for and identify infection
- X ray (RADIOGRAPHY) to examine structures
- BIOPSY to evaluate any suspicious lesions

TREATMENT OPTIONS

The underlying condition is the focus of treatment. Some treatment strategies include
- Vitamin supplementation for deficiencies
- Antibiotics such as amoxicillin for any bacterial infection
- Antifungals such as ketoconazole or nystatin for fungal infection
- Denture adjustment for traumatic injury or irritation
- Surgery, chemotherapy, or radiation for ORAL CANCER

Tongue pain is an unusual symptom but often an important one. It is not the same as generalized mouth pain; it is usually more specific.

TREMBLING

Although most tremors are either barely noticeable or a mere nuisance, some can become disabling.

Trembling is an involuntary, rhythmic, visible shaking or quivering of all or part of the body. Most commonly affected are the hands, head, and voice; less commonly affected are the legs and trunk. Typically, tremors occur only during waking hours and cease during sleep.

CAUSES

By far the most common cause of tremor is essential tremor, also called *benign tremor* or *familial tremor* (because some patients can inherit it) or *senile tremor* (when a benign tremor begins in old age).

Other causes are

- PARKINSON DISEASE
- Diseases that involve the cerebellum (the back part of the brain that is largely responsible for coordination), such as inherited diseases, degenerative diseases, MULTIPLE SCLEROSIS, STROKES, tumors, and alcoholism
- Alcohol withdrawal after several days (or more) of heavy drinking
- A forearm tremor that occurs during prolonged writing
- Diseases that produce weakness such as MULTIPLE SCLEROSIS or STROKES
- Chorea, which is frequently confused with tremor, especially in the initial stages when there are involuntary, arrhythmic, rapid jerks
- Other causes not associated with disease states, such as anxiety, stress, and FATIGUE
- Stimulant beverages, such as coffee, tea, and sodas, and other caffeine-containing foods
- Nicotine in cigarettes and nicotine patches

Tremor may also be a side effect of some medicines, such as

- Drugs used in the treatment of lung conditions such as ASTHMA or EMPHYSEMA (theophylline or albuterol inhalers)
- Valproic acid and sodium valproate compound used in the treatment of epilepsy
- Lithium, a medication used in the treatment of manic illness
- Antipsychotics and antidepressants such as fluoxetine, sertraline, and paroxetine
- Too much thyroid hormone, either as part of a

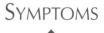
disease state (HYPERTHYROIDISM) or if administered in excess to patients undergoing treatment for HYPOTHYROIDISM

APPROACH

A MEDICAL HISTORY would focus on
- Drug use
- Alcohol use
- Family history

These points can be very useful. The results of a PHYSICAL EXAMINATION, particularly a neurologic examination, and the characteristics of the tremor—whether it occurs only while at rest or only during purposeful movement—usually provide adequate information to make a diagnosis.

TREATMENT OPTIONS

For essential tremor, propranolol, a drug otherwise used in the treatment of heart disease and HYPERTENSION, is the treatment of choice, although the patient's response is often incomplete.

Other drugs to treat essential tremor include primidone and alprazolam (a sedative drug related to diazepam).

URINATION, FREQUENT

A person's bladder habits can change over time without having a discernable medical cause, but sudden changes in bladder function or habit warrant medical evaluation.

Frequent urination is commonly defined as the need to urinate more often than every two hours. It is a disturbing symptom and can affect lifestyle and cause sleep problems.

CAUSES

Frequent urination may result from
- BLADDER INFECTION or bladder tumor
- Enlarged prostate (PROSTATE, ENLARGED)
- Neurologic disease or aging

Urinary frequency may also occur in the absence of a specific identifiable cause and may be related to subtle changes in a person's response to bladder sensations.

APPROACH

The diagnostic approach to urinary frequency involves a careful MEDICAL HISTORY of symptoms and habits. A PHYSICAL EXAMINATION may focus on prostate problems in men.

The adequacy of bladder emptying may be assessed by an ULTRASOUND examination of the bladder or by catheterization to determine how much urine is left in the bladder after voiding. In some cases, a urodynamic study, which measures responses of the bladder to filling and the behavior of the bladder during urination, may be performed.

URINALYSIS is performed in all patients to rule out infection, and in some cases urine CYTOLOGY or cystoscopy (a form of ENDOSCOPY) may be performed to rule out the presence of a bladder tumor.

TREATMENT OPTIONS

Treatment depends on the cause:
- In men with a large obstructing prostate (PROSTATE, ENLARGED), medical therapy may be used to alleviate symptoms, or surgical therapy may be recommended to remove the prostatic obstruction.
- In patients with neurologic disease or age-related changes in bladder function, medication may be used to reduce the irritative symptoms.
- In patients with BLADDER INFECTION, antibiotic therapy can usually clear the infection.
- In patients with BLADDER STONES or a tumor, surgical removal may be an option.

URINATION, PAINFUL

Dysuria is the medical term for painful urination. Although sometimes caused by irritation, painful urination is usually a sign of an infection. These infections are rarely serious, but a physician should be consulted if the condition persists, especially if it is associated with FEVER or BACKACHE.

CAUSES

The most common cause of painful urination is a bacterial infection of the lower urinary tract, the urethra, or the bladder (BLADDER INFECTION). It is important to treat this infection promptly to prevent it from ascending the urinary tract to the kidneys, which can be more serious. Other causes of painful urination include

- Sexually transmitted diseases
- Prostatitis
- Yeast infections
- Atrophic VAGINITIS
- KIDNEY STONES

APPROACH

In order to diagnose the cause of painful urination, a careful MEDICAL HISTORY needs to be taken about the symptom and any associated symptoms, such as

- A change in urine appearance (URINE, ABNORMAL APPEARANCE)
- A change in bladder habits (URINATION, FREQUENT)
- FEVER
- BACKACHE
- Penile or VAGINAL DISCHARGE

The PHYSICAL EXAMINATION includes palpation of the bladder as well as pounding on the back to determine if there is any tenderness over the kidneys. Additionally, a URINALYSIS will be performed. Other procedures may include a pelvic examination or urethral swabs for CULTURE.

TREATMENT OPTIONS

Treatment of the underlying cause should alleviate the symptom. Most causes of persistent, painful urination are from infections (see BLADDER INFECTION), which are treated with antibiotics. KIDNEY STONES can be resolved by medical or surgical means (see ULTRASONIC LITHOTRIPSY).

> Painful urination is most frequently caused by infections that are rarely serious and usually subside with antibiotic treatment.

URINE, ABNORMAL APPEARANCE

Although a sudden change in the appearance of one's urine can be an alarming symptom, it is not usually an ominous one.

Abnormal appearance of the urine is most commonly caused by the presence of blood in the urine or the presence of infection. Blood in the urine may turn the urine pink or red depending on the concentration of blood. Cloudy urine, sometimes emitting a foul odor, may indicate infection.

CAUSES

Some of the possible conditions that could cause urine to change appearance include
- BLADDER STONES
- KIDNEY STONES
- Severe BLADDER INFECTION
- Bladder tumors
- Kidney tumors
- Other diseases of the lower urinary tract such as atrophic VAGINITIS affecting the opening for urine
- Certain diseases affecting the function of the kidneys such as glomerulonephritis
- Infection such as malaria
- Crystals in the urine that are benign

APPROACH

The MEDICAL HISTORY of the patient, including onset and duration of the symptom, gives important clues for diagnosis. The single most important test is the URINALYSIS, in which the doctor performs a microscopic examination of the urine to determine whether blood or pus cells are present.

Depending on the findings on URINALYSIS, tests such as an intravenous pyelogram (a form of RADIOGRAPHY) of the kidney or cystoscopy (a form of ENDOSCOPY) of the bladder may be performed to look for a source of bleeding in the kidneys or bladder .

If infection is suspected, a urine CULTURE may be performed.

TREATMENT OPTIONS

Treatment for blood in the urine depends on finding the cause and then treating it appropriately. For tumors, surgery may be required. KIDNEY STONES and BLADDER STONES can be removed with certain procedures (see ULTRASONIC LITHOTRIPSY). Infections are usually cleared with antibiotics.

VAGINAL BLEEDING

Although some vaginal bleeding is usually not an ominous sign, excessive bleeding can be a medical emergency. If the bleeding soaks through a regular sanitary napkin within 30 minutes, a physician should be notified. Also, if bleeding is associated with DIZZINESS or FAINTING OR FAINTNESS, immediate evaluation is necessary. Postmenopausal women should always have unexpected bleeding evaluated.

A woman should keep a good record of her menstrual history to aid in the evaluation of vaginal bleeding.

CAUSES

In postmenopausal women, vaginal bleeding may be attributable to
*   Atrophic VAGINITIS
*   Uterine prolapse
*   Endometrial polyps
*   UTERINE CANCER
*   Vaginal cancer
*   CERVICAL CANCER
*   Systemic bleeding disorders

In premenopausal women, the above causes are possible, but bleeding may also be attributable to
*   MENSTRUAL IRREGULARITIES
*   Complications of pregnancy (often unsuspected)
*   ENDOMETRIOSIS
*   PELVIC INFLAMMATORY DISEASE
*   VAGINITIS
*   Endometrial hyperplasia
*   HYPERTHYROIDISM or HYPOTHYROIDISM
*   OVARIAN CYST
*   OVARIAN CANCER
*   Rare endocrine disorders such as Cushing syndrome

APPROACH

A MEDICAL HISTORY, including a complete menstrual history and a pelvic examination, are probably the first steps in evaluating vaginal bleeding. A BLOOD COUNT to check for ANEMIA and BLOOD TESTS to test for thyroid function, pregnancy (if it is at all possible), and other problems may also be performed.

Further tests may include
*   Hysteroscopy (a form of ENDOSCOPY)
*   A BIOPSY of the uterine lining (endometrium)
*   DILATION AND CURETTAGE for cases in which biopsy is not easily obtainable

VAGINAL DISCHARGE

A small amount of discharge, especially in the middle days between periods, is normal and related to ovulation.

Normal vaginal discharge can sometimes lead women to try products like sprays and douches that may create a problem. If any blood is present, it should be evaluated (see V<small>AGINAL BLEEDING</small>).

C<small>AUSES</small>

- V<small>AGINITIS</small> from lack of estrogen or from infection with yeast or *Trichomonas* or *Chlamydia* bacteria not normally present in large numbers
- Irritation from products such as douches, sprays, or contraceptive foam
- P<small>ELVIC INFLAMMATORY DISEASE</small>
- Foreign bodies including intrauterine devices (IUDs), cervical caps, tampons, or diaphragms
- Cervical, uterine, or vaginal polyps or cancer (see C<small>ERVICAL CANCER</small>; U<small>TERINE CANCER</small>)
- O<small>VARIAN CYSTS</small>
- Urethral infection (B<small>LADDER INFECTION</small>)

A<small>PPROACH</small>

A M<small>EDICAL HISTORY</small> would focus on the use of any materials inserted into the vagina, presence of a F<small>EVER</small>, sexual contacts, and changes in contraceptive pills or devices. Recent antibiotic use commonly alters the bacterial balance of the vagina and may lead to infection.

P<small>HYSICAL EXAMINATION</small>, especially pelvic and abdominal examination, is useful in determining a diagnosis. Laboratory tests could include C<small>ULTURES</small>, microscopic examination of secretions, and a P<small>AP SMEAR</small>. If intrauterine, tubal, or ovarian problems are suspected, B<small>IOPSY</small> and U<small>LTRASOUND</small> may be used.

T<small>REATMENT OPTIONS</small>

Antifungal creams such as clotrimazole and antibiotics such as metronidazole—or other prescription medications—may be recommended, depending on the underlying cause.

VISION DISTURBANCES

Vision can be defined in many ways. Aside from the ability to read the newspaper or street signs, vision can be the ability to perceive color, to see at night, or to see out of the corner of the eye. A disturbance in vision can mean any disruption in the above or the perception of light flashes or sparks and the appearance of floaters in the eyes.

CAUSES

Different types of visual disturbances have different causes. For example, flashes of light suggest something may be tugging at or tearing the retina.

Floaters are noted when some opacity is floating in the interior of the eye. This could simply be some spot of localized degeneration, but it could also be blood or inflammatory material.

A reduction in central vision may simply mean that spectacles need updating to reflect a change that has occurred within the focusing elements of the eye. Nearsightedness usually progresses until age 30 and may not begin until the mid-20s. At around age 40, the ability to focus up close decreases to the point of causing symptoms. Reading glasses may be needed shortly after the initial observation of change.

Some systemic diseases, such as DIABETES with high blood sugar, can induce a nearsighted shift. A reduction in night vision may occur after laser treatment for eye disease related to DIABETES.

Retinitis pigmentosa causes a chronic, progressive, and permanent loss of night vision. Visual obscuration from CATARACT also may reduce visual function at night. CATARACT is a reversible cause of central vision loss, while macular degeneration causes permanent reduction in central visual function.

The sudden loss of side vision may occur in retinal detachment or in blockage of blood vessels within the retina. A STROKE involving the visual pathways could also cause this symptom. Episodic loss of vision may be due to bits of material within the arteries temporarily blocking blood flow in the retina.

MIGRAINE HEADACHE may initially be experienced as a blurring of side vision. This usually passes within 20 minutes. The gradual perception of a side vision abnormality could be related to GLAUCOMA or a tumor within the eye. It could also be caused by CATARACT.

Early treatment of vision disturbances may reduce the chance of progressive or permanent sight loss.

Loss of color vision is usually caused by an abnormality in the function of the optic nerve that transmits the visual message to the brain. Inflammation, poor circulation to the nerve, or a drop in the speed at which the signal can be sent, may make colors appear washed out. Inherited color vision problems do not occur suddenly and are usually present from birth.

Any eyedrop, drug, or eye disease that causes the pupils to decrease in size will limit the amount of light that enters the eye, thereby decreasing night vision. Pilocarpine, a common GLAUCOMA drop, reduces pupil size.

APPROACH

Visual problems that clear with a blink or that clear when glasses are used are generally not of a serious nature. However, a change in visual function that is not simply remedied should prompt a call to the doctor. A MEDICAL HISTORY is necessary, including information about

- The onset of the symptom (sudden or gradual)
- The duration of the symptom
- The number of episodes
- The timing of the most recent episode
- Whether both eyes were involved
- Any associated symptoms such as HEADACHE, eye redness or EYE PAIN, weakness, or NUMBNESS

The examination will include a measurement of visual acuity. It is important to bring one's best pair of spectacles to the examination. Side vision testing may also be done. The ability of the pupils to react to light will be checked. Careful examination with the microscope, including a measurement of eye pressure, is necessary. The pupils will probably be dilated, so it's helpful to bring sunglasses and perhaps a friend or relative to drive home. Dilation is needed to get the best possible view of the inside of the eye, including the retina and optic nerve.

TREATMENT OPTIONS

Treatment will depend on the cause of the problem. Treatment may be as simple as a new pair of glasses or use of tear-supplement drops. The key to treatment is prompt evaluation. Early treatment may reduce the chance of progressive or permanent sight loss.

VOMITING

Vomiting is a very common and typically transient or self-limited symptom. Its occasional occurrence should not cause alarm. More serious instances that may demand medical attention include

- Persistent vomiting (lasting more than two days)
- Vomiting associated with severe ABDOMINAL PAIN
- Vomiting associated with severe HEADACHES
- Vomiting of undigested food that was eaten many hours earlier
- Vomiting of foul- or feculent-smelling material
- Vomiting associated with a significant amount of blood

CAUSES

The most common causes of vomiting, which are typically self-limited and resolve in a matter of hours, are most often related to

- Dietary indiscretion
- Overindulgence in food or drink, especially too much alcohol
- Simple food poisoning

Other causes of vomiting include

- GASTROENTERITIS, which is due to a viral infection and is typically associated with a low-grade FEVER, generalized muscle aches and pains, and some DIARRHEA. It usually resolves in a few days
- Stomach or INTESTINAL OBSTRUCTION, PANCREATITIS, and gallbladder disease (see GALLSTONES; CHOLECYSTITIS AND CHOLANGITIS)
- Neurologic illness that ranges from MIGRAINE HEADACHES to problems within the brain that elevate spinal fluid pressure (rare)
- Pregnancy, especially in the early stage ("morning sickness")

APPROACH

Evaluation is needed only for those rare cases of persistent, prolonged, or recurrent vomiting. A description of the specific circumstances may point to the need for more diagnostic evaluation.

Although some cases of vomiting demand medical attention, most are due to overindulgence in food or drink or to simple food poisoning and resolve in a matter of hours.

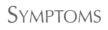
The PHYSICAL EXAMINATION will focus on signs of dehydration, BLOOD PRESSURE TESTING and pulse while lying down and standing up, the degree of moisture in the skin and mouth, and abnormalities of the abdomen and rectum. At times, a neurologic examination or evaluation of the eyes and retina will be done.

Laboratory tests will be ordered only if the preliminary examination is abnormal. These may include BLOOD COUNT, serum electrolytes, and serum amylase (see BLOOD TESTS).

Further tests may include

- X rays (RADIOGRAPHY) of the abdomen if INTESTINAL OBSTRUCTION is suspected
- COMPUTED TOMOGRAPHY or MAGNETIC RESONANCE IMAGING of the brain if neurologic disease is suspected
- Barium X rays (RADIOGRAPHY) of the intestine and ULTRASOUNDS or COMPUTED TOMOGRAPHY of the abdomen in unclear cases

TREATMENT OPTIONS

Most episodes of vomiting resolve within a short period of time and are not caused by a persistent medical problem. Food intake should be limited to clear liquids, such as soft drinks, juices, and broth, until the problem resolves and the patient feels up to eating regular food. Physicians may prescribe antinausea medications, including

- Chlorpromazine
- Prochlorperazine
- Promethazine
- Thiethylperazine
- Metoclopramide
- Trimethobenzamide

WEIGHT GAIN

Concern about weight is ubiquitous. But for all the worry, there is no absolute value of weight that is desirable. Tables that list "ideal" body weights, adjusted for body build, age, sex, and height, are readily available but not always useful for individuals.

Although many people find it difficult to accept, almost all instances of increased body weight relate to increased caloric intake, decreased caloric expenditure because of decreased physical activity, or a combination of both factors. Problems stemming from a slow metabolism rarely explain weight gain.

Rapid fluctuation in weight (on the order of one to two pounds per day) is almost always due to fluid retention and is quite commonly noted premenstrually in women.

CAUSES

Increased caloric intake, coupled with decreased activity, accounts for the overwhelming majority of cases of progressive weight gain. Illnesses that result in rapid weight gain from fluid and salt accumulation within the body include

- CONGESTIVE HEART FAILURE
- Cirrhosis of the liver
- Nephrotic syndrome of the kidney (see KIDNEY FAILURE)

These diseases are frequently associated with other symptoms, including

- Abdominal distension and ABDOMINAL SWELLING
- Swelling of the legs (ANKLE SWELLING)
- BREATHING DIFFICULTY

An underactive thyroid gland (HYPOTHYROIDISM) may result in weight gain on occasion.

APPROACH

The patient's weight is adjusted for body build, height, sex, and age to determine whether the weight gain is normal or excessive. The weight should be taken in the same manner each time, preferably without clothes or shoes. A dietary history should be reviewed to estimate caloric intake on a daily basis. Some sense of energy expenditure can be ascertained by reviewing job responsibilities, hobbies, and exercise habits.

In most cases, progressive weight gain is due to increased caloric intake accompanied by decreased physical activity.

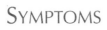

Abnormal fluid retention can be detected from the PHYSI-CAL EXAMINATION by examining the heart, neck, lungs, abdomen, and legs. If abnormalities are suspected because of findings from the PHYSICAL EXAMINATION, the following are more extensive tests that may be performed:

- The heart may be assessed with ELECTROCARDIOGRA-PHY or chest X ray (RADIOGRAPHY).
- The liver may be assessed with blood liver function tests (see BLOOD TESTS) or ULTRASOUND examination of the liver itself.
- The kidneys may be assessed with URINALYSIS.
- The thyroid gland may be assessed with blood thyroid function tests (see BLOOD TESTS).

TREATMENT OPTIONS

Weight gain due to increased caloric intake can be treated by dietary restrictions in fat and total calories as well as an exercise program. Quick fixes such as crash diets almost never work in the long term. Programs that result in permanent lifestyle adjustments are the only ones with the potential for long-term success.

Fluid overload states can be treated with salt restriction and diuretics such as hydrochlorothiazide.

Appetite suppressant pills, although touted by lay advertisers, are usually ineffective in the long term.

WEIGHT LOSS

Unexpected weight loss—that is, weight loss not related to dieting or increased exercise—can represent serious illness. Weight loss should be interpreted within the context of a patient's usual weight. Physicians begin to worry seriously about an underlying illness when weight loss reaches approximately ten percent of the individual's stable weight.

CAUSES

Decreased intake of food is obviously the most common cause of weight loss; dietary changes, such as a reduction in total fat intake, can easily explain weight loss. If the dietary changes are associated with a poor appetite (see APPETITE, LOSS OF), substantial weight loss may point to DEPRESSION, PANCREATIC CANCER, STOMACH CANCER, some other undiscovered malignancy, or AIDS.

At times, patients lose weight despite maintaining or even increasing their dietary intake. In this instance, an overactive thyroid gland (HYPERTHYROIDISM) or DIABETES needs consideration. Diseases of the small intestine or pancreas that interfere with complete digestion and absorption of food may lead to weight loss, although changes in bowel habits or even DIARRHEA are usually present as well.

Anorexia nervosa may be a cause of weight loss in young women (see APPETITE, LOSS OF).

APPROACH

General nutritional information, MEDICAL HISTORY, PHYSICAL EXAMINATION, and baseline laboratory tests—BLOOD COUNT, screening chemistries (see BLOOD TESTS), and OCCULT BLOOD TESTING—will determine the need for additional testing. Testing would be directed toward abnormalities noted on the general evaluation.

TREATMENT OPTIONS

Many oral nutritional supplements are commercially available and can be used without harm in an effort to gain weight. The first step, however, is to determine whether weight loss is a sign of a medical problem and whether weight gain is necessary for the patient.

Small fluctuations in weight are not unusual, but progressive weight loss without an obvious explanation merits some concern.

ILLNESSES

AIDS

In the United States, there are between 1 and 1.5 million people infected with the human immunodeficiency virus (HIV), the virus that causes AIDS; worldwide, as many as 20 million people are infected. AIDS—which stands for *acquired immunodeficiency syndrome*—affects all races and ethnic groups as well as people of all ages.

CAUSES

AIDS is caused by infection with HIV. There are two types of HIV: type 1 and type 2. HIV type 1 is the only virus that causes AIDS in the United States. However, infection with HIV type 2 occurs in Africa.

The groups at highest risk for HIV infection are
- Gay and bisexual men
- Injection drug users
- Hemophiliacs
- Children born to mothers with HIV
- Sexually active heterosexuals

Transmission of HIV by blood transfusion is extremely rare in the United States.

SYMPTOMS

After exposure to HIV, some patients develop an *acute retroviral syndrome* characterized by FEVER, RASH, and swollen lymph nodes. This is often indistinguishable from other viral illnesses.

The patient is generally without symptoms, though, for several years until the immune system deteriorates. At that time, symptoms suggestive of HIV infection include
- WEIGHT LOSS greater than ten percent of total body weight
- DIARRHEA for longer than one month
- FEVER for longer than one month
- COUGH for longer than one month
- Skin RASH
- Recurrent SHINGLES
- Oral thrush (yeast infection in mouth)
- Swollen glands all over the body

Unfortunately, these symptoms are not specific to HIV infection and can mimic other infections or cancer.

Few infections are associated with as much panic and misinformation as infection with the human immunodeficiency virus—the virus that causes AIDS. But without a cure, education and prevention are the best weapons with which to fight it.

DIAGNOSIS

HIV infection can be detected by a BLOOD TEST. If the first screening test is positive, a second is performed for confirmation. More sophisticated testing can be performed in research studies or at many university medical centers.

A positive result on an HIV test is not, however, a diagnosis of AIDS. An HIV-infected person is considered to have AIDS only when he or she develops any one of a number of diseases that occur in individuals with abnormalities in their immune system. In addition, when the patient's T-cell count (a measure of the immune system's function) falls below 200 (the normal range is 750 to 1,250), the patient is considered to have AIDS.

COMPLICATIONS

The complications related to infection with HIV are the result of infections that develop due to deteriorating immune function. These include

- PNEUMONIA
- Tuberculosis
- Meningitis

Patients with HIV infection also have an increased risk of developing cancer.

Patients with HIV should contact their physician if they develop

- A high FEVER
- Severe or persistent HEADACHE
- VOMITING
- BREATHING DIFFICULTY
- Persistent DIARRHEA
- VISION DISTURBANCES
- Significant WEIGHT LOSS

The complexity of this syndrome prohibits a more detailed explanation of the complications. All patients with HIV disease should be closely monitored by a physician with experience treating AIDS patients.

TREATMENT

SELF TREATMENT:

While there is no cure for AIDS, there are many things that patients can do to help prolong their life. Common sense dictates that patients with HIV infection should eat well-balanced meals, exercise regularly, and get plenty of sleep. Tobacco and illicit drug use should be stopped. Alcohol is acceptable in moderation, unless it interacts with a medication the patient is taking. There is no benefit to megadoses of vitamins, but a daily multivitamin is acceptable.

MEDICAL TREATMENT:

There are many drugs that can be used to treat patients with HIV. The antiviral medications that are commonly used are zidovudine (AZT), didanosine (ddI), zalcitabine (ddC), and stavudine (d4T). There are several other experimental medications that are undergoing clinical evaluations. Additional therapy for HIV and its associated complications is beyond the scope of this book and should be discussed with a health care provider.

SURGICAL TREATMENT:

None, except for cases in which there is a surgical treatment for a secondary condition, such as an enlarged spleen or cancer.

PREVENTION

The best way to avoid HIV is by prevention. This means that condoms should be worn during intercourse and needles should not be shared. There is no evidence that HIV is transmitted via casual contact.

There are many medications that can prevent infections in patients already infected with HIV. A sulfamethoxazole and trimethoprim combination can be used to prevent PNEUMONIA; isoniazid can be used to prevent tuberculosis; and fluconazole is effective in preventing fungal infections.

Once again, the preventive measures for patients with AIDS are in constant evolution and should be discussed with a physician.

ALZHEIMER DISEASE

Alzheimer disease is a degenerative disorder of the brain that causes the progressive loss of intellectual abilities. The disease usually affects memory (see MEMORY PROBLEMS) and at least one other cognitive domain such as language, attention, visual-perceptual skills, reasoning, judgment, or behavior.

CAUSES

The underlying cause of Alzheimer disease is unknown, but there have been recent advances in understanding the disorder. It appears that the disease is probably several diseases that cause similar changes in the metabolism of the brain.

Heredity may play a role; several genetic markers have been linked to the disease.

Although aluminum poisoning was once thought to be a factor, recent studies have not supported that theory.

SYMPTOMS

The initial symptoms of the disease are usually subtle and may not be recognized at all by the affected person. Family members are often the first to notice increasingly frequent MEMORY PROBLEMS. Often the individual will
- Display a lack of interest in work or social activities
- Neglect or have difficulty with routine tasks
- Become withdrawn

Signs of more advanced disease include
- Confusion
- Need for assistance eating or dressing
- INCONTINENCE

DIAGNOSIS

Diagnosis of memory disorders almost always begins with a detailed MEDICAL HISTORY and a PHYSICAL EXAMINATION, including a complete neurologic and mental status assessment. A mental status examination is a detailed review of various cognitive functions to check performance of attention, memory, language, visual-spatial function, abstract reasoning, insight, behavior, and judgment.

BLOOD TESTS and a BLOOD COUNT can be useful to check for metabolic disturbances, systemic infections, and nutrient deficiencies.

> Alzheimer disease is the most common cause of dementia, accounting for up to 80 percent of all cases.

Further tests can include
* ELECTROENCEPHALOGRAPHY
* COMPUTED TOMOGRAPHY
* MAGNETIC RESONANCE IMAGING
* LUMBAR PUNCTURE

Sometimes, cognitive and PHYSICAL EXAMINATIONS are repeated over the course of several months to determine if the disease is progressing.

The diagnosis of Alzheimer disease is made by finding the characteristic pattern of symptoms in the absence of any other causes after a reasonable search.

COMPLICATIONS

DEPRESSION is often associated with the disease, and overall life expectancy decreases because of a number of factors. Inability to care for oneself and reduced mental function can precipitate problems ranging from vitamin deficiencies to automobile accidents.

TREATMENT

SELF TREATMENT:

None.

MEDICAL TREATMENT:

At this time, there are no good treatments available; no medication has been shown even to slow the disease significantly. The only drug approved for use in Alzheimer disease is tacrine, but its effects are modest at best. Other medications used to treat associated disorders are
* Antidepressants such as sertraline
* Mild sedatives such as low doses of haloperidol used sparingly
* Antianxiety drugs such as lorazepam

SURGICAL TREATMENT:

None.

PREVENTION

There seems to be a protective effect in education; studies show that the risk of developing dementia is two to five times more likely in those with little or no education.

ANEMIA

> The course of anemia can be reversed with medical treatment, but severe, untreated cases can be dangerous.

Anemia is a condition in which the blood has a reduced number of red blood cells. These cells are responsible for carrying oxygen from the lungs to all body tissues, so a reduced number of them leads to less efficient oxygen distribution.

CAUSES

The multiple causes of anemia can be divided into two main categories: decreased production of red blood cells in the bone marrow and increased destruction or loss of red blood cells. Decreased production is seen in

- Deficiencies of vitamin B_{12}, folate, or iron
- Bone marrow disorders such as LEUKEMIA
- Chronic inflammatory disorders such as RHEUMATOID ARTHRITIS
- Thalassemia

Increased destruction is seen in

- Hereditary diseases such as sickle-cell disease
- Infections
- Use of drugs such as methyldopa
- Autoimmune disorders (LUPUS ERYTHEMATOSUS)
- Blood loss

SYMPTOMS

- FATIGUE
- BREATHING DIFFICULTY
- Pallor
- Fast heart rate
- CHEST PAIN
- DIZZINESS
- Blood in stool (RECTAL BLEEDING) or in vomit
- Excessive menstruation (MENSTRUAL IRREGULARITIES)
- Jaundice
- Dark-colored urine (URINE, ABNORMAL APPEARANCE)

DIAGNOSIS

Anemia is diagnosed with tests such as

- Complete BLOOD COUNT
- BLOOD TESTS for vitamin B_{12}, folate, and iron to check for deficiencies

- Blood tests for hemoglobin electrophoresis to check for hereditary diseases
- Blood tests to check for red cell destruction and evidence of chronic diseases
- Stool and urine samples to check for the presence of blood (occult blood testing; urinalysis)

If no diagnosis can be made, a bone marrow biopsy may be performed.

Complications

In cases of severe or rapidly developing anemia, body organs may be damaged from a lack of oxygen. This can result in stroke, heart attack, kidney failure, liver failure, and in severe cases, death.

Treatment

SELF TREATMENT:

Iron supplements are recommended for women with heavy menstrual periods. A diet consisting of vegetables, fruits, and meats should provide enough of the necessary nutrients to prevent anemia.

MEDICAL TREATMENT:

Medical therapy is dependent on the underlying cause. Usually, treatment of the underlying cause or of the chronic disease will reverse the anemia. In cases of severe anemia, blood transfusions can be given. Iron can be given in cases of chronic blood loss, and erythropoietin is helpful in patients with kidney failure.

SURGICAL TREATMENT:

Surgical intervention may be needed to treat sources of blood loss such as colon polyps or tumors.

Prevention

- A well-balanced diet with adequate iron and vitamins is helpful.
- Avoid exposure to solvents such as benzene and insecticides, which can damage the bone marrow.

ANEURYSM

> An aneurysm is a balloonlike swelling in the wall of a blood vessel. Rupture and clot formation in the area of the defect are a serious danger.

An aneurysm is a weak spot in the wall of a blood vessel. Common locations for an aneurysm include the small blood vessels, such as those in the brain, and the largest blood vessels, such as the aorta as it travels from the heart, through the chest, and into the abdomen.

Aneurysms in and of themselves are not a serious danger, but the very real potential for rupture and clot formation at the site is life-threatening.

CAUSES

Most aneurysms of the aorta are caused by ATHEROSCLEROSIS. Less often, infections or hereditary diseases can also contribute to aneurysm formation. Aneurysm formation in the blood vessels in the brain also appears to have some hereditary factor, but it can be associated with other diseases, as well.

High blood pressure (HYPERTENSION) increases the stress on the weak spot of the blood vessel wall causing the aneurysm to increase in size like a balloon and increasing the risk of rupture.

SYMPTOMS

Aneurysms are usually without symptoms until a catastrophe occurs. Occasionally, an aneurysm in the brain will cause HEADACHES before it ruptures.

In the aorta, an aneurysm can also go completely unnoticed until disaster strikes, but in rare cases, it can cause
- CHEST PAIN or discomfort
- Hoarseness
- SWALLOWING DIFFICULTIES
- Persistent COUGH

For an aortic aneurysm in the abdomen, a throbbing so-called *pulsatile mass* may be an indicator.

Usually, when an aortic aneurysm ruptures, there is sudden severe pain, severe drop in blood pressure, and even loss of consciousness. Even with emergency surgery, aortic aneurysms are associated with a very high mortality.

DIAGNOSIS

An aortic aneurysm in the abdomen can usually be diagnosed in a PHYSICAL EXAMINATION by feeling the abdominal pulsatile mass.

An aneurysm in the chest can be suspected by marked differences in BLOOD PRESSURE TESTS and pulse between the right and left arm. Chest X ray (RADIOGRAPHY) can also be useful in the diagnosis of an aortic aneurysm in the chest.

Aneurysms in the brain can be detected by
- COMPUTED TOMOGRAPHY
- MAGNETIC RESONANCE IMAGING
- Angiography (a form of RADIOGRAPHY)

Angiography may be needed to detect or confirm the presence of an aneurysm in all three locations. ULTRASOUND may also be useful.

COMPLICATIONS

The two major complications associated with aneurysm are rupture, in which the walls of the blood vessel actually break at the site of the aneurysm, and clot formation, in which the widened space of the aneurysm provides a place where blood can start to coagulate. Depending on the size of the vessel, rupture can lead to serious internal bleeding or damage to surrounding tissue. A clot, particularly in an aortic aneurysm, can break off and travel farther down the blood stream causing gangrene in the leg or internal abdominal organs.

WARNING SIGNS:
Sudden rupture in the brain leads to
- Extremely severe HEADACHE
- NECK PAIN
- Neurologic weakness

Rupture in the abdomen or chest results in
- Severe pain, often in the back near the rupture site
- Extremely low blood pressure
- Loss of consciousness
- Shock

TREATMENT

SELF TREATMENT:

Limitations in exercise may be necessary to decrease the chance of temporarily elevated blood pressure that could cause rupture.

MEDICAL TREATMENT:

Medical therapies include beta-blockers such as propranolol to lower blood pressure and stress on the blood vessel wall. Nimodipine is sometimes prescribed for a ruptured aneurysm in the brain.

SURGICAL TREATMENT:

Surgical therapy may be necessary when an aneurysm is identified but has not yet ruptured. The timing of surgery for aortic aneurysm is based on the speed at which the aneurysm is expanding and its size at the time of detection. Aneurysms can be managed surgically by removal and repair with Dacron or other techniques to reinforce the walls of the vessel (see ANEURYSM REMOVAL).

Recently, special prosthetic devices called *stents* delivered to the area of weakness by a catheter threaded through the blood vessels have been used with increasing frequency. This technique is a less invasive alternative to open surgical repair.

PREVENTION

Prevention of aneurysm formation and progression includes controlling the risk factors for ATHEROSCLEROSIS and HYPERTENSION. Strategies include

- Avoiding smoking
- Following a low-fat, low-cholesterol diet
- Limiting intake of sodium
- Participating in regular exercise (if so advised by a physician)
- Diligently taking all prescribed blood pressure medication

ANGINA

The heart muscle gets its blood from the coronary arteries; when this blood flow is momentarily interrupted or limited, the heart muscle doesn't get the food and fuel it needs, and the CHEST PAIN of angina is the result.

CAUSES

The most common cause of angina is ATHEROSCLEROSIS. Much less common causes include spasms of the coronary arteries or disease of the smallest branches of these vessels. Spasms can be triggered by
- Nicotine in cigarettes
- Cold air
- Emotional stress
- Cocaine and other stimulant drugs

The risk factors for ATHEROSCLEROSIS include
- HYPERTENSION
- Smoking
- High blood cholesterol level (HYPERLIPIDEMIA)
- DIABETES
- Male gender (Men are more susceptible than women.)
- Family history of the disease

SYMPTOMS

Angina is most commonly described as a pressure, squeezing, or heavy sensation in the center of the chest. Less often, it can be an achy feeling or burning. The discomfort is sometimes experienced in other locations, including the left or right side of the chest, the upper abdomen, the neck, the jaw, and the arms. The discomfort is usually precipitated by some type of physical effort and is relieved with rest. An angina attack commonly lasts approximately one to two minutes.

DIAGNOSIS

The diagnosis of angina is usually made from the characteristic symptoms and the individual's MEDICAL HISTORY and risk factors for ATHEROSCLEROSIS. ELECTROCARDIOGRAPHY performed *during* the pain usually shows some abnormalities but can be totally normal in between episodes. A CARDIAC STRESS TEST can usually help sort out atypical symptoms. A CARDIAC CATHETERIZATION or angiogram (RADIOGRAPHY) may be necessary.

Angina is a discomfort or pain usually located in the center of the chest and caused by a lack of blood flow to the heart muscle. Although not life-threatening in itself, it can progress to more serious heart problems.

COMPLICATIONS

Angina can progress to unstable angina or directly to a myocardial infarction (HEART ATTACK).

WARNING SIGNS:

- Longer episodes of pain
- More frequent episodes
- Episodes precipitated more easily
- Episodes less responsive to medications

TREATMENT

SELF TREATMENT:

(See Prevention below.)

MEDICAL TREATMENT:

NITROGLYCERIN is the most commonly used drug to treat or prevent episodes of angina. Calcium channel blockers, such as diltiazem and nifedipine, and beta-blockers, such as atenolol and metoprolol, are also used to prevent episodes.

Aspirin and drugs to reduce blood cholesterol levels, such as cholestyramine and lovastatin, are also helpful in treating underlying coronary artery ATHEROSCLEROSIS.

SURGICAL TREATMENT:

Procedures to clear blockages and improve blood flow in the coronary arteries include

- CORONARY ARTERY BYPASS GRAFT SURGERY
- Percutaneous transluminal coronary ANGIOPLASTY

PREVENTION

- Avoid smoking
- Eat a low-fat, low-cholesterol diet
- Control HYPERTENSION with a low-sodium diet and diligent use of prescribed medication
- Regular exercise as recommended by a physician
- Estrogen replacement therapy for postmenopausal women (probably)
- Adequate vitamin E intake (possibly)

ARRHYTHMIA

A normal heart rhythm is regular and beats between approximately 50 and 100 times per minute during periods of rest—faster during periods of exertion. A heart rhythm that is abnormal is an arrhythmia. When the heart rhythm is too slow, it's called *bradycardia,* and when the rhythm is too fast, it's called *tachycardia.* Rhythm abnormalities can be either intermittent (called *paroxysmal*) or persistent.

CAUSES

The heart's rhythm is controlled by electrical impulses originating from areas in the heart called *nodes.* Disruptions in the normal rhythm can be caused by
- Scar tissue in the electrical system of the heart or in other parts of the heart muscle
- Degenerative changes in heart tissue
- Side effects of certain drugs—for example, erythromycin combined with terfenadine, or caffeine or cocaine
- Coronary artery disease (ATHEROSCLEROSIS and other conditions)
- MYOCARDITIS
- Excessive thyroid hormone
- Potassium and magnesium deficiency

SYMPTOMS

Many people with rhythm abnormalities do not have any symptoms. When someone does have symptoms, palpitations are one of the most common feelings. More serious rhythm abnormalities cause
- FAINTING OR FAINTNESS
- DIZZINESS
- Light-headedness
- BREATHING DIFFICULTY

The most severe rhythm disturbances can lead to sudden cardiac death.

DIAGNOSIS

Many rhythm abnormalities can be detected by a careful PHYSICAL EXAMINATION, especially of the pulse and neck veins.

Almost everyone will experience a heart rhythm abnormality— whether it's a skipped beat or a minor palpitation. Most of these occurrences are not serious. However, persistent rhythm problems can be dangerous.

The most definite diagnosis is by ELECTROCARDIOGRAPHY, which can be performed in many ways: Some individuals may wear Holter monitors, portable recorders usually worn for a 24-hour period. Longer-event monitors and even subcutaneous implants to monitor the heart rhythm are used in selected cases to capture and record an intermittent arrhythmia.

Electrophysiologic studies using pacing catheters are commonly used today both to detect and even treat rhythm abnormalities.

COMPLICATIONS

The most serious rhythm abnormalities can lead to unconsciousness, FAINTING OR FAINTNESS, and if prolonged, sudden cardiac death. Rhythm disturbances may also lead to the formation of emboli (see PULMONARY EMBOLISM and STROKE).

TREATMENT

SELF TREATMENT:

A physician may teach a patient certain "vagal maneuvers" in order to turn off an intermittent arrhythmia. This technique can trigger the nervous system to terminate certain types of rhythm abnormalities. These maneuvers include straining, gagging, or putting one's face in a bowl full of ice water. These should be attempted, however, only when a physician has directed one to do so.

Stress reduction may also help certain types of rhythm disturbances. Emotional stress can both precipitate rhythm disturbances and make someone more distressed by otherwise innocent rhythm disturbances.

MEDICAL TREATMENT:

Drug therapy may be necessary in extremely bothersome rhythm disturbances, such as palpitations that persistently keep someone from sleeping, or in otherwise harmless rhythm disturbances that are distressing despite reassurance. Drugs are usually reserved for serious rhythm abnormalities that have led to symptoms of FAINTING OR FAINTNESS or warning signs of sudden cardiac death.

Commonly used drugs include
- Procainamide
- Amiodarone
- Verapamil
- Propranolol
- Digoxin

Because some of these drugs can actually aggravate rhythm problems, drug therapy is generally reserved for the most serious disturbances. Anticoagulation drugs such as warfarin can also be used to cut down the chance of emboli in certain types of rhythm abnormalities, such as ATRIAL FIBRILLATION.

SURGICAL TREATMENT:

Electronic PACEMAKER INSERTION is commonly used to treat heart rhythms that are too slow and are causing distressing symptoms.

Some cases of tachycardia can be treated with a special catheter technique in which part of the faulty electrical system is destroyed. Some tachycardias that can lead to sudden cardiac death have a high rate of recurrence; in survivors, recurrences have been successfully treated with specialized pacemaker-like devices called implantable defibrillators.

Occasionally, open heart surgery is necessary to control some types of serious tachycardia.

PREVENTION

A generally heart-healthy lifestyle that may decrease the chance of rhythm disturbances includes
- Regular exercise
- Not smoking
- Avoiding excessive amounts of alcohol and caffeine
- Avoiding illegal drug use (especially cocaine)

ASTHMA

> Although asthma can be quite severe and problematic for some sufferers, most do not have debilitating disease, and symptoms are controllable.

Asthma is a chronic inflammation disorder of the bronchial tubes that causes excess mucus formation, muscular constriction, and variable degrees of reversible airflow obstruction, resulting in incomplete emptying of the lung and lung over-inflation. Unlike chronic bronchitis (BRONCHITIS, CHRONIC) though, asthma appears to be episodic in nature, and it can often be set off by various triggers such as allergens, cold air, and exercise.

CAUSES

The exact cause of asthma is not completely understood. It seems to have a genetic component because people with a family history of the disease have a greater risk of eventually developing it.

Other factors that may precipitate asthma in susceptible individuals include
- Childhood exposure to allergens such as warm-blooded animals and dust
- Exposure to tobacco smoke
- Certain respiratory infections
- Occupational exposure to plastics and some inorganic chemicals

SYMPTOMS

In the classic case of asthma, the patient experiences recurrent episodes of
- Wheezing
- BREATHING DIFFICULTY
- COUGH
- Chest tightness, particularly at night and in the early morning

Not every case is the classic case, and various combinations of these symptoms are possible in individual cases. Some patients, for example, experience COUGH alone; others experience BREATHING DIFFICULTY only during exercise or only at certain times of the year.

DIAGNOSIS

Asthma can usually be diagnosed from the symptoms and the MEDICAL HISTORY. A PHYSICAL EXAMINATION provides support for the diagnosis.

Other tests include measurements of lung function using a spirometer or peak flow meter (see PULMONARY FUNCTION TESTING). People with asthma have lower peak flow readings than people without asthma, especially after exercise.

Another common test for asthma is the methacholine challenge. It is a test of bronchial wall inflammation in the presence of the chemical methacholine. In people with asthma, methacholine causes a drop in lung function, which can be reversed with medication.

COMPLICATIONS

All patients with asthma are at risk of developing a severe asthma attack that can lead to respiratory failure—a disorder called *status asthmaticus*. Attacks of status asthmaticus can come on suddenly, or more commonly, the symptoms develop over a number of days until the patient ends up in the emergency room with respiratory distress. Regardless of the circumstance, status asthmaticus is a life-threatening disorder that can require mechanical ventilation in an intensive care unit.

Overinflated lungs may rupture, allowing air to escape into the chest cavity and compressing the lung tissue because the air can get in, but it can't get back out—a potentially life-threatening condition called *pneumothorax* that may require immediate treatment.

Because medication is used on a long-term basis in asthma, cumulative side effects can cause problems. Long-term steroid use can lead to

- WEIGHT GAIN
- Muscle loss
- Bone thinning (OSTEOPOROSIS)
- CATARACT
- High blood pressure (HYPERTENSION)
- Cushing syndrome

TREATMENT

SELF TREATMENT:

Avoiding asthma triggers, such as smoke or specific pollutants, and caring for general health, such as ensuring proper nutrition, are appropriate measures. Contact with pets may need to be limited.

MEDICAL TREATMENT:

For patients with infrequent symptoms, inhaled medications such as albuterol or metaproterenol provide adequate control.

For patients with more severe symptoms (episodes one to two times per week), specific treatment of bronchial wall inflammations is recommended. Inhaled anti-inflammatory medications such as steroids (beclomethasone), nedocromil sodium, or cromolyn sodium are effective. Nonsteroidal medication is preferred for children because steroids can retard growth. Theophylline, a bronchodilator, may have useful anti-inflammatory effects as well.

SURGICAL TREATMENT:

None.

PREVENTION

Primary prevention—preventing the development of asthma—includes altering the environment of those at risk for the disease, such as infants of asthmatic parents. Decreasing exposure to allergens, such as dust mites and warm-blooded pets, and to tobacco smoke can help. Vaccinations for children can prevent respiratory infections that may precipitate asthma.

Secondary prevention—preventing attacks in those who already have asthma—includes avoiding triggers, including some food additives, some drugs (beta-blockers) used to treat HYPERTENSION and GLAUCOMA, and anti-inflammatory agents such as aspirin and ibuprofen. Vaccinations and frequent hand washing can limit respiratory tract infections.

ATHEROSCLEROSIS

In atherosclerosis, also commonly called hardening of the arteries, fat and sometimes calcium deposits build up on the inner wall of blood vessels. Although the condition can affect blood vessels anywhere in the body, the vessels in which atherosclerosis causes the most noticeable problems include the coronary arteries, which feed the heart muscle, the carotid and vertebral arteries, which feed the brain, and the iliac and femoral arteries, which feed the legs.

CAUSES

Although the exact cause of atherosclerotic build-up in the blood vessels is not known, certain risk factors for atherosclerosis have been identified, including
* High blood pressure (HYPERTENSION)
* Smoking
* High blood cholesterol level (HYPERLIPIDEMIA)
* DIABETES
* Male gender
* Family history of the disease

SYMPTOMS

Atherosclerosis can be quite silent, causing no noticeable symptoms at all for long periods of time while deposits build up on the walls of blood vessels. Ultimately, though, the progressive occlusion of the blood vessels by fat and calcium deposits can lead to symptoms. Gradually progressive symptoms can stem from the slowly diminishing blood flow to the area, or sudden serious symptoms can appear when there is a sudden total blockage, or occlusion, of the blood vessel.

When a localized deposit of cholesterol and fats (called atherosclerotic *plaque*) ruptures and causes a blood clot to form, the blood vessel can become completely blocked and the flow of blood stopped. The specific symptoms of such an occurrence depend on the location of the affected blood vessels:
* If the arteries to the brain are affected, then the common symptoms include those of a transient ischemic attack—brief episodes of weakness in an arm or leg, difficulty speaking, or loss of vision in one eye—or STROKE.
* If the coronary arteries are affected, then symptoms related to ANGINA or HEART ATTACK can result.

Atherosclerosis is a condition that can lead to some of the biggest killers, including heart attacks and stroke.

- If the blood vessels to the bowels are affected (mesenteric ischemia), severe ABDOMINAL PAIN after meals can be a manifestation (especially in older people).
- If the vessels of the legs are affected, a reproducible, consistent ache that occurs most commonly in the back of the calf when walking and that is relieved with rest (a symptom known as *claudication*) is the most common manifestation.

DIAGNOSIS

Atherosclerosis can be diagnosed on the basis of typical symptoms. Sometimes a PHYSICAL EXAMINATION reveals a decreased circulation; examination of the pulses or listening for a turbulent flow (called *bruits*) can also provide clues.

Diagnostic tests include

- CARDIAC STRESS TEST to evaluate signs of atherosclerosis to the heart
- Carotid artery blood-flow studies (including ULTRASOUND) for evidence of decreased flow or blockages to the brain and legs
- Angiography (CARDIAC CATHETERIZATION and RADIOGRAPHY) of the affected area to show signs of narrowing caused by atherosclerosis

COMPLICATIONS

The complications of atherosclerosis are related to the area in which the circulation is affected. The most serious ones are

- STROKE—if the blood vessels in the brain are affected
- HEART ATTACK—if the coronary arteries are affected
- Gangrene—if the blood vessels of an extremity are affected

TREATMENT

SELF TREATMENT:

- Avoidance of smoking
- A low-fat, low-cholesterol diet
- Regular exercise

MEDICAL TREATMENT:

Because blockages are a dangerous consequence of atherosclerosis, drug therapy is aimed at promoting good blood flow. To this end, calcium-channel blockers, such as diltiazem and nifedipine, are sometimes prescribed. Nitroglycerin is commonly used to treat or prevent episodes of ANGINA caused by atherosclerosis. Beta-blockers, such as atenolol and metoprolol, are also used to help compensate for a lack of blood flow.

Aspirin, warfarin, and ticlopidine are sometimes used to decrease the chance of blood clots forming on a ruptured atherosclerotic plaque.

In recent years aggressive attempts to lower blood cholesterol levels have been shown to slow and even reverse progressive plaque buildup in the blood vessels to the brain, heart, and legs. Drugs such as simvastatin, lovastatin, cholestyramine, and niacin have been the most frequently used for this purpose.

SURGICAL TREATMENT:

Surgical procedures designed to treat more advanced cases of atherosclerosis include

- CORONARY ARTERY BYPASS GRAFT SURGERY
- Percutaneous transluminal ANGIOPLASTY
- CAROTID ENDARTECTOMY
- Peripheral vascular surgery (using veins to bypass blockages in the legs)

PREVENTION

- Avoidance of smoking
- Low-fat, low-cholesterol diet
- Control of HYPERTENSION
- Regular exercise
- Estrogen replacement therapy for postmenopausal women (probably)
- Adequate vitamin E intake (possibly)

ATRIAL FIBRILLATION

The frequency of atrial fibrillation increases with age; a few percent of people over 65 experience the condition.

Atrial fibrillation is an irregular heartbeat caused by rapid chaotic discharge of the upper chambers of the heart (called the *atria*). These erratic signals travel through the heart's electrical system to the bottom chambers (called the *ventricles*), leading to a rapid and irregular pulse.

CAUSES

Atrial fibrillation is most commonly related to some underlying heart disease, such as

- Hypertensive heart disease related to long-standing high blood pressure (see HYPERTENSION)
- HEART VALVE DISEASE
- Ischemic heart disease (such as prior HEART ATTACK)

Other causes include HYPERTHYROIDISM and excessive alcohol consumption that can cause heart rhythm and heart muscle problems.

SYMPTOMS

Atrial fibrillation in many cases can be completely without symptoms for years at a time. When it does cause symptoms, it may be noted as palpitation or an awareness of one's own heartbeat. Unfortunately, one of the complications of atrial fibrillation is sometimes the first sign to be noticed.

DIAGNOSIS

A PHYSICAL EXAMINATION that reveals a randomly irregular pulse may signal the presence of atrial fibrillation. The diagnosis is usually confirmed by ELECTROCARDIOGRAPHY.

COMPLICATIONS

The complications of atrial fibrillation include formation of blood clots in the atria that can travel to various parts of the body including the brain (leading to a STROKE or a transient ischemic attack), the abdominal organs (for example, the bowels), or the extremities (causing a suddenly cold and painful pulseless arm or leg and possibly gangrene). This complication is called an *embolism*.

Because atrial fibrillation is a less efficient form of heart function, it may also lead to a worsening of CONGESTIVE HEART FAILURE or ANGINA.

TREATMENT

SELF TREATMENT:

Lifestyle changes that decrease the underlying causes of atrial fibrillation (HYPERTENSION, alcoholism, or coronary artery disease) are the most helpful. Measures include

- Low-salt diet
- Moderate exercise
- Avoidance of alcohol
- Avoidance of other risk factors for ATHEROSCLEROSIS

MEDICAL TREATMENT:

Pharmaceutical treatment can help control the heart rate with digoxin, verapamil, and beta-blockers such as propranolol. Attempts to convert the heart rhythm to a more normal rhythm (called a *sinus* rhythm) may include the use of the drugs quinidine, procainamide, or amiodarone.

Drugs can also be useful in the control of potential embolic complications. The drugs warfarin and aspirin reduce the blood's clotting ability, thus decreasing the chance of blood-clot formation in the atria and the risk of embolism.

Another medical therapy is electrical cardioversion, which involves using electrical paddles in a monitored setting to convert the atrial fibrillation to a normal sinus rhythm.

SURGICAL TREATMENT:

Surgical therapies are rarely used to treat atrial fibrillation, but some persistent and severe atrial rhythm abnormalities that do not respond to drug treatment may warrant surgery. Certain electrical oblation techniques involving catheters passed through blood vessels to the heart or open heart surgery to change the electrical pathways within the heart can be used to treat these rare severe cases.

PREVENTION

- Avoidance of excessive alcohol consumption
- Appropriate treatment of strep throat infection to decrease the chance of rheumatic heart disease and HEART VALVE DISEASE
- Measures to decrease the risk of ATHEROSCLEROSIS
- Weight control and adherence to a low-salt diet

BLADDER INFECTION

Bladder infections are almost always bacterial infections. In women, these infections can recur sporadically, and although they are often uncomfortable and inconvenient, they are rarely dangerous.

In men, bladder infections are often a signal of some underlying urologic problem.

CAUSES

Bladder infections are usually caused by bacteria migrating up the urethra to the bladder. Often bacteria from other parts of the body are involved; bacteria that normally live in the digestive tract, for example, are frequently implicated in bladder infections because of the close proximity of the anus and the urethra, especially in women. Recurrent infections in women may sometimes be associated with sexual intercourse (see Prevention below).

In men, a bladder infection is usually caused by an infection of the prostate gland that has spread to the bladder or by bacteria trapped in the bladder by an enlarged prostate (PROSTATE, ENLARGED).

SYMPTOMS

The symptoms of a bladder infection include
* Frequent and often urgent need to urinate (URINATION, FREQUENT)
* Burning sensation upon urination (URINATION, PAINFUL)
* Lower back pain (occasionally)
* FEVER (occasionally)
* Blood in the urine (rarely, and usually seen in women only)

DIAGNOSIS

Bladder infection can usually be suspected from the symptoms, but the definitive diagnosis of bladder infection relies primarily on two basic tests
* URINALYSIS
* Urine CULTURE

COMPLICATIONS

Left untreated, bladder infection can lead to kidney infection, which can, in turn, progress to BLOOD POISONING, KIDNEY STONES, and kidney damage.

TREATMENT

SELF TREATMENT:
Drinking plenty of fluids can help.

MEDICAL TREATMENT:
The main weapons used to fight bladder infection are antibiotics such as
- Trimethoprim
- Ampicillin
- Sulfamethoxazole
- Ofloxacin

For men whose infection is associated with an underlying urologic problem such as an enlarged prostate (PROSTATE, ENLARGED), the underlying condition is also treated.

SURGICAL TREATMENT:
None.

PREVENTION

- Drinking plenty of fluids and not delaying urination help to flush the bladder regularly.
- Front-to-back wiping with toilet tissue can prevent contamination of the urethra by bacteria from the anal area.
- For women who experience recurrent bladder infections associated with sexual intercourse, urinating immediately after intercourse may prevent some infections.

BLADDER STONES

The urine produced by the kidneys and stored in the urinary bladder contains various inorganic minerals that can, under certain circumstances, precipitate and form stones.

Bladder stones are conglomerates of minerals that form in the urinary bladder for various reasons. The stones can vary considerably in size and shape and can cause severe discomfort.

CAUSES

Although the exact cause of stones is quite often never determined, stones most commonly form when the bladder does not empty completely, allowing time for minerals in the urine to coalesce. This condition can be brought on by an obstruction or by an anatomic abnormality that allows the urine to pool.

BLADDER INFECTIONS can change the chemical nature of the urine, contributing to stone formation. Less often, the stones can be a result of KIDNEY STONES that have passed down the ureter and lodged in the bladder.

There may be a hereditary tendency to develop bladder stones; people with a family history of bladder stones appear to have an increased chance of developing them.

SYMPTOMS

The symptoms are relatively obvious and include
*   Sharp pain in the bladder region (lower ABDOMINAL PAIN) that can come in waves
*   Sudden, painful interruption of flow during urination

The pain of bladder stones is sometimes associated with
*   Profuse sweating (SWEATING, EXCESSIVE)
*   VOMITING and nausea
*   Blood in the urine (URINE, ABNORMAL APPEARANCE)

DIAGNOSIS

Besides the tell-tale symptoms, diagnosis can include
*   X ray (RADIOGRAPHY) of the bladder
*   ULTRASOUND of the bladder

COMPLICATIONS

- Bladder stones can set the stage for a BLADDER INFEC-
TION.
- Prolonged obstruction of the urinary tract can lead
to kidney damage.

TREATMENT

SELF TREATMENT:
(See Prevention below.)

MEDICAL TREATMENT:
(See Prevention below.)

SURGICAL TREATMENT:
If the stones are not passed, they are removed surgically
with either an open surgical technique or with a cystoscope—
a flexible tube that passes up through the urethra. The latter
procedure is less expensive and requires no incision, but
might not be appropriate for all kinds of stones.

PREVENTION

Adequate fluid intake ensures proper hydration and may
discourage stone formation.

Drugs such as hydrochlorothiazide and allopurinol may be
used to prevent additional stone formation, depending on the
type of stone and the likelihood of recurrence. This preventive therapy is not appropriate for all patients, however.

BLOOD POISONING

Blood poisoning is a nonmedical term used to describe patients who have a serious bacterial infection that is causing widespread reaction in the body.

The technical term for blood poisoning is *septicemia*, or *sepsis*. The danger of septicemia can be caused by the rampant infection itself or by toxins being released by the bacteria and spread through the blood. By definition, the whole body is affected because the blood distributes the bacteria and toxins throughout the body.

CAUSES

An infection in any one portion of the body that gets out of control and spreads throughout the body is the cause of blood poisoning. Examples of conditions that can lead to septicemia include

- Ruptured appendix in appendicitis
- Ruptured gallbladder (see CHOLECYSTITIS AND CHOLANGITIS)
- Kidney infection
- PELVIC INFLAMMATORY DISEASE
- Gangrene
- Tooth abscess

Immunosuppressive drugs such as prednisone and diseases such as DIABETES and LEUKEMIA that interfere with the body's immune system can also precipitate septicemia.

SYMPTOMS

Any one symptom is not sufficient to label a patient as having blood poisoning. However, the increasing number and constellation of them does. These symptoms include

- Shaking chills
- High FEVER
- Fast heart rate
- Confusion or other symptoms of mental impairment such as MEMORY PROBLEMS
- Low blood pressure
- General malaise (a feeling of being unwell)

DIAGNOSIS

Diagnosis is based on the symptoms. Additional tests that may be helpful include white blood cell count (see BLOOD COUNT) and blood CULTURES looking for bacteria.

In severely ill patients with low blood pressure, additional measurements may be made with a catheter threaded up to the right side of the heart (see CARDIAC CATHETERIZATION). The additional cardiovascular measurements may further confirm a picture of sepsis and aid in the proper treatment.

COMPLICATIONS

Very low blood pressure can progress to shock, with multiple organ failure and even death. Organs that can fail during sepsis are the kidneys, lungs and, less often, the liver. Also, any underlying heart disease would be aggravated during the period of low blood pressure because of the extreme stress sepsis puts on the heart.

TREATMENT

SELF TREATMENT:

A person with symptoms of septicemia requires prompt medical attention; however, general measures include reducing the FEVER with acetaminophen and maintaining adequate hydration by drinking enough fluids.

MEDICAL TREATMENT:

Generally, broad-spectrum antibiotics such as gentamicin and large volumes of intravenous fluids are the initial treatments for sepsis. Temporary measures to assist with any organ failure may be necessary, including drugs such as furosemide to maintain urine flow, oxygen to assist the lungs, and drugs such as dopamine to help the heart.

Occasionally, if sepsis progresses to total KIDNEY FAILURE or respiratory failure, mechanical devices such as dialysis or mechanical ventilation may be required on a temporary basis.

SURGICAL TREATMENT:

Surgical drainage may be required of the original source of the infection, such as a ruptured appendix, a ruptured gallbladder, or an abscess located elsewhere in the body.

PREVENTION

Prompt attention to bacterial infections can generally prevent them from progressing to blood poisoning. For certain high-risk individuals, vaccinations are appropriate such as pneumococcal vaccine for older adults or patients with significant heart or lung disease or DIABETES.

BOIL

Boils are usually more unsightly than dangerous, but they can precipitate dangerous complications, especially if treated improperly.

A boil, also called a *carbuncle*, is an infection of the follicle of a hair. Accordingly, they occur only in areas of the skin that have hair follicles. Areas of the skin that are subject to friction and perspiration are common sites of boils, including the neck, face, underarms, skin folds, and buttocks.

As the boil progresses, the infected hair follicle becomes a firm, deep-seated, inflammatory bump (or nodule). It can be warm and tender and usually is red. It may eventually drain pus, especially if manipulated.

CAUSES

Boils are caused by infection of the hair follicle by the bacteria *Staphylococcus aureus*.

SYMPTOMS

A boil is a firm, warm, tender, deep-seated, red nodule in a hair-bearing region of the skin. The nodule may drain pus or feel like it has liquid inside of it. If the nodule drains the pus, the tenderness usually improves rapidly, and the nodule may resolve itself over several days.

DIAGNOSIS

A physician can usually recognize a boil, or carbuncle. The diagnosis may be confirmed by sampling the pus and performing a gram stain and CULTURE to identify *Staphylococcus aureus*. Sometimes a BIOPSY is performed on the lesion to confirm that it is, in fact, just a boil.

COMPLICATIONS

- The infection of the hair follicle may spread to involve surrounding soft tissue and even bone.
- A chronic deeper infection involving fibrotic firm connective tissue may occur; this is called a *furuncle* and can be difficult to eradicate.
- A diffuse infection of the skin around the hair follicle may occur. This is called cellulitis.
- Sometimes the bacteria in the infected hair follicle can spread to the blood stream (sepsis, or BLOOD POISONING) and cause a systemic infection involving other organs.

TREATMENT

SELF TREATMENT:

- Moist warm compresses should be applied to the boil to encourage it to drain spontaneously.
- The patient should make every effort to avoid manipulating the boil or squeezing it.
- After the boil ruptures and releases its contents, the area can be soaked with aluminum acetate solution for one hour two to four times a day.
- An over-the-counter ointment containing polymyxin B sulfate and bacitracin (such as Polysporin) applied between soaks can be helpful.
- The lesion should be washed with an antibacterial soap (such as Hibiclens) daily, and the patient should wash his or her hands very well with the same soap after changing dressings.

MEDICAL TREATMENT:

Systemic antibiotics against *Staphylococcus aureus*, such as penicillin or dicloxacillin, are usually the first medical treatments indicated. For patients who are allergic to penicillin, clindamycin and erythromycin are good alternative antibiotics. Unresponsive or recurrent boils can be treated with rifampin, another antibiotic.

All of the above self-treatment measures should be instituted by the physician if the patient has not yet started them.

SURGICAL TREATMENT:

Boils can be lanced and drained by a physician, but warm, moist compresses accomplish the same thing and allow the lesion to drain spontaneously with minimal trauma to the tissues.

PREVENTION

- Washing and changing clothes, towels, and bed linens frequently
- Use of antibacterial soap in areas of previous boil eruption
- Meticulous hygiene and daily bathing

BREAST CANCER

About one in ten women will get breast cancer at sometime in their life, usually between the ages of 50 and 70.

Breast cancer is a cancer that originates in the breast tissue of women and men. It can spread to the lymph nodes under the arm before diagnosis. With advanced disease, metastasis can be seen in many body organs, including bone, brain, lung, liver, and skin.

CAUSES

Risk factors for developing breast cancer include
- Early onset of menses or late menopause
- First pregnancy after age 30
- Family history of the disease
- Radiation exposure

Possible risk factors include
- High-fat diet
- Excessive alcohol intake
- Estrogen replacement therapy
- Oral contraceptive use

SYMPTOMS

Breast cancer is usually manifest as a painless lump anywhere in the breast or under the arm (see BREAST PAIN OR LUMPS). Occasionally, its symptoms can be more subtle, such as
- An inverted nipple
- Bloody discharge from the nipple
- Changes in the skin overlying the breast making it resemble the skin of an orange

DIAGNOSIS

Any BREAST PAIN OR LUMPS felt on PHYSICAL EXAMINATION by a woman or her physician, and any lumps found on mammography (RADIOGRAPHY) should be considered for BIOPSY. Lumps seen on mammography but not palpable on examination can be located by ULTRASOUND or mammogram for BIOPSY.

If a diagnosis of breast cancer is established, staging tests include
- Liver function tests (see BLOOD TESTS)
- Alkaline phosphatase test to check for bone disease (see BLOOD TESTS)
- Chest X ray (RADIOGRAPHY)
- Bone scan (NUCLEAR MEDICINE)

COMPLICATIONS

Complications of breast cancer are related to areas of metastasis:

- Metastasis to bone can cause pain, bone fractures, or elevated calcium levels in the blood.
- Metastasis to the brain or spinal cord can cause seizures, HEADACHES, weakness, NUMBNESS, or confusion.
- Metastasis to the lungs can cause BREATHING DIFFICULTY, CHEST PAIN, or swelling of the face and neck.

TREATMENT

SELF TREATMENT:

- A well-balanced diet should be maintained.
- Once a diagnosis of breast cancer is made, all estrogen medication should be stopped, including birth control pills.

MEDICAL TREATMENT:

Many women will require additional drug therapy after surgery to prevent breast cancer from returning. Either tamoxifen (a hormonal pill) or chemotherapy (intravenous medication) may be recommended, depending on the type of tumor. More advanced breast cancer is also treated with chemotherapy or hormonal therapy.

SURGICAL TREATMENT:

Two alternative initial treatments for breast cancer are

- Lumpectomy with lymph node dissection followed by radiation therapy to the breast
- Mastectomy (MASTECTOMY, PARTIAL; or MASTECTOMY, MODIFIED RADICAL)

PREVENTION

Early detection of breast cancer by regular breast self-examination and regular mammography (RADIOGRAPHY) screening is important. A low-fat diet and moderate alcohol intake may be important. Some researchers theorize that exercise for preadolescent girls may be helpful as it delays the age of onset of menstruation.

BRONCHITIS, CHRONIC

Chronic bronchitis
is distinguished
from acute
bronchitis by its
duration and cause.
The acute condition
is an inflammation
of the bronchial
tubes caused by an
infection; the
chronic condition
causes ongoing
symptoms even
without infection.

Chronic bronchitis is a condition of the lung characterized by excess mucus in the bronchial tubes and a COUGH present on most days. In patients with chronic bronchitis, there is an increase in the number and size of mucus-secreting glands in the bronchial tubes.

Because the condition is so closely associated with smoking, people with chronic bronchitis often have EMPHYSEMA as well.

CAUSES

The most important cause of chronic bronchitis is smoking. The greater the extent and duration of smoking, the greater the likelihood of developing bronchitis. Other causes include occupational exposures to chemicals and exposure to air pollutants. There are also cases that have no apparent cause. Infections generally do not cause chronic bronchitis but can aggravate the condition.

SYMPTOMS

The hallmarks of chronic bronchitis are
- Persistent COUGH
- Excess mucus
- BREATHING DIFFICULTY
- Wheezing (occasionally)
- ANKLE SWELLING in cases of heart strain

Respiratory symptoms tend to wax and wane, resulting in "good days" and "bad days." The coughing and mucus production are often worst first thing in the morning.

DIAGNOSIS

The diagnosis of chronic bronchitis is made from the characteristic symptoms and a characteristic MEDICAL HISTORY that includes a long history of smoking. PHYSICAL EXAMINATION often reveals wheezes and a prolonged expiratory phase during breathing similar to but not as pronounced as that seen in ASTHMA and EMPHYSEMA. Other tests include
- PULMONARY FUNCTION TESTING
- Chest X rays (RADIOGRAPHY)
- Testing of blood oxygen and carbon dioxide levels (see BLOOD TESTS)

COMPLICATIONS

Patients with chronic bronchitis tend to minimize their symptoms by adopting a sedentary lifestyle, resulting in general deconditioning and WEIGHT GAIN—both of which can aggravate BREATHING DIFFICULTY.

Because the condition can lead to decreased levels of oxygen in the blood and a subsequent constriction of pulmonary blood vessels, chronic bronchitis can lead to heart strain and symptoms of CONGESTIVE HEART FAILURE.

Infections are particularly dangerous in chronic bronchitis and can lead to life-threatening PNEUMONIA.

TREATMENT

SELF TREATMENT:

- Quitting smoking
- Embarking on a sensible exercise program
- Washing hands frequently to decrease the risk of infection

MEDICAL TREATMENT:

- Oxygen for patients whose blood-oxygen level is too low
- Inhaled bronchodilators such as albuterol and ipratropium bromide and oral bronchodilators such as theophylline to improve airflow
- Corticosteroids (prednisone) to reduce swelling and inflammation in the bronchial tubes
- Antibiotics to address infections promptly
- Guaifenesin to loosen mucus

INFLUENZA vaccine given in the fall can protect against the usual outbreak of INFLUENZA seen in the winter months. Pneumococcal vaccine offers protection against one of the most common causes of PNEUMONIA.

SURGICAL TREATMENT:

None.

PREVENTION

Avoidance of smoking and exposure to smoke and pollutants is the most important preventive step.

BURSITIS

Bursitis is an inflammatory condition of the small fluid filled sacs (called *bursas*) overlying prominent parts of the skeleton. A bursa normally consists of a thin sac with lining cells that decrease the gliding friction of tendons or other soft tissues as they move and rub against each other. In bursitis, the inflamed lining cells increase the fluid production and cause swelling and tension.

Patients who have bursitis in an area may have recurrent episodes, as the lining cells become more susceptible to pressure or friction.

> Bursitis can usually be attributed to some overuse or injury, but not all cases have an obvious cause.

CAUSES

Bursitis is frequently caused by minor trauma or overuse in the area of the bursa or by adjacent tendons. Repeated physical activities, such as swinging a tennis racket or sweeping, can cause bursitis.

There are also medical conditions, such as gout, that cause inflammatory changes in joints and tendons throughout the body that can involve the bursas.

SYMPTOMS

Patients may notice pain and swelling in the area and painful motion as they use a particular joint. The overlying skin may become red or feel warm. Bursitis is most commonly seen in the shoulders, elbows, wrist, lateral area of the hip, knees, and ankles.

DIAGNOSIS

Diagnosis of bursitis is generally made clinically by combining the patient's recent activity history with the findings of a PHYSICAL EXAMINATION; the findings are usually similar to those noted by the patients themselves.

Occasionally, fluid can be removed for testing, primarily when there is concern that the bursa might be infected. X rays (RADIOGRAPHY) may be helpful in evaluating the painful joint, but the film will not show the bursa itself.

COMPLICATIONS

The main complication of bursitis is an infection of the bursa. The bursa is frequently just under the skin, and it is possible that skin bacteria could cause an infection.

TREATMENT

SELF TREATMENT:
- Decreasing the activity involving the joint gives the inflammation time to go down.
- Over-the-counter anti-inflammatory and analgesic medication such as ibuprofen can reduce pain and inflammation.

MEDICAL TREATMENT:
- Splinting may help the joint rest by limiting its motion.
- Anti-inflammatory and analgesic medication such as ibuprofen and naproxen can reduce pain and inflammation.

SURGICAL TREATMENT:
In severe or recurrent cases, bursal drainage (in which the fluid is drawn out of the swollen bursa) and bursectomy (in which the affected bursa is removed) are options.

PREVENTION

Many times, bursitis is caused by repetitive overuse or minimal traumas associated with sports or work. Early recognition of overuse problems and treatment with rest and anti-inflammatory medications may resolve the problem before serious problems arise.

CARDIOMYOPATHY

When a disease of the heart muscle affects its ability to pump blood normally, the term *cardiomyopathy* is used.

There are three basic categories of cardiomyopathy based on the cause and the mechanical difficulty with the heart muscle: 1) the heart balloons out in size (dilated); 2) the heart thickens excessively (hypertrophic); or 3) the heart loses its ability to relax between heartbeats and refill for the next contraction (restrictive).

CAUSES

A wide variety of causes have been identified, although many cases do not have any apparent cause. Common causes include

- Advanced HYPERTENSION or coronary artery disease (ATHEROSCLEROSIS)
- Familial hypertrophic cardiomyopathies
- Chronic excessive alcohol intake (alcoholism)
- Vitamin deficiencies (for example, thiamin)
- Viral infections causing MYOCARDITIS
- Pregnancy-related cardiomyopathy

Obesity and DIABETES may also contribute to the problem. In some cases, medications such as thyroid hormone may contribute to the problem and need to be regulated.

SYMPTOMS

Many times, some decrease in heart muscle performance is without symptoms. In more advanced stages, signs of CONGESTIVE HEART FAILURE (BREATHING DIFFICULTY, ANKLE SWELLING) or symptoms from complications may be the first clue.

DIAGNOSIS

A MEDICAL HISTORY and PHYSICAL EXAMINATION compatible with CONGESTIVE HEART FAILURE would be the initial step in diagnosis. A chest X ray (RADIOGRAPHY) and ELECTROCARDIOGRAPHY provide additional information. The absence of other causes of CONGESTIVE HEART FAILURE, such as HYPERTENSION, ATHEROSCLEROSIS, HEART VALVE DISEASE, or pericardial or congenital heart disease, increases the likelihood of a primary heart muscle problem. An echocardiogram (ULTRASOUND) or NUCLEAR MEDICINE study can confirm a cardiomyopathy. In some cases, CARDIAC CATHETERIZATION, angiography (RADIOGRAPHY), and BIOPSY may be needed.

COMPLICATIONS

Cardiomyopathy may lead to ARRHYTHMIAS (ventricular tachycardia, heart block), causing FAINTING OR FAINTNESS or even cardiac arrest. When young people in athletic events die unexpectedly, this is often the cause. Dilated heart muscles may allow blood clots to form along the inner walls of the heart, and these may break off and travel to the brain or limbs, causing a STROKE or gangrene.

TREATMENT

SELF TREATMENT:
(See Prevention below.)

MEDICAL TREATMENT:
- Control of hypertension with medication such as hydrochlorothiazide
- Treatment of CONGESTIVE HEART FAILURE with medications such as digoxin, furosemide, and ACE inhibitors (enalapril)
- In selected cases of MYOCARDITIS, immunosuppressive treatment with medication such as prednisone
- The suspension, at least on a trial basis, of medications that may aggravate CONGESTIVE HEART FAILURE, such as steroids, beta-blockers (atenolol, propranolol), disopyramide, and verapamil

SURGICAL TREATMENT:
- Heart transplant or related surgery may be warranted in advanced refractory cases where the prognosis is otherwise poor.
- Occasionally, CORONARY ARTERY BYPASS GRAFT SURGERY may help in very carefully selected patients.

PREVENTION

- Control of HYPERTENSION
- Treatment of ATHEROSCLEROSIS
- Avoidance of excessive alcohol intake
- Maintenance of a healthy weight
- Other strategies to prevent ATHEROSCLEROSIS (not smoking, low-fat diet, regular exercise)

CARPAL TUNNEL SYNDROME

Carpal tunnel syndrome is a grouping of symptoms involving the median nerve in the wrist and hand. Symptoms include NUMBNESS, tingling, weakness, and pain in the palm side of the wrist and hand, which are innervated by the median nerve. Symptoms in the fingers are most frequently noted in the thumb-side fingers (thumb, index finger, and middle finger).

> Carpal tunnel syndrome can affect anyone, but the most commonly affected group is women in their 30s and 40s.

CAUSES

Carpal tunnel syndrome is caused by a decrease in the local blood supply to the median nerve as it moves through a tunnel-like area in the wrist. The nerve shares the tunnel with the flexor tendons of the wrist (the tendons of muscles that flex the wrist and fingers), and may be under pressure if the tendons swell from overuse.

Swelling of the soft tissues caused by increased fluid volume (particularly in pregnancy) may also increase the pressure in the carpal tunnel and decrease the blood supply to the nerve.

SYMPTOMS

The symptoms of carpal tunnel syndrome include
- NUMBNESS and tingling on the thumb side of the hand, including the thumb, index finger, and middle finger
- Weakness of thumb-side grip strength
- Pain in the hand and wrist that may worsen with repetitive motions or increase when the wrist is flexed

DIAGNOSIS

The diagnosis of carpal tunnel syndrome includes noting the symptoms and finding NUMBNESS or weakness on PHYSICAL EXAMINATION. These findings may be determined by sensory testing and by objective measurements of grip and finger strength. Several tests may briefly increase the pressure on the median nerve and provoke the symptoms.

Definitive evidence of nerve compression with slowing of the nerve signals of the median nerve can be demonstrated with electrical testing (electromyography) in which electrodes are attached to the forearm.

COMPLICATIONS

Episodic NUMBNESS and tingling complaints can resolve with time; prolonged and continuous loss of sensory abilities and motor strength may suggest more severe compression of the nerve, which can lead to permanent nerve damage and chronic symptoms.

TREATMENT

SELF TREATMENT:
Avoidance of repetitive activities that cause symptoms may help reduce inflammation.

MEDICAL TREATMENT:
- Anti-inflammatory medications such as ibuprofen and naproxen
- Wrist splints to keep the wrists in a neutral position
- Injection of anti-inflammatory medications to decrease swelling

Women who have symptoms associated with pregnancy may not need treatment because the condition can resolve after delivery when fluid volume returns to normal; however, splints may relieve discomfort if needed.

SURGICAL TREATMENT:
CARPAL TUNNEL RELEASE may be appropriate for certain intractable cases.

PREVENTION

Carpal tunnel syndrome is considered a chronic overuse condition; interrupting continuous activities with a break or varying hand and wrist positions frequently during repetitive tasks may be helpful.

CATARACT

A cataract is an opacity, or clouding, of the crystalline lens of the eye that reduces visual function.

> The lens of the eye, which helps to focus light onto the retina, is usually clear, but the clouding effect of a cataract scatters the incoming light, causing blurred vision.

CAUSES

Cataracts are usually associated with aging, but they can also occur in patients with certain diseases such as DIABETES. Drugs such as steroids and cortisone taken orally or topically can induce cataracts. Cataracts can also occur after trauma to the eye or in association with a chronic inflammation.

SYMPTOMS

Cataract causes VISION DISTURBANCES including
- Altered color vision
- Diminished side vision or night vision
- Double vision in the affected eye

DIAGNOSIS

The diagnosis is made after a careful eye examination in which a microscope is used to examine the lens of the eye.

COMPLICATIONS

GLAUCOMA and inflammation can occur in rare cases.

TREATMENT

SELF TREATMENT:
None.

MEDICAL TREATMENT:
Pupil-dilating eye drops that allow the patient to see around the cloudy part of the lens.

SURGICAL TREATMENT:
CATARACT REMOVAL is indicated in some patients.

PREVENTION

Cataracts can be prevented in some cases by
- Promptly treating ocular inflammation
- Using eye protection in hazardous situations

CERVICAL CANCER

The cervix is that part of the uterus that protrudes into the vagina and dilates during labor. Cervical cancer can be formed from either the cells on the outside surface of the cervix (squamous cells) or the cells inside the cervical canal (glandular or adenocarcinoma cells).

CAUSES

Malignant cells in the cervix are thought to arise from a particular event or exposure. Risk factors associated with pre-malignant changes that can go on to form cancer include
- Early sexual intercourse
- Multiple sexual partners
- Infection with certain types of human papilloma virus (genital warts)
- Tobacco use

In addition, women who were exposed prenatally to a substance called diethylstilbestrol (DES)—a drug that until 1971 was given to some pregnant women to help prevent miscarriage—are at increased risk for a rare type of cervical cancer.

SYMPTOMS

Premalignant changes usually cause no symptoms. Once the cancer becomes invasive, however, patients may notice
- Unusual VAGINAL DISCHARGE, which may or may not be malodorous
- Bleeding or spotting after intercourse

Advanced cancer may be associated with
- Pain in the back or leg
- Blood in the urine
- Loss of urine through the vagina

DIAGNOSIS

Fortunately, there is a long premalignant phase for most cervical cancers. PAP SMEARS are screening tests for the presence of abnormal cells on the cervix. Once a PAP SMEAR is found to be abnormal, colposcopy is performed. This involves looking at the cervix with a special microscope and using special solutions such as acetic acid to highlight and visualize the areas of abnormality (see ENDOSCOPY).

Once these areas are seen, a BIOPSY may be performed to obtain a sample for pathologic analysis. Depending on the

Cervical cancer is preceded by a precancerous condition that is usually detectable only by Pap smear. This simple test, then, allows women to catch and treat cervical cancer before it becomes malignant.

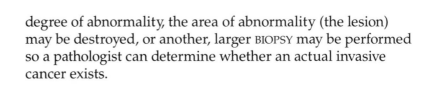

degree of abnormality, the area of abnormality (the lesion) may be destroyed, or another, larger BIOPSY may be performed so a pathologist can determine whether an actual invasive cancer exists.

COMPLICATIONS

Allowing the cancer to progress without therapy will likely result in life-threatening bleeding and blockage of the urine flow from the kidneys to the bladder resulting in KIDNEY FAILURE and death.

TREATMENT

SELF TREATMENT:

None.

MEDICAL TREATMENT:

Medical therapy for cervical cancer is reserved for patients with cancer that has spread. Chemotherapy is used but is not as effective as either surgery or radiation therapy.

SURGICAL TREATMENT:

A radical HYSTERECTOMY with removal of the lymph nodes from the pelvis is performed for patients with early cancer. Once the cancer has spread beyond the cervix to the tissue next to the uterus, radiation therapy is necessary.

PREVENTION

Cervical cancer has a long premalignant phase that can be treated with minimal surgical therapy and retention of reproductive function. However, in order for this to occur, the patient must have regular pelvic examinations and PAP SMEARS performed by a physician experienced in interpreting the results. The frequency of the examinations should be based on the individual woman's risk factors.

Lifestyle changes to help prevent the development of premalignant changes include

- Sexual abstinence unless in a mutually monogamous relationship
- Avoidance of smoking
- Use of barrier methods of contraception

CHOLECYSTITIS AND CHOLANGITIS

Cholecystitis is an inflammation in the gallbladder; the condition can be chronic or acute. Chronic cholecystitis is the inflammation that is found with symptomatic GALLSTONES. Acute cholecystitis is a complication of GALLSTONES that causes infection in the gallbladder wall and bile.

Cholangitis is an inflammation in the bile duct system. It is most often due to bacteria, but it can be viral, parasitic, or chemical in nature.

CAUSES

The cause of chronic cholecystitis is not known, but mechanical irritation of the gallbladder or intermittent obstruction of the gallbladder by GALLSTONES are suspected.

Acute cholecystitis results when a GALLSTONE obstructs the duct emptying the gallbladder. Infection begins in the bile behind the stone and extends into the gallbladder wall.

Acute cholangitis occurs when bile contains bacteria and when the pressure increases in the bile duct system. Increased pressure can be caused by several factors, including obstruction of the bile duct by a GALLSTONE; a bile duct narrowing; or a tumor of the bile duct, of the first part of the intestine (the duodenum), or of the pancreas (PANCREATIC CANCER), which the bile duct traverses to reach the intestine.

SYMPTOMS

Chronic cholecystitis causes
- Intermittent attacks of upper right ABDOMINAL PAIN
- Nausea and VOMITING
- Indigestion
- Increased flatulence

Acute cholecystitis causes
- Unremitting upper right ABDOMINAL PAIN
- FEVER
- Nausea and VOMITING

The symptoms of acute cholecystitis may be very similar to chronic cholecystitis, but the symptoms do not resolve spontaneously. They progress and worsen with time.

Acute cholangitis typically causes
- Jaundice
- Upper right ABDOMINAL PAIN
- FEVER

Cholecystitis and cholangitis are discussed together because the gallbladder and the bile ducts are connected, and infection in one can spread to the other.

However, most patients have only one or two of the three symptoms.

Sometimes acute cholangitis can be very severe, in which case it is called *toxic cholangitis*. In this condition, the patient experiences confusion and very low blood pressure. This is a life-threatening event and requires emergency treatment.

DIAGNOSIS

Chronic cholecystitis is diagnosed from the history of the symptoms and by documenting the presence of GALLSTONES with ULTRASOUND of the gallbladder. If ULTRASOUND is not helpful, X rays (RADIOGRAPHY) can be used.

Acute cholecystitis may be diagnosed by the symptoms, a PHYSICAL EXAMINATION, and by documenting the presence of GALLSTONES with ULTRASOUND of the gallbladder. NUCLEAR MEDICINE tests can be very useful in the diagnosis.

With both chronic and acute cholecystitis, blood levels of enzymes produced by the liver and bilirubin are measured (see BLOOD TESTS) to exclude liver disease and jaundice due to stones in the common bile duct.

Acute cholangitis is suspected from the symptoms and from elevated levels of liver enzymes and bilirubin (see BLOOD TESTS). Diagnostic tests are then directed toward defining the cause of the cholangitis. Endoscopic retrograde cholangiography is a test in which a flexible scope is passed from the mouth through the stomach and into the duodenum to find the opening of the common bile duct (see ENDOSCOPY). A small tube is then placed into the opening and radiologic dye is injected while X rays (RADIOGRAPHY) are taken. COMPUTED TOMOGRAPHY of the abdomen is useful in some cases to exclude a tumor in the area of the bile duct, such as a PANCREATIC CANCER.

COMPLICATIONS

- Chronic cholecystitis can develop into acute cholecystitis.
- GALLSTONES can pass into the common bile duct causing jaundice (and possibly cholangitis) or PANCREATITIS.
- Acute cholecystitis can lead to perforation of the gallbladder with abscess formation or to generalized infection in the abdomen (peritonitis).

- Acute cholangitis can lead to systemic infection in the circulatory system (BLOOD POISONING). This is a life-threatening condition.
- Patients with bile duct obstruction and acute cholangitis become very dehydrated and experience circulation impairment leading to critically low blood pressure and possibly KIDNEY FAILURE.

TREATMENT

SELF TREATMENT:
Avoiding fatty meals may be helpful, but patients with symptomatic GALLSTONES should seek medical advice.

MEDICAL TREATMENT:
Asymptomatic GALLSTONES do not require treatment. The risk of observation is no higher than that of treatment.

Symptomatic GALLSTONES should be treated; the risk of complications increases significantly once symptoms are present. The orally administered bile salts, ursodeoxycholate or chenodeoxycholate, dissolve cholesterol GALLSTONES in selected patients. Dissolution requires 12 to 24 months, and stones recur in the majority of patients. Unfortunately, most patients have stones that are not amenable to this treatment.

SURGICAL TREATMENT:
For cholecystitis, GALLBLADDER REMOVAL can be performed. Antibiotics are usually administered in conjunction with the procedure.

For cholangitis, options include
- Endoscopic retrograde cholangiography (see page 120), papillotomy (increasing the size of the bile duct opening to allow the stone to pass), and removal of stones
- Direct operative bile duct drainage with or without removal of stone from the duct
- Stone removal using ULTRASONIC LITHOTRIPSY

PREVENTION

Early treatment of symptomatic GALLSTONES is the best preventive measure.

COLON POLYP

A colon polyp is a small outgrowth of tissue in the large bowel, or colon. It can resemble a pea or sometimes a small mushroom on a stalk. Polyps can be made up of various types of tissue, some of which carry no malignant potential and some that do. If the tissue of the polyp is an adenoma, it may represent an increased risk for COLORECTAL CANCER. Hyperplastic polyps do not carry risk for COLORECTAL CANCER.

CAUSES

The cause of colon polyps is unclear, although there may be genetic explanations for polyps in some patients, especially those with a family history of colon polyps or COLORECTAL CANCER. Polyps may occur frequently in the population, and perhaps it is only those people with a certain genetic profile or those who have large or multiple polyps that are at increased risk for the development of COLORECTAL CANCER.

SYMPTOMS

Polyps are usually too small to cause any symptoms; often they are only discovered during routine screenings by a physician. At times, especially if the polyp is larger, it can cause visible RECTAL BLEEDING or microscopic bleeding that can be detected only by an OCCULT BLOOD TESTING of stools.

DIAGNOSIS

Because there are often no readily apparent symptoms, the diagnosis of colon polyps can require several tests, including
- OCCULT BLOOD TESTING of stool samples for hidden blood
- Sigmoidoscopy or colonoscopy—forms of ENDOSCOPY in which a flexible lighted instrument can view the rectum or entire colon
- X-ray barium studies of the large bowel (also called lower gastrointestinal [GI] series or barium enema; see RADIOGRAPHY)

COMPLICATIONS

The most important complication of a polyp is the development of a COLORECTAL CANCER. If there is a strong family his-

> A polyp can develop in any area of the large bowel, although it most often affects the lower part of the large bowel or colon.

tory of COLORECTAL CANCER or colon polyps, especially in parents or siblings, patients are advised to seek medical advice regarding screening for colon polyps. This is especially important if there is a history of COLORECTAL CANCER occurring at an age younger than 50 in close family members.

WARNING SIGNS:
- Visible RECTAL BLEEDING
- Change in the nature or frequency of bowel movements
- Development of iron-deficiency ANEMIA

TREATMENT

SELF TREATMENT:
None.

MEDICAL TREATMENT:
Some preliminary research suggests that aspirin or aspirin-like substances may inhibit the growth of polyps, but this treatment option remains experimental.

SURGICAL TREATMENT:
RECTAL OR COLON POLYP REMOVAL can usually be accomplished through a flexible instrument called a *sigmoidoscope* or *colonoscope* placed into the rectum and colon (see ENDOSCOPY). In the rare case when the polyp is very large, however, more traditional surgery may be needed to remove the polyp.

PREVENTION

- Avoidance of smoking may reduce the risk of abnormal growths in the colon.
- Diets high in soluble fiber and low in fat may carry some protection against the development of colon polyps.
- Periodic screening (every three to five years) with colonoscopy (ENDOSCOPY) may be needed once an adenoma type of polyp is discovered. Because this type of polyp can recur and does carry some risk of developing into COLORECTAL CANCER, regular surveillance is important.

COLORECTAL CANCER

One in every 20
people living in the
United States
contracts cancer of
the large intestine.

Most cancers of the colon originate in the left side of the colon. These cancers are usually discovered during routine screening sigmoidoscopy (a form of ENDOSCOPY) or after tests are performed to investigate changes in the pattern of the bowels (see RECTAL BLEEDING; OCCULT BLOOD TESTING).

CAUSES

The incidence of cancer of the colon is higher in families with hereditary polyp syndromes, in which family members have multiple polyps in the colon (COLON POLYP). The COLON POLYPS in this condition have a high chance of becoming malignant. Some of the syndromes can also be associated with the development of other forms of cancer.

Patients with ULCERATIVE COLITIS or CROHN DISEASE also have an increased risk of developing colorectal cancer.

A diet high in fat has also been identified as a risk factor in the development of colorectal cancer.

SYMPTOMS

Symptoms may include
- Change in the pattern of the bowels, such as in frequency, caliber, color, consistency, and smell (see STOOL, ABNORMAL APPEARANCE)
- Red streaks or dark jellylike stool related to bleeding (see RECTAL BLEEDING)
- Pain with bowel movements in rectal cancer
- Generalized ABDOMINAL PAIN or WEIGHT LOSS in advanced disease

DIAGNOSIS

Some of the symptoms noted above will prompt the performance of a sigmoidoscopy or a colonoscopy, a form of ENDOSCOPY in which a scope is introduced into the rectum and colon and any suspicious lesions can be tested by BIOPSY or excised.

Following a diagnosis of a malignancy, COMPUTED TOMOGRAPHY of the abdomen is performed to define the extent of disease and to check if the cancer has spread to other organs.

COMPLICATIONS

Potential complications of cancer of the colon or rectum include
- Bleeding resulting in ANEMIA or iron loss
- INTESTINAL OBSTRUCTION
- Bowel perforation
- ABDOMINAL PAIN, WEIGHT LOSS, and ABDOMINAL SWELLING in advanced disease

TREATMENT

SELF TREATMENT:
A well-balanced diet will assist in the maintenance of a stable weight during treatment for this malignancy.

MEDICAL TREATMENT:
Treatment with chemotherapy after surgery in some stages of colon cancer, and the combination of chemotherapy and radiation before surgery in rectal cancer, have led to a higher rate of survival.

SURGICAL TREATMENT:
Early on, before cancer develops, RECTAL OR COLON POLYP REMOVAL is a preventive surgery.

Resection of colon and rectal cancers offers the only chance for cure of this cancer (see SIGMOID COLON REMOVAL; COLOSTOMY). Removal of the tumor that has spread to the liver, when this is the only site to which it has spread, may also cure this cancer.

PREVENTION

The maintenance of a low-fat diet and careful follow-up with routine screening sigmoidoscopies or colonoscopies for suspicious lesions lead to the prevention, early discovery, and potential cure of these cancers. This is especially important for patients at high risk of developing this cancer, such as patients with familial polyp syndromes (see COLON POLYP) or ULCERATIVE COLITIS.

CONGESTIVE HEART FAILURE

> Congestive heart failure is a condition in which the heart cannot pump efficiently enough to keep up with the body's circulatory demand.

When the heart does not pump enough blood to meet the needs of the body, the kidneys begin to retain fluid. In an attempt to make the heart catch up with circulatory demands, the adrenal glands release hormones that cause the blood vessels to constrict and the heart to increase its rate of pumping. The constriction of blood vessels caused by the adrenal glands may contribute to the worsening of heart failure over time by increasing the workload on the heart because of the increased resistance.

In some cases, the heart contracts well but fails to fill adequately (called stiffness) in between heartbeats, leading to a backup of blood and congestion in the lungs, liver, and legs. The fluid retention causes congestion leading to many of the symptoms of heart failure.

CAUSES

Anything that damages the heart's ability to contract or fill well in between heartbeats can lead to congestive heart failure. Major causes include
- HEART ATTACK (myocardial infarction)
- HEART VALVE DISEASE
- HYPERTENSION
- CARDIOMYOPATHY
- Congenital heart disease
- Pericardial diseases

SYMPTOMS

FATIGUE and progressive shortness of breath (BREATHING DIFFICULTY) with exertion are early signs of congestive heart failure. The shortness of breath may be associated with a COUGH or with wheezing. Fluid accumulation may lead to visible swelling in the legs (edema; see ANKLE SWELLING) and a loss of appetite from congestion in the liver (see APPETITE, LOSS OF).

As the process progresses, the patient may wake up hours after falling asleep and have to sit up to breathe or even spend the night in a chair to breathe easier.

DIAGNOSIS

Diagnosis can involve many facets. An individual's MEDICAL HISTORY and description of certain symptoms, such as shortness of breath, provide many important clues. A PHYSICAL EXAMINATION may reveal signs of congestion, including distended neck veins and fluid in the lungs, liver, and legs. A heart examination also may detect valve problems and signs of stiffness or weakness.

The chest X ray (RADIOGRAPHY) may confirm a diagnosis of congestive heart failure. An ELECTROCARDIOGRAPHY and echocardiography (ULTRASOUND) may help determine the cause. Ultimately, a CARDIAC CATHETERIZATION may be part of the diagnostic process.

COMPLICATIONS

The weakened heart is prone to ARRHYTHMIAS that could lead to FAINTING OR FAINTNESS or even sudden cardiac death. Because blood is allowed to pool, clots are more likely to form both in the heart and in the veins in the legs. These clots can travel to the brain causing a STROKE or to the lungs causing a PULMONARY EMBOLISM.

TREATMENT

SELF TREATMENT:

Physical activity may initially have to be limited, but in many cases, cautious mild exercise can be resumed when recommended and supervised by a physician. Salt intake should be restricted, and alcohol should be avoided.

MEDICAL TREATMENT:

Treatment varies depending on the underlying circulatory or cardiac problem and the immediate cause that brought on the current episode of congestive failure (for example, medication or diet problems).

Drugs that are commonly used include
- Diuretics (such as furosemide) to reduce fluid accumulation
- Digitalis (digoxin) to strengthen the heartbeat and improve heart rhythm

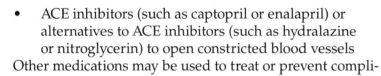

- ACE inhibitors (such as captopril or enalapril) or alternatives to ACE inhibitors (such as hydralazine or nitroglycerin) to open constricted blood vessels

Other medications may be used to treat or prevent complications, including

- Anticoagulants, such as warfarin
- Antiarrhythmics, such as procainamide and amiodarone

Drugs may also be needed to treat the underlying causes of heart failure such as HYPERTENSION and HYPERLIPIDEMIA.

SURGICAL TREATMENT:

- Open heart surgery can repair or replace a faulty valve (HEART VALVE REPLACEMENT) or bypass blocked vessels (CORONARY ARTERY BYPASS GRAFT SURGERY).
- Balloon catheter procedures (ANGIOPLASTY) may be used to open arteries or valves.
- Heart transplantation may be the best alternative for some advanced cases.

PREVENTION

- Avoidance of smoking (see ATHEROSCLEROSIS and HEART ATTACK)
- Avoidance of excessive alcohol intake (see CARDIOMYOPATHY)
- Appropriate treatment of strep throat infections to prevent heart valve and muscle damage from rheumatic heart disease
- With the advice and help of a physician, control of the problems that can otherwise progress to congestive heart failure (for example HYPERTENSION, HYPERLIPIDEMIA, and ATHEROSCLEROSIS)
- A diet low in salt, fat, and cholesterol

CONSTIPATION

Constipation has different meanings for different people. The term can mean that stools are too small, too hard, too difficult to pass, or too infrequent. Patients may also experience a sense of straining and incomplete evacuation. The popular belief that one should have a daily bowel movement is not true. Patterns of bowel movements can be quite variable, and it is completely normal for some people to have a bowel movement only every five to seven days.

CAUSES

The cause of constipation is frequently related to temporary changes in lifestyle or habits. Travel, changes in diet, and a reduction in normal activity can all bring on a case of constipation, as can the use of some medications. On the more serious side, underlying metabolic and endocrine diseases, such as DIABETES or HYPOTHYROIDISM, can result in constipation. Neurologic problems in which there is nerve damage in the muscle groups related to the bowel may also result in constipation. Rarely, constipation can be caused by narrowing of the intestines or by an INTESTINAL OBSTRUCTION.

SYMPTOMS

- Hard, rounded, pebblelike bowel movements
- Incomplete, difficult, or painful evacuation
- Sense of rectal fullness with inability to pass stool

DIAGNOSIS

If constipation is limited and occasional and there are no other symptoms, no testing may be necessary. However, if the problem is persistent or severe, the following diagnostic tests may be in order
- BLOOD TESTS to check thyroid function and calcium or magnesium levels
- Sigmoidoscopy (a form of ENDOSCOPY of the rectum)
- X-ray barium studies of the large bowel (also called a lower gastrointestinal [GI] series or barium enema; see RADIOGRAPHY)
- Tests of motor function (anorectal motility)
- Tests of colonic transit using radio-opaque markers that the patient swallows

Constipation is not a disease, but it can be a symptom of many diseases. Overall, it is a very common condition, affecting all age groups and both sexes.

COMPLICATIONS

Complications are rarely seen with simple constipation. In the elderly or bedridden, however, an impaction may develop in which the stool becomes so hard that it physically obstructs the large bowel (INTESTINAL OBSTRUCTION) and can lead to lower ABDOMINAL PAIN, ABDOMINAL SWELLING, and occasionally VOMITING.

TREATMENT

SELF TREATMENT:
- Regular daily exercise
- A diet that is high in fiber (breads, cereals, and fresh fruits and vegetables)
- Adequate fluid intake (at least eight 8-ounce glasses of fluid per day)

MEDICAL TREATMENT:
If dietary and lifestyle measures do not help, laxatives or small-volume rectal enemas can be used. Patients should only very rarely use stimulant laxatives or enemas because, over time, these medications can paradoxically cause the large bowel to become even more sluggish and less responsive. Bulking agents (for example, psyllium, methylcellulose, calcium polycarbophil) that increase the volume and soften the consistency of stools are safe for long-term use and are the recommended agents to treat constipation.

SURGICAL TREATMENT:
Surgical treatment of constipation is very rare and used only for specific problems of constipation, such as Hirschsprung disease (congenital absence of nerve fibers in the rectum) or INTESTINAL OBSTRUCTION or narrowing.

PREVENTION

The best preventive measure is to ensure adequate bulk and fiber in the diet. Although the dosage requirements are not well studied, increasing soluble fiber to approximately 20 grams daily—either in the diet or by supplementing with bulking agents such as psyllium, methylcellulose, and calcium polycarbophil—is a good strategy.

CROHN DISEASE

Crohn disease is an inflammatory disease of the intestine that can involve the lower part of the small intestine, the large intestine, and other parts of the digestive tract. Crohn disease tends to be patchy in its distribution and may skip large areas of the intestine. Inflammation, however, does involve all layers of the intestinal wall—from the inner lining to the outside wall. When Crohn disease involves the lower part of the small intestine, it is called *ileitis*, or *regional enteritis*.

Crohn disease, sometimes called granulomatous colitis, can afflict people of all ages, but tends to be a disease of the young.

CAUSES

Crohn disease is a chronic illness and its cause remains unknown. It is *not* caused by emotional stress, food, or by anything transmitted from person to person. Research suggests that Crohn disease may result from an immunologic imbalance; the interaction of an infectious agent with the body's immune system might trigger the immune system, and the stimulated immune system then causes constant or intermittent intestinal inflammation.

SYMPTOMS

There are many varied symptoms associated with Crohn disease, including
- ABDOMINAL PAIN, frequently in the right lower abdomen, especially after meals
- DIARRHEA
- Sores or recurrent BOILS in the anus
- Fissures or drainage in the anus
- Joint pain
- Loss of appetite (APPETITE, LOSS OF)
- WEIGHT LOSS
- Skin fistulae (abnormal openings from the intestine to the skin)
- Frequent canker sores of the mouth

DIAGNOSIS

There is no single test that provides a clear diagnosis of Crohn disease, but screening BLOOD TESTS can provide clues. In addition to a thorough PHYSICAL EXAMINATION, barium X rays of the lower bowel and barium X rays of the stomach and small intestine are generally performed (see RADIOGRAPHY). Sigmoidoscopy or colonoscopy—forms of ENDOSCOPY that permit direct examination and BIOPSY of the large bowel through a lighted flexible tube or video camera—are very frequently used in the diagnosis of Crohn disease and similar disorders.

COMPLICATIONS

On rare occasion, the inflammation in Crohn disease can be severe enough to cause an abscess outside the bowel wall in the abdomen. This complication results in high FEVER and persistent ABDOMINAL PAIN. The inflammation may also burrow through the intestine and cause abnormal connections (fistulae) with other organs such as

- Other parts of the intestinal system
- The skin
- The vagina
- The urinary bladder

If the inflammation does not respond to treatment, there may be enough intestinal scarring in some patients to cause a stricture or narrowing of the intestine. This condition can lead to INTESTINAL OBSTRUCTION with persistent ABDOMINAL PAIN and intractable VOMITING.

Occasionally, the liver and bile ducts are affected by an inflammatory condition called *sclerosing cholangitis*. This process is primarily detected by abnormal liver enzymes noted on BLOOD TESTS.

TREATMENT

SELF TREATMENT:

Good nutrition is essential. While specific foods play no role in causing Crohn disease, soft, bland foods may be better tolerated and cause less discomfort when the disease is active. If patients have substantial narrowing of the intestine, such poorly digestible foods such as nuts, raw fruits, and raw vegetables should be limited.

Emotional stress can influence the course of Crohn disease, and the family and medical professionals involved with these patients should be ready to provide understanding and support.

MEDICAL TREATMENT:

Several pharmaceutical options are available to decrease symptoms including

- Sulfasalazine
- Corticosteroids such as prednisone and methylprednisolone (pill and enema formulations)
- Azathioprine
- Metronidazole
- Mesalamine (pill and enema formulations)
- Olsalazine
- 6-mercaptopurine

SURGICAL TREATMENT:

Surgery for Crohn disease is reserved only for complications that do not respond to conservative treatment. Surgery is never curative, but it may allow for prolonged symptom-free periods. Usually, surgery involves removing a diseased segment of the bowel and two healthy ends of bowel are reattached (anastomosis).

At times, an abscess within the rectum, skin, or abdomen needs to be drained. If the abscess is in a "favorable" location, it sometimes can be drained by a radiologist using imaging such as ULTRASOUND or COMPUTED TOMOGRAPHY to guide a needle or catheter to the abscess, thus avoiding open surgery.

PREVENTION

Medical therapy has not been proved unequivocally to be of benefit in preventing flare-ups of Crohn disease, but some physicians feel that there is a benefit to long-term treatment with such agents as

- Sulfasalazine
- Azathioprine
- Mesalamine
- 6-mercaptopurine
- Corticosteroids (in small doses)

DEHYDRATION

Dehydration is a lack of water and salt in the tissues and bloodstream that can affect the entire body. The kidneys are particularly vulnerable to damage when there is not enough water to use in the elimination of wastes.

CAUSES

The causes include any excessive fluid loss or decreased fluid intake. Excessive losses can result from

- VOMITING
- DIARRHEA
- High FEVER causing excessive sweating (SWEATING, EXCESSIVE)
- Excessive loss of fluid through the kidneys because of diuretic medication or, occasionally, certain types of kidney disease or DIABETES

SYMPTOMS

Some of the earliest signs are increased thirst and dry mouth. As dehydration progresses, the skin may become wrinkled. Blood pressure may decrease and confusion and coma can develop.

Except when the kidneys are to blame for the dehydration, the kidneys usually attempt to save fluid, leading to a marked decrease or absence of urination.

DIAGNOSIS

The patient's MEDICAL HISTORY and a PHYSICAL EXAMINATION, including BLOOD PRESSURE TESTING while laying and standing, can make the diagnosis of dehydration. BLOOD TESTS, including kidney function and mineral balance tests, can confirm the diagnosis and help estimate its severity.

COMPLICATIONS

With moderate dehydration, kidney function may be impaired. With more extreme dehydration, drops in blood pressure can cause shock, loss of consciousness, and even death.

TREATMENT

SELF TREATMENT:

An appropriate amount of liquid, particularly electrolyte solutions, can treat mild dehydration. (See Prevention below.)

MEDICAL TREATMENT:

More severe dehydration may need to be treated with intravenous fluids. If an underlying condition such as DIABETES, a kidney disorder, or a gastrointestinal disorder has led to the dehydration, then a specific treatment for that problem will also help.

SURGICAL TREATMENT:

None.

PREVENTION

In general, one should drink at least eight eight-ounce glasses of fluid per day to stay well hydrated.

In some cases of excessive fluid loss from heavy sweating (SWEATING, EXCESSIVE) or DIARRHEA, increasing fluid intake can prevent severe dehydration. A number of electrolyte solutions are commercially available or can be made up for adults by adding one teaspoon of sugar and one-half teaspoon of salt to one pint of water.

DEPRESSION

> Depression is the most common psychiatric disorder. It affects 10 to 25 percent of women and 5 to 12 percent of men at some point in their lives.

People of all ages can suffer from depression, but the highest rates occur in people 25 to 45 years old. The rate of depression is not affected by ethnic group, education, income, or marital status.

CAUSES

The main cause of depression is not known. There is a genetic association, and relatives of people who have had depression, manic-depression, or obesity are at higher risk.

Alcohol or drug abuse can cause symptoms of depression, as can certain prescription medications such as prednisone and some blood pressure medications.

Various medical conditions, such as HYPOTHYROIDISM, systemic infections, CONGESTIVE HEART FAILURE, autoimmune diseases, cancers, and neurologic disorders, can also cause symptoms of depression.

A difficult or tragic life circumstance may bring on depression, but often there is no triggering life event.

SYMPTOMS

The main symptoms of depression are either a depressed, saddened mood or the inability to enjoy things normally enjoyed. Other common symptoms include
- Sleep problems or sleeping too much
- Eating too little or too much (see APPETITE, LOSS OF)
- Difficulty concentrating or making decisions
- FATIGUE
- Feelings of guilt or worthlessness
- Feeling either physically slowed down or sped up
- Recurrent thoughts of death or wanting to be dead

DIAGNOSIS

Diagnosis is based on the presence of a combination of the common symptoms in the absence of a medical disorder, a medication side effect, or substance abuse that can adequately explain the symptoms. There is no specific test that can be used to detect depression.

COMPLICATIONS

The most severe complication of depression is suicide, the possibility of which makes depression a potentially fatal illness. Less severe but more common are impairments of one's ability to work and interact socially. Missed days of work, inefficiency at work, lost jobs, arguments with family and friends, divorce, and social isolation are all potential complications of depression.

TREATMENT

SELF TREATMENT:

*   Reducing or eliminating use of alcohol, prescription sedatives, or recreational drugs
*   Eating properly
*   Getting regular exercise
*   Using the appropriate therapies for any medical conditions

MEDICAL TREATMENT:

Psychotherapy and antidepressant medication can be used individually or together. Both have proved effective in the treatment of depression. The medicines most commonly used for depression are the selective serotonin-reuptake inhibitors (SSRIs) such as fluoxetine and the tricyclic antidepressants such as amitriptyline.

Severe depression that is not manageable with medication is occasionally treated with electroconvulsive therapy.

SURGICAL TREATMENT:

None.

PREVENTION

Depression is difficult to anticipate, but those who have a family history should be acquainted with the symptoms. Suicide is preventable by seeking professional help promptly at the first hint of suicidal thoughts. Strong suicidal impulses warrant an immediate visit to an emergency department.

DERMATITIS

Dermatitis includes erythema (redness), pin-point vesicles (little tiny water blisters under the skin), scale, and severe itching. Poison ivy is a classic example of acute contact dermatitis.

Dermatitis is not a single disease. It is a pattern of skin inflammation that can be due to a number of causes. Another word for dermatitis is *eczema*. When eczema is chronic and long-standing, skin may have other changes, and the pin-point vesicles may be much less obvious or even absent. Other changes include increased or accentuated skin lines (due to scratching), darkening of the skin, and sometimes a thickening or heaping up of the skin in the area.

CAUSES

Eczema can be caused by an external source or an internal source. External sources are those substances, such as poison ivy, that get on the patient's skin and either directly irritate it or cause an allergic reaction.

Internal reasons for eczema are probably genetic in nature. One kind of common eczema is seen in some families and is associated with ASTHMA and hay fever; it is called *atopic eczema*.

Many people have hand eczema that has no discernible cause. Some of these people may have poor hand-care habits, which lead to irritation of the hands or exacerbate the intrinsic problem. Some of these people have atopic eczema that is limited to the hands.

There are, however, some patients who have an allergy to something that gets on their hands and have true allergic eczema. These people may need ALLERGY TESTING to know which chemicals cause an allergic reaction, so that they may avoid these substances.

SYMPTOMS

- Hands that are easily irritated by a number of external agents such as soaps, detergents, fruit juices, vegetables, and oils
- ITCHING
- Red, scaly skin
- Pin-point tiny water blisters (see RASH) in groups just under the skin of the most severely involved areas

DIAGNOSIS

It is important to rule out or isolate an external cause with a careful MEDICAL HISTORY, usually via directed questions from a physician who is aware of the common culprits such as nickel, ethylenediamine, paraphenylenediamine, dichromates, parabens, vulcanizing ingredients, rubber products, formaldehyde, fabric softeners, and fragrances. Selected patch testing (ALLERGY TESTING) should be performed to confirm the suspected allergy. Sometimes a product use test is in order.

Fungal infections need to be ruled out by examining the scale with a microscope. Sometimes a CULTURE must be performed to make the determination.

Sometimes an already existing eczema may be infected by bacteria—a so-called *infectious eczematoid*—usually the bacteria *Staphylococcus aureus* or, less commonly, *Streptococcus* organisms. This infection can be confirmed by CULTURE.

New onset eczema in a middle-aged to elderly person with no obvious explanation may indicate cutaneous T-cell lymphoma and Sezary syndrome. In this situation, the patient must undergo BIOPSY at multiple sites of the eczema and the specimens are sent to a dermatopathologist to rule out lymphoma (see LYMPHOMA, NON-HODGKIN).

Sometimes chronic eczema can change so much in appearance from the patient's scratching, manipulations of the skin, and trials of topical agents that the eczema may have the features of a whole other group of skin diseases such as PSORIASIS. In these cases, a BIOPSY to rule out these other diseases may be needed.

COMPLICATIONS

Secondary infection is common, possibly causing an acceleration of the eczema, ITCHING (painful at times), pus pockets under the scale, glazing of blood and pus over the scale, red skin, and even oozing.

TREATMENT

SELF TREATMENT:

Cool wet compresses applied for one or two hours, three to five times a day can be helpful in alleviating the itching and redness. Applying hydrocortisone cream to the areas, followed by wet compresses over the cream, is often very effective, too.

Over-the-counter antihistamines, such as diphenhydramine or chlorpheniramine, taken approximately every six hours can help to take the edge off the ITCHING.

Topical preparations related to benzocaine or antihistamines can be helpful, but there is a relatively high incidence of contact allergy associated with these agents. Therefore, it is recommended that these agents be avoided if possible.

MEDICAL TREATMENT:

Low-, medium-, and high-potency topical steroids such as triamcinolone are the cornerstone of the treatment of skin eczemas. In general, cool wet compresses applied over the topical steroids are a highly effective adjunct.

If an acute eczema is very weepy or infected, aluminum acetate solution soaks are very effective. For acute eczemas, topical steroid creams are advisable over ointments because the latter may occlude the weeping lesion and trap the inflammatory material being extruded.

Sometimes, a very brief course of oral corticosteroids is in order in addition to intensive topical care.

SURGICAL TREATMENT:

None.

PREVENTION

Avoiding substances that induce repeated irritation, redness, or ITCHING of the skin is the best preventive strategy for contact dermatitis. Good hygiene habits and prompt attention to skin problems can decrease the risk of complications.

DIABETES

Insulin, a hormone produced by the pancreas gland, helps blood sugar (the body's fuel) enter the cells and provide energy. In diabetes, the blood sugar, or glucose, cannot get into the cells properly. There are probably a number of mechanisms of diabetes, but two general types are recognized: type I diabetes (called insulin-dependent diabetes or juvenile diabetes) and type II diabetes (called non-insulin-dependent diabetes or adult-onset diabetes).

In insulin-dependent diabetes, the pancreas does not produce enough insulin. Because the blood sugar cannot get into the cells without the insulin, sugar levels rise in the bloodstream. In adult-onset (non–insulin-dependent) diabetes, the pancreas gland generally produces a reasonable amount of insulin, but the insulin is poorly timed and the body's cells seem to be resistant to insulin's effects. This also leads to elevated blood sugar levels.

CAUSES

Insulin-dependent diabetes is probably related to the immune system attacking the pancreas gland, making it unable to produce as much insulin. Other diseases such as PANCREATITIS can also attack the pancreas gland. Of course, surgical removal of the pancreas, which is required for conditions such as PANCREATIC CANCER, will lead to a lack of insulin production.

Genetic causes are fairly important in non–insulin-dependent diabetes. Obesity and receiving high levels of cortisone or drugs like prednisone can also increase the risk.

SYMPTOMS

The most common symptoms related to high blood sugar levels are frequent urination (URINATION, FREQUENT) and excessive thirst. The appetite may be increased, but despite this, WEIGHT LOSS will still occur when diabetes is out of control. High sugar levels also cause VISION DISTURBANCES. When blood sugar levels are extremely high, patients may experience
- Nausea and VOMITING
- Confusion
- Weakness
- Coma in severely neglected cases

Complications of diabetes can also cause symptoms.

Diabetes is a relatively common problem that leads to excessively high levels of blood sugar.

DIAGNOSIS

An elevated blood sugar level is the most common way of diagnosing diabetes in a patient with a MEDICAL HISTORY and PHYSICAL EXAMINATION consistent with the disease. BLOOD TESTS that look for prolonged elevations of blood sugar can also be done and further support the diagnosis in cases in which the blood sugar results are unclear. In men, URINALYSIS can also detect inappropriate amounts of glucose in the urine characteristic of diabetes.

COMPLICATIONS

Diabetes affects many parts of the body. After years of high blood sugar levels, almost all parts of the body may be damaged. The main parts of the body that are affected are

- The eyes
- The kidneys
- The nervous system

Eye problems include excessive growth of small blood vessels in the retina (the back part of the eye) that can lead to VISION DISTURBANCES and blindness. People with diabetes are more likely to get GLAUCOMA, too.

Nervous system problems can take years to develop and usually cause

- NUMBNESS
- Sudden weakness
- Shooting pains, particularly in the legs

After years of diabetes, the kidneys begin to leak protein and can progressively fail (KIDNEY FAILURE), leading to the need for dialysis. These complications usually take 10 to 20 years to develop.

People with diabetes are also predisposed to

- ATHEROSCLEROSIS
- HEART ATTACK
- Claudication (a pain in the calf that appears when walking and is relieved by rest)

TREATMENT

SELF TREATMENT:

Self-care is crucial in the treatment of diabetes. Careful control of diet is very important and can minimize or eliminate the need for medication.

For patients who are overweight, appropriate weight loss may lead to resolution of diabetes and eliminate or minimize the need for medications.

MEDICAL TREATMENT:

Regular insulin injections are generally required for insulin-dependent diabetes.

For non–insulin-dependent diabetes, medication may be necessary. Oral hypoglycemic drugs such as glipizide, glyburide, chlorpropamide, or metformin can be used alone or in combination with insulin.

For difficult cases, insulin may be injected with a pump placed under the skin that can allow for more frequent dosing and potentially tighter control. It is becoming more and more clear that tight control—that is, attempting to keep blood sugar levels as normal as possible—can significantly decrease the chance of complications.

SURGICAL TREATMENT:

None.

PREVENTION

Avoiding excess weight decreases the chance of adult-onset diabetes.

For people who already have diabetes, preventive measures can help avoid complications. Periodic eye exams can be helpful in detecting problems before they lead to more severe VISION DISTURBANCES. Patients should be attentive to numbness and circulatory problems in the legs; otherwise, these conditions can lead to injuries and infection that can progress undetected. A daily foot self-exam can be helpful in catching skin breakdown early and avoiding severe infections and gangrene.

DIVERTICULAR DISEASE

Diverticula can be found in the majority of patients over the age of 55 and often cause no symptoms, but they can cause complications.

Diverticula are small marble-sized outpockets in the wall of the large bowel. When uncomplicated and asymptomatic, their presence is described as *diverticulosis*. When complicated by infection or inflammation, patients develop symptoms, and the condition is called *diverticulitis*. By far, the most common site within the large bowel for diverticula is the left or sigmoid colon.

CAUSES

Diverticula form in clefts of muscle where nourishing blood vessels penetrate the wall of the large bowel. With advancing age, the elasticity of the colon wall decreases, rendering the tissue less flexible and reducing its tensile strength. As pressure builds within the large bowel from muscle contraction, the weakest point of the large bowel muscle wall (the cleft with the blood vessel) balloons outward, forming the diverticulum.

Diverticular disease is an illness of the developed world and its refined carbohydrate diet. It is virtually unknown in developing countries where insoluble cereal fiber is the primary dietary constituent. This suggests that increased stool weight, increased stool consistency, and faster transit (reducing intestinal wall tension) protect against the development of diverticular disease.

SYMPTOMS

Uncomplicated diverticulosis usually causes no symptoms, but at times, the patient may experience some mild cramping or bloating in the left lower part of the abdomen (see ABDOMINAL PAIN; ABDOMINAL SWELLING).

When stool or indigestible material gets caught in the diverticulum, inflammation and infection may develop. This condition can cause

- Severe ABDOMINAL PAIN, usually in the left lower abdomen
- Acute CONSTIPATION
- More rarely, DIARRHEA
- FEVER and chills, if the inflammation is severe enough

DIAGNOSIS

Diverticular disease is usually diagnosed with barium X rays of the large bowel (RADIOGRAPHY) or with sigmoidoscopy or colonoscopy (forms of ENDOSCOPY). If a patient experiences severe ABDOMINAL PAIN or FEVER it may be best, in certain cir-circumstances, to delay diagnostic studies until the inflammation settles down.

Diverticulosis develops in many people, and the mere presence of these pockets on a diagnostic study such as an X ray does not indicate a significant problem. The findings should always be interpreted with the patient's symptoms in mind.

COMPLICATIONS

If the inflammation within a diverticulum is severe enough, it may result in perforation of the colon, the formation of an abscess within the wall of the large bowel, or even an abscess in the abdomen itself.

Since the diverticula tend to form where blood vessels penetrate the wall of the large bowel, these blood vessels at times may rupture, causing serious RECTAL BLEEDING. (The bleeding tends to be painless because there is little inflammation involved with this complication.)

Fortunately, inflammation of the diverticulum usually results in THROMBOSIS of these blood vessels, reducing the risk of bleeding.

TREATMENT

SELF TREATMENT:

When symptoms are intermittent and chronic, prevention is in order (see Prevention below).

When the symptoms are acute and painful, especially if there is FEVER, avoiding solid food and restricting the diet to clear liquids may make the episode less uncomfortable by easing the stress placed on the digestive tract.

MEDICAL TREATMENT:

Medications that can be useful in the treatment of diverticular disease include

- Antispasmodic or anticholinergic drugs, such as dicyclomine or hyoscyamine
- Stool softeners and bulking agents such as psyllium, docusate, and methylcellulose
- For bacterial infection, antibiotics such as amoxicillin, clavulanic acid, clindamycin, trimethoprim, metronidazole, and sulfonamide antibiotics

SURGICAL TREATMENT:

In severe cases of diverticulitis, removal of the affected part of the large bowel may be needed. If surgery is done in an emergency, patients may require a temporary COLOSTOMY with reconnection of the bowel at a future date.

PREVENTION

The best preventive measure is insuring adequate fiber in the diet. Although the dosage requirements are not well studied, the propensity for diverticular disease may be reduced by increasing soluble fiber intake to approximately 20 to 30 grams daily either with high-fiber foods such as

- Fresh fruits and vegetables
- Bran cereals
- Unprocessed bran
- Whole-grain products

or with fiber supplements such as

- Psyllium
- Methylcellulose
- Calcium polycarbophil

Avoiding nuts, popcorn, and foods with small seeds and pits may also help. Although it has not been clearly proved, these foodstuffs may get caught in the diverticula and lead to inflammatory problems.

EMPHYSEMA

Emphysema is a condition of the lung characterized by permanent enlargement of the air sacs (called *alveoli*). The alveoli are located at the ends of the bronchial tubes and are bunched in groups like a bunch of grapes.

In healthy people, oxygen crosses the thin elastic walls of the alveoli into the bloodstream, and carbon dioxide from the blood enters the air sac to be exhaled. In emphysema, the walls of the alveoli are damaged or dissolved, creating a larger air sac—essentially a hole. This damage and the tendency of smaller bronchial tubes to collapse more easily interfere with the exhalation of air, trapping air in the enlarged air sacs. The next breath is taken on top of this trapped air, resulting in overinflation of the lung.

CAUSES

Cigarette smoking is *the* major cause of emphysema. The risk of developing emphysema is directly related to the amount and duration of smoking. Most patients have smoked at least an average of one pack of cigarettes per day for 30 years before developing symptoms in their 50s or 60s.

In rare cases, emphysema can occur in young adults who have an inherited deficiency of a protein called *alpha$_1$-antitrypsin* that protects healthy lung tissue.

Rare environmental exposures, such as inhaled cadmium, may also result in emphysema.

ASTHMA does not cause emphysema.

SYMPTOMS

Emphysema results in gradual development of BREATHING DIFFICULTY. With mild to moderate disease, BREATHING DIFFICULTY occurs only during significant exertion, but as the disease progresses, BREATHING DIFFICULTY occurs with less and less exertion. Finally, the symptom occurs when the patient is at rest. In the initial stages, the symptom is often masked by the patient's increasingly sedentary lifestyle.

COUGH, excess mucus, and wheezing are features of chronic bronchitis (BRONCHITIS, CHRONIC) or respiratory tract infection, both of which may coexist with emphysema.

> In more than 80 percent of the cases, emphysema is directly attributable to cigarette smoking.

DIAGNOSIS

Emphysema is suspected in patients with a significant history of cigarette smoking who develop BREATHING DIFFICULTY in their 50s or 60s. PHYSICAL EXAMINATION usually reveals an enlarged chest (barrel-shaped) due to lung overinflation and possibly the overdevelopment of the muscles of the neck and chest trying to compensate for BREATHING DIFFICULTY. Breath sounds may be found to be diminished, and there is a delay in the exhalation of air.

Other tests that may be used to confirm the diagnosis include

- Chest X ray (RADIOGRAPHY)
- COMPUTED TOMOGRAPHY of the chest
- PULMONARY FUNCTION TESTING

COMPLICATIONS

The increasingly sedentary lifestyle adopted by many emphysema patients can result in general deconditioning, leading to even more BREATHING DIFFICULTY. WEIGHT GAIN may result from the lifestyle changes, especially if patients are receiving corticosteroid treatment; however, emphysema can also cause WEIGHT LOSS, perhaps because of the increased labor of breathing.

Many patients experience psychological complications such as DEPRESSION from the isolation of a sedentary lifestyle and episodes of panic during periods of breathlessness, which can be alarming.

The disease has secondary effects on the heart. It becomes increasingly difficult for the right ventricle to pump blood through the diseased lungs, resulting in right heart failure in severe cases (see CONGESTIVE HEART FAILURE).

Occasionally, the air sacs may rupture, allowing air to escape into the chest cavity—a condition called *pneumothorax*. This condition can cause the lung to collapse because air can enter the chest cavity but it can't get back out, leading to serious BREATHING DIFFICULTY and requiring emergency treatment.

Routine respiratory tract infections can produce serious problems for people with emphysema. PNEUMONIA is life-threatening for emphysema patients.

TREATMENT

SELF TREATMENT:

Self treatment consists of
- Quitting smoking
- Embarking on a sensible exercise program
- Ensuring proper nutrition to maintain ideal body weight
- Washing hands frequently to decrease the risk of infection

MEDICAL TREATMENT:

Drug therapy may involve
- Oxygen for patients whose blood oxygen level is not adequate
- Inhaled bronchodilators such as albuterol and ipratropium bromide and oral bronchodilators such as theophylline to improve airflow
- Corticosteroids (prednisone) to reduce swelling and inflammation in the bronchial tubes
- Antibiotics to treat infections promptly
- Mucolytic agents such as guaifenesin to loosen mucus

INFLUENZA vaccine given in the fall can protect against the usual outbreak of INFLUENZA seen in the winter months. Pneumococcal vaccine offers protection against one of the most common causes of PNEUMONIA.

SURGICAL TREATMENT:

In select patients, a surgical procedure known as *volume-reduction surgery* may be beneficial (see LUNG RESECTION).

PREVENTION

Avoidance of smoking and exposure to smoke and pollutants is the most important preventive step.

ENDOMETRIOSIS

Endometriosis is the condition in which tissue from the inner lining of the uterus (the endometrium) becomes implanted outside the uterus. The areas most commonly affected include the ovaries, the ligaments supporting the uterus, and the space behind the uterus called the *posterior cul-de-sac*. Occasionally the bowel and the bladder can also be involved.

CAUSES

The specific cause of endometriosis is unclear, but theories include
- Endometrial tissue flows out through the fallopian tubes at the time of menstruation and becomes implanted outside the uterus.
- Embryonic cells that are present from birth are transformed into endometrial implants through hormone stimulation.
- Poor immune response allows the misplaced cells to grow outside the uterus.

Most investigators believe that the cause of endometriosis is a combination of all three.

Risk factors of endometriosis include
- Family history of the disease
- Short cycles and heavy flow (see MENSTRUAL IRREGU-LARITIES)
- Nulliparity (having never given birth to a live infant)

SYMPTOMS

Although many women with endometriosis are symptom free, for those who have symptoms, the most common are
- Painful periods, especially if pain begins after years of pain-free menstruation
- Painful intercourse, especially in instances of deep penetration
- Lower back pain (BACKACHE)
- Infertility, with no other obvious cause

DIAGNOSIS

Diagnosis is based on
- Clinical history—MEDICAL HISTORY and reported symptoms
- Findings on PHYSICAL EXAMINATION
- Findings at the time of surgery (Surgery—either open surgery or surgery using ENDOSCOPY—is the only definitive means of diagnosis of endometriosis.)

COMPLICATIONS

Complications include
- Acute and/or chronic ABDOMINAL PAIN
- Infertility

TREATMENT

SELF TREATMENT:
Over-the-counter pain relievers such as acetaminophen and ibuprofen can be used for milder symptoms.

MEDICAL TREATMENT:
Nonsteroidal anti-inflammatory drugs (naproxen, ibuprofen) are often used for relief of symptoms. Danazol, progestin, and leuprolide may help to shrink the tissue.

SURGICAL TREATMENT:
Surgical removal (using either ENDOSCOPY or open technique) of the tissue may be necessary for severe symptoms that do not otherwise respond to medical treatment. Removal may help improve fertility.

PREVENTION

No preventive strategies exist, but routine pelvic examinations done at the time of PAP SMEARS may detect endometriosis early, which can be helpful in family planning.

FIBROCYSTIC BREAST DISEASE

The nodules associated with fibrocystic breast disease are problematic because they make breast examination difficult and because they can mimic the findings of breast cancer. They do not, however, increase a woman's risk of breast cancer.

Fibrocystic breast disease refers to a group of entities which cause breast pain, breast masses, and breast cysts in women. Although the symptoms can be quite variable, most women with fibrocystic changes of the breast have some degree of pain related to their menstrual cycles. Their breasts also develop areas of nodularity and firmness that are difficult to distinguish from breast tumors.

Some women develop large palpable fluid-filled cysts that can resolve spontaneously. When they do not, aspiration of the fluid with a fine needle can distinguish a breast cyst from a solid mass suspected of being BREAST CANCER.

CAUSES

The cause of fibrocystic changes of the breast are not known, but it appears to run in families, and there is probably a hereditary predisposition to the condition.

Dietary factors including high-fat and high-sodium diets have been implicated.

SYMPTOMS

Patients note pain in their breasts, often related to their menstrual cycle. Episodes of pain are most often intermittent, waxing and waning, and although troublesome, do not interfere with daily activities. However, many women become quite concerned because they believe that the pain is a symptom of a more serious problem, especially BREAST CANCER. (This fear is unfounded, as BREAST CANCER is manifest by a *painless* mass.) A minority of women have constant, severe pain that does impact greatly on their life.

Patients may also notice change in the consistency and nodularity of part or all of their breast tissue. Discrete masses are also common.

DIAGNOSIS

The diagnosis of fibrocystic breast disease is a clinical one based on the patient's symptoms and PHYSICAL EXAMINATION.

Mammography (a form of RADIOGRAPHY) is useful in excluding BREAST CANCER, but fibrocystic changes in the breast can make mammographic interpretation more difficult.

Aspiration of a suspicious mass with a fine needle to see if it contains fluid or to obtain aspirate for CYTOLOGY can be quite helpful. A fluid-filled cyst that disappears when aspirated requires no further evaluation.

If a mammogram and aspiration are not able to establish that a lump is due to fibrocystic changes, the lump should undergo surgical BIOPSY. The pathologist can then distinguish the finding of cancer from those of fibrocystic changes.

COMPLICATIONS

None.

TREATMENT

SELF TREATMENT:
Patients should perform regular breast self-examinations. Significant changes or the development of a discrete breast lump should be evaluated by a physician.

Women with pain may find relief by
- Finding reassurance from her doctor that she does not have a serious problem
- Wearing supportive, but not tight, clothing
- Taking aspirin and ibuprofen for severe pain
- Taking vitamin E (400 to 800 IU per day)

About half of the women affected obtain relief if they avoid caffeine and too much sodium, but it takes several months before relief is noted.

MEDICAL TREATMENT:
Danazol has been used to treat pain associated with fibrocystic disease. It is rarely used today because it causes side effects such as development of male characteristics (hair pattern, voice change, and MENSTRUAL IRREGULARITIES).

SURGICAL TREATMENT:
Surgical therapy is usually limited to BIOPSY of suspicious lesions.

PREVENTION

There is no known way to prevent the condition, but symptoms can sometimes be avoided or lessened (see Self Treatment above).

FIBROID TUMORS

Fibroid tumors, also known as leiomyoma or myoma, are small benign growths in the uterus. The growths look like white marbles growing in the uterus; they are only rarely found in other parts of the body.

CAUSES

Fibroids are overgrowths of smooth muscle cells. While no specific cause is known, they are thought to grow in response to certain hormones. For many years, estrogen, the major female hormone, was believed to be the culprit. More recently, though, studies have shown progesterone to be the stimulating hormone.

SYMPTOMS

A large percentage of women with fibroids have no symptoms. However, depending on their size and location, fibroids can cause symptoms, including

- ABDOMINAL SWELLING and a heavy feeling when fibroids are large (Some women complain that their clothes no longer fit at the waistline.)
- CONSTIPATION when the fibroids press on the intestines
- Frequent urination (URINATION, FREQUENT) when the fibroids press on the bladder
- MENSTRUAL IRREGULARITIES such as bleeding between periods
- ABDOMINAL PAIN, MENSTRUAL IRREGULARITIES (heavy bleeding), and pain during sexual intercourse

It is very rare for fibroids to be a cause of infertility. During pregnancy they may cause uterine contractions but generally do not cause premature labor.

DIAGNOSIS

The diagnosis of uterine fibroids is usually made during a pelvic examination by a primary care physician or a gynecologist and may be confirmed by ULTRASOUND. Fibroids may also be discovered during abdominal surgery, such as cesarean section or appendectomy, or during hysteroscopy (a form of ENDOSCOPY) performed to assess abnormal VAGINAL BLEEDING.

> Fibroids are common benign tumors. One third to one half of all women have them at some point in their lives.

COMPLICATIONS

The complications of fibroids relate to the symptoms they cause. Large fibroids may compress other intra-abdominal organs such as the ureter, which carries urine from the kidneys to the bladder.

Fibroids may also prevent the detection of other medical problems. For example, a uterus enlarged by fibroids hides growths on the ovaries (such as OVARIAN CANCER) or confuses a physician's attempts to discover the cause of intestinal complaints of CONSTIPATION or increased gas. ANEMIA can result from fibroids that cause excessive blood loss.

TREATMENT

SELF TREATMENT:

None.

MEDICAL TREATMENT:

Some medications can alleviate symptoms for a short amount of time, but they do not cure fibroids. Nonsteroidal anti-inflammatory drugs such as ibuprofen can help with pain and bleeding. Leuprolide given in monthly injections for three to six months may decrease fibroid size and symptoms. However, these effects reverse when the medicine is stopped; therefore it is only given preoperatively to facilitate surgery.

SURGICAL TREATMENT:

HYSTERECTOMY is the operation to remove the entire uterus, thus removing fibroids as well.

FIBROID TUMOR REMOVAL (called *myomectomy*) is a procedure to remove the fibroids from the uterus, which is then repaired and left in place. Myomectomy is generally performed in younger women who desire future fertility. It is not recommended for women who have completed childbearing as fibroids will grow back, requiring surgery again in the future.

PREVENTION

There are no known methods to prevent the development of fibroid tumors.

GALLSTONES

Gallstones are concretions of cholesterol, bile pigments, and calcium salts that precipitate from bile in the gallbladder. Gallstones sometimes pass into the bile duct, which drains bile from the liver into the intestine. Less commonly, stones form in the bile duct instead of the gallbladder.

Gallstones occur in as many as ten percent of the population, but most cases are without symptoms.

CAUSES

Gallstones are common in patients with no predisposing factors, but there are populations at higher risk, including
- Women, especially after multiple pregnancies
- Obese patients
- Native Americans

Dietary factors clearly influence gallstone formation and the high-fat, high-cholesterol diet consumed in Western society is associated with a high incidence of gallstones.

SYMPTOMS

Gallstones usually cause no symptoms. However, the characteristic symptoms, referred to as *biliary colic,* include
- Indigestion
- Flatulence
- Mild to severe intermittent attacks of upper right ABDOMINAL PAIN
- Nausea and VOMITING

Biliary colic may also be associated with pain in the right shoulder. Pain from gallstones is sometimes felt in the middle of the abdomen or chest. Gallstones can also mimic symptoms of ULCER disease or a HEART ATTACK.

DIAGNOSIS

Symptomatic gallstones can usually be suspected from the patient's description of the symptoms. Gallstones are most often documented by ULTRASOUND of the gallbladder. If ULTRASOUND is not helpful, an X-ray test (RADIOGRAPHY) in which the patient is given an iodinated agent that collects in the gallbladder may be performed. Other radiographic tests are required in selected patients to eliminate peptic ULCER disease.

Blood levels of enzymes produced by the liver and bilirubin are measured to exclude jaundice due to stones in the common bile duct and liver disease (see BLOOD TESTS).

COMPLICATIONS

- Acute cholecystitis (see CHOLECYSTITIS AND CHOLANGITIS) results in unremitting ABDOMINAL PAIN similar to biliary colic and FEVER.
- Obstructive jaundice can be caused by gallstones in the common bile duct. Infection is then a possibility (see CHOLECYSTITIS AND CHOLANGITIS).
- Common bile duct stones may also cause PANCREATITIS. Gallstone PANCREATITIS ranges from a very mild, self-limiting problem to a life-threatening disease.

TREATMENT

SELF TREATMENT:

Although gallstone formation and growth are related to dietary factors, the exact dietary causes of gallstones have not been defined, and recommendations are not yet available.

MEDICAL TREATMENT:

Asymptomatic gallstones require no treatment. The risk of observation is less than that of medical or surgical treatment. Symptomatic gallstones should be treated; the risk of complications increases significantly once symptoms begin.

The orally-administered bile salts, ursodeoxycholate or chenodeoxycholate, dissolve cholesterol gallstones in selected patients. Unfortunately, most patients have stones that are not amenable to this treatment, dissolution requires from 12 to 24 months, and stones recur in the majority of patients.

Gallstones have also been fragmented with sound waves (ULTRASONIC LITHOTRIPSY). Again, this has only been effective in a minority of patients, and recurrence rates are high.

SURGICAL TREATMENT:

GALLBLADDER REMOVAL.

PREVENTION

No reliable method of prevention is yet available.

GASTROENTERITIS

Gastroenteritis is any acute inflammation of the lining of the stomach and small intestines. Although it can cause many difficult symptoms, it is usually not serious.

CAUSES

Viruses, such as rotavirus and Norwalk virus, are the most common causes of gastroenteritis, but bacteria can also be the agent. Some bacteria, such as *Shigella, Campylobacter, Yersinia*, and *Aeromonas* species, can directly invade the intestine, causing ulceration, DIARRHEA, and VOMITING. Other bacteria, such as *Salmonella* species, *Vibrio cholerae* (the cause of cholera), and toxigenic *Escherichia coli*, or *E. coli* (the cause of traveler's diarrhea), cause disease by stimulating the intestine to secrete excessive amounts of fluid. Still other bacteria, such as *Staphylococcus*, are lumped into the category of food poisoning and produce a toxin that induces a short-lived illness.

SYMPTOMS

- Nausea and VOMITING
- DIARRHEA
- FEVER
- ABDOMINAL PAIN or cramps
- HEADACHE
- Muscle aches

DIAGNOSIS

Most episodes of gastroenteritis are self-limited and not dangerous and do not need laboratory investigation. The symptoms are quite typical and strongly suggest the diagnosis. However, if the illness is severe or prolonged, stools may be examined for the presence of infection. CULTURE of the stool can be used to identify the responsible organism if bacteria are involved.

COMPLICATIONS

Gastroenteritis tends to run its course in three to five days and complications are rare. DEHYDRATION from the VOMITING and DIARRHEA may be a problem in the aged or very young.

> Gastroenteritis is an inclusive term for many types of intestinal infections. It is a very common illness, affecting all age groups, but especially young people.

On very rare occasion in bacterial gastroenteritis, bacteria can invade the bloodstream and cause a severe systemic infection (see BLOOD POISONING).

TREATMENT

SELF TREATMENT:

Drinking plenty of clear liquids ensures proper hydration. Liquids should contain some sodium; soft drinks, juices, or bouillon are good choices. Beverages with caffeine or alcohol should be avoided. Avoiding solid food will prevent stimulation of the intestine and lessen the symptoms of VOMITING and DIARRHEA.

Over-the-counter medications, such as bismuth subsalicylate, pectin, phosphorated carbohydrate solution, and attapulgite, can be somewhat helpful.

MEDICAL TREATMENT:

Prescription agents include
- Antinausea medication (prochlorperazine, promethazine, trimethobenzamide, metoclopramide, or thiethylperazine)
- Antidiarrheal medication (diphenoxylate and atropine combination or loperamide)
- Antispasmodic, or anticholinergic medication (dicyclomine)
- Antibiotics (trimethoprim, ampicillin, or ciprofloxacin)

SURGICAL TREATMENT:

None.

PREVENTION

The unique instance of traveler's diarrhea associated with travel to underdeveloped countries can sometimes be prevented by the use of antibiotics or bismuth subsalicylate during the visit to an area at high risk. The benefits of this approach should be discussed with medical professionals before travel.

GINGIVITIS

Gingivitis is preventable and completely reversible once the cause of the inflammation is eliminated, but it can lead to irreversible damage if not attended to.

Gingivitis is inflammation of the gum tissue, or gingiva, that surrounds the teeth. If left unchecked, gingivitis can mature into the more destructive form of gum disease, PERIODONTITIS, in which actual bone loss around the teeth occurs.

CAUSES

Gingivitis is caused by a number of factors, including
- Plaque (collections of bacteria)
- Tartar
- Systemic disease such as DIABETES
- Hormonal changes
- Certain medicines such as oral contraceptives
- Dry mouth

Stress and smoking have also been shown to contribute to this disease process. In the majority of cases, however, the primary cause of gingivitis is accumulation and retention of plaque around the necks of the teeth.

SYMPTOMS

Bleeding is the cardinal sign of gingivitis. This bleeding is easily seen after flossing; blood in the rinse water or on the toothbrush after use can also reveal the condition. Direct examination of the gingiva itself can lead to discovery of blood around the crevice of the gum. Bad breath or a bad taste in the mouth can also be a warning that gingivitis is present.

DIAGNOSIS

Clinical evaluation of the mouth is the chief means of confirming whether a patient has gingivitis. The clinician evaluates the tissue, looking for signs of swelling, puffiness, redness, and a smooth shiny surface—all characteristics of gingivitis. The insertion of a probe in the gum cuff around the tooth with bleeding in the crevice upon removal is also a clinical sign of gingivitis.

COMPLICATIONS

The single most significant adverse outcome of gingivitis is progression into PERIODONTITIS. This subsequent disease process causes loss of bone and deepening of the gingival pockets around the teeth. Moreover, this secondary disease is not reversible like gingivitis. When the early warning signs of gingivitis are noted, an appointment with a dentist for a thorough cleaning is the best remedy.

TREATMENT

SELF TREATMENT:

The best treatment for gingivitis is prevention. If the tooth surface is clean and clear of plaque, the gum tissue will remain healthy. The tooth surface will remain clean if brushed after every meal and if the teeth are flossed daily. In conjunction with oral home care, a cleaning by a dental professional every six months will help ensure that all areas of the teeth remain tartar free. If gingivitis is present, a visit for a professional cleaning will clear up the inflammation.

MEDICAL TREATMENT:

Some people accumulate more plaque than others do in spite of their efforts at good oral hygiene. Various mouthwashes (most notably, Listerine) are effective in reducing the amount of plaque-causing bacteria. A prescription drug, chlorhexidine, inhibits the ability of bacteria to bind to the tooth. Chlorhexidine is also a mouth rinse, but its use must be monitored because, like most medications, it may produce side effects.

SURGICAL TREATMENT:

Generally, a professional cleaning is enough to eliminate the gingival inflammation and allow for the return of the gum to its normal contour and shape. When, however, the source of the gingivitis is exacerbated by systemic disease, hormonal changes, or adverse medication effects, removal of the tissue (PERIODONTAL SURGERY) is occasionally indicated.

PREVENTION

As in most aspects of good oral health, the most important, cost-effective, and time-saving way to avoid gingivitis is with daily flossing, brushing after eating, and dental visits every six months.

GLAUCOMA

Glaucoma is the number one cause of blindness in the United States, but it is treatable if discovered early.

Glaucoma is an eye condition that results from elevated fluid pressure in the eye. The optic nerve, which carries the visual information from the eye to the brain, is prone to permanent damage when the eye pressure is elevated. The amount of damage is related to

- The degree of pressure elevation
- The length of time the pressure has been elevated
- The underlying health of the nerve

CAUSES

The front of the eye is filled with a clear fluid called aqueous. Normal eye pressure is maintained because of a balance between aqueous produced in the eye and aqueous leaving the eye through its outflow mechanism. Glaucoma is usually caused by a defect or obstruction in this fluid outflow mechanism. Because fluid continues to be produced, but is unable to exit the eye, the eye pressure goes up.

Risk factors for the development of glaucoma include a family history of the condition, glaucoma in the other eye, and nearsightedness.

DIABETES, HYPERTENSION, and other diseases that affect circulation of blood to the optic nerve, such as ATHEROSCLEROSIS, make it more susceptible to pressure damage.

Ocular injuries and chronic inflammation of the eye can damage the fluid outflow mechanism, resulting in elevated pressure. Farsightedness, an abnormally small eye, progressive CATARACT, or other abnormalities can block the fluid outflow apparatus. Finally, advancing age is associated with an elevation in the pressure within the eye.

SYMPTOMS

In the majority of cases, glaucoma causes painless loss of peripheral vision. The patient is often unaware of this irreversible loss in vision until it is so severe that it encroaches on the line of sight.

In the relatively rare cases of sudden elevations in eye pressure, a patient may notice

- Aching EYE PAIN
- Blurred vision (see VISION DISTURBANCES) with haloes around street lights
- Redness of the eye

DIAGNOSIS

The ophthalmologist makes the diagnosis of glaucoma by detecting an elevated intraocular pressure in the presence of glaucomatous optic nerve damage and loss of side vision on visual field testing.

COMPLICATIONS

The risk of undetected glaucoma is progressive loss of side vision. Ultimately, total blindness can result. In the majority of cases, there are no warning signs such as pain, redness, or blurred vision. For this reason, it is recommended that patients over 40 have their eye pressure measured at least every two years. When risk factors for glaucoma are present, closer monitoring is warranted.

TREATMENT

SELF TREATMENT:
Except for seeking professional evaluation as soon as possible, there is no self treatment for glaucoma.

MEDICAL TREATMENT:
Medical treatment consists of eyedrops and/or pills. The drops are used to improve the outflow or decrease the production of aqueous fluid. Some drops have both capabilities. The pills act to reduce production of the fluid. The ophthalmologist and patient together determine the right combination of medications such as acetazolamide and pilocarpine to control the eye pressure.

SURGICAL TREATMENT:
- A laser can be used to improve the outflow function or to improve the circulation of aqueous fluid within the eye.
- Glaucoma filter surgery creates a new outflow capability by bypassing the natural path.

PREVENTION

In most cases there is no way to prevent glaucoma. The key is early detection with regular ophthalmologic examination.

HEART ATTACK

Heart disease kills more than 500,000 people in the United States every year. Most of these deaths are attributable to heart attacks. Many people who have a heart attack never make it to the hospital, but of those who do, generally 90 to 95 percent are able to return home.

A heart attack (called a *myocardial infarction*) occurs when the heart muscle is damaged. Usually this damage is a result of a lack of blood flow to the affected area. Without the blood supply, the muscle does not get the oxygen it needs, and part of it dies.

CAUSES

The main cause of the lack of blood flow to an area of the heart muscle is coronary artery disease (ATHEROSCLEROSIS). Rarely, a spasm of the coronary artery—the blood vessels feeding the heart muscle—can cause a lack of blood flow temporarily, long enough to cause a clot to form and block the flow entirely. Spasm has been seen under conditions of severe emotional stress and drug abuse (including cocaine use and cigarette smoking).

The general risk factors for ATHEROSCLEROSIS, and hence heart attack, include

- Smoking
- High blood pressure (HYPERTENSION)
- DIABETES
- Increased blood cholesterol levels (HYPERLIPIDEMIA)
- Family history of heart disease

Men are more prone to heart disease than women, but after menopause, a woman's risk soon equals that of a man's.

SYMPTOMS

Approximately one-third of heart attacks cause no symptoms at all and may be detected incidentally by ELECTROCARDIOGRAPHY done for some other purpose. Symptoms generally include CHEST PAIN, which can be a pressure or heaviness or a squeezing type of pain in the center of the chest, but the pain can also be located as high as the jaw or as low as the upper abdomen. It can be in the right or left arm. ANGINA is a similar feeling and usually precedes a heart attack by weeks or years. The pain of a heart attack, however, generally lasts significantly longer, ranging from approximately 20 minutes to a few hours. Associated symptoms include

- Nausea
- BREATHING DIFFICULTY
- Profuse sweating

In the elderly, the symptoms can be more vague and can include sudden weakness and FAINTING OR FAINTNESS.

DIAGNOSIS

BLOOD TESTS are often used to detect signs of heart muscle damage by measuring the levels of certain enzymes in the blood. ELECTROCARDIOGRAPHY almost always reveals something abnormal. Echocardiography (ULTRASOUND) can reveal an area of the heart muscle that is not functioning normally because of a heart attack. Certain NUCLEAR MEDICINE studies can also show damage to the heart muscle. Ultimately, a CARDIAC CATHETERIZATION may be performed to locate the blocked artery and document the heart muscle damage.

COMPLICATIONS

A heart attack is very serious in itself, but it can also precipitate further life-threatening problems including
- CONGESTIVE HEART FAILURE
- Mitral regurgitation (a form of HEART VALVE DISEASE)
- Sudden cardiac death

TREATMENT

SELF TREATMENT:

The safest thing to do when one suspects that he or she is having a heart attack is to call 911 or other local emergency services. There is no way to self-treat a heart attack.

After a heart attack, a survivor may be involved in rehabilitation which can assist him or her in getting back to work and in reducing the risk of future heart attacks. The American Heart Association can also link people to support groups if necessary.

MEDICAL TREATMENT:

Many different drugs are used in the early hours and days of a heart attack. The most dramatic include the thrombolytic drugs—streptokinase and tissue plasminogen activator (TPA)—which help dissolve the blood clots that usually interfere with the blood flow to the heart muscle and cause the heart attack. For these drugs to be most effective, they need to be given within four to six hours of the onset of symptoms. This highlights the need for prompt medical attention if a heart attack is suspected.

Drugs comonly prescribed for heart attack include
- Nitroglycerin
- Beta-blockers such as atenolol and metoprolol
- Morphine
- Heparin
- Aspirin

Because ARRHYTHMIAS may develop during a heart attack, certain medications such as lidocaine may be necessary. Defibrillation by medical personnel, in which an electrical charge is used to restore a steady rhythm to the heart muscle, may be necessary to treat sudden cardiac death.

SURGICAL TREATMENT:

Surgery is rarely needed in the early phase of a heart attack; however, emergency CORONARY ARTERY BYPASS GRAFT SURGERY may be needed to improve the blood flow to the heart and to treat some of the complications of a heart attack.

Emergency percutaneous transluminal coronary ANGIOPLASTY may also be used in the early hours of a heart attack. PACEMAKER INSERTION is occasionally needed to treat the complications of a heart attack.

In select patients, under rare circumstances when a very large amount of heart muscle has been damaged, cardiac transplantation may be the best option.

PREVENTION

Avoidance of smoking is the single most powerful preventive measure. Also important is
- Control of high blood pressure (HYPERTENSION)
- Control of blood cholesterol levels with a low-fat, low-cholesterol diet and possibly drug therapy
- Regular aerobic exercise

Aspirin therapy for patients at significant risk for coronary artery disease and hormone replacement therapy for some postmenopausal women can also be useful in preventing heart attacks.

HEART VALVE DISEASE

Heart valves are, in a sense, one-way doors between the different chambers and exits of the heart. These valves can become damaged during the development of the fetus (in which case it is called *congenital* heart valve disease) or, more commonly, in childhood or adult life (called *acquired* heart valve disease). The disease can result in two types of problems: 1) if a valve becomes narrowed by scarring or a buildup of calcium deposits, it can partially block the flow of blood to the body and is said to be *stenotic*; or 2) if a valve becomes weak and leaky, it can allow blood to flow backward and is said to be *insufficient* or *regurgitant*.

CAUSES

Congenital heart valve disease is a result of either genetic abnormality or some problem during the pregnancy. Acquired valve disease can result from many factors including infections (such as rheumatic heart disease or endocarditis) and degenerative causes. HYPERTENSION, coronary artery disease (ATHEROSCLEROSIS), and other conditions such as CARDIOMYOPATHY that weaken the heart muscle can also cause a valve to malfunction.

SYMPTOMS

- Progressive BREATHING DIFFICULTY, fluid retention (ANKLE SWELLING), FATIGUE, and FAINTING OR FAINTNESS (symptoms similar to CONGESTIVE HEART FAILURE)
- Persistent unexplained FEVERS (possibly caused by heart valve infection—endocarditis)
- Heart rhythm abnormalities or palpitations (ARRHYTHMIA)

DIAGNOSIS

A physician can detect most cases by careful PHYSICAL EXAMINATION of the heartbeat and pulse, especially by listening with a stethoscope. A certain ULTRASOUND technique called *Doppler echocardiography* can identify and assess the severity of valve disease. CARDIAC CATHETERIZATION and angiocardiography may ultimately be needed to confirm the diagnosis of valve disease.

There are four valves in the heart: the aortic, the mitral, the pulmonic, and the tricuspid. These valves ensure that blood flows through the heart in the proper direction.

COMPLICATIONS

Blood clots can form near the malfunctioning valve and then travel in the bloodstream to other parts of the body, potentially causing STROKE or, rarely, PULMONARY EMBOLISM.

Damaged valves can become infected (endocarditis) when bacteria are present in the bloodstream—an occurrence sometimes associated with recent dental work.

Valve malfunction can lead to CONGESTIVE HEART FAILURE.

TREATMENT

SELF TREATMENT:

Severe disorders may require restrictions on activity. Checking with a physician before any surgical procedure, including dental work, is important because of the risk of valve infection; prophylactic antibiotics may reduce this risk.

MEDICAL TREATMENT:

A physician may prescribe
- Antibiotics such as penicillin to treat infected valves
- Anticoagulant drugs such as aspirin and warfarin to remove risk of clot formation
- Drugs that remove the workload of the heart and resistance to forward flow of blood (nifedipine, ACE inhibitors such as enalapril and captopril)
- Drugs to treat congestive heart failure (digoxin, diuretics such as hydrochlorothiazide and furosemide)

SURGICAL TREATMENT:

- HEART VALVE REPLACEMENT or heart valve repair
- Balloon expansion of a narrowed valve (a form of ANGIOPLASTY)

PREVENTION

- Appropriate treatment of strep throat infections significantly decreases the risk of rheumatic heart disease and, therefore, heart valve damage.
- Control of HYPERTENSION and avoidance of excessive alcohol consumption can help prevent damage to the heart muscle and subsequent valve malfunction.

HEMORRHOIDS

Hemorrhoids are varicose veins in the lower rectum or anal canal. There are two types of hemorrhoids: internal hemorrhoids, which form in the lower rectum, and external hemorrhoids, which form at the end of the anal canal.

CAUSES

Hemorrhoids are frequently associated with CONSTIPATION. The straining during bowel movements puts pressure on the blood vessels of the area, thus slowing blood flow and causing the veins to swell. In developed countries, where a low-fiber diet is common, the population is more susceptible to hemorrhoids because adequate fiber can speed elimination and prevent CONSTIPATION and straining.

There may be a hereditary predisposition to hemorrhoids, but shared dietary habits could account for some of the apparent familial connections.

In women, hemorrhoids often develop or worsen during pregnancy. This occurs because the growing fetus presses on the pelvic veins.

SYMPTOMS

Hemorrhoids may cause
- ITCHING and mild perianal discomfort (Severe anal pain indicates another problem or complications of hemorrhoids.)
- Most commonly, painless, bright red RECTAL BLEEDING with bowel movements (Blood may be noted in the toilet water and coating the stool; it never mixes with the stool, however.)
- A soft mass that protrudes from the anus, called a *prolapsed* hemorrhoid

DIAGNOSIS

The diagnosis is made on the basis of the symptoms and a PHYSICAL EXAMINATION. A rectal examination should be performed and followed by examination of the anal canal and lower rectum with an anoscope (a form of ENDOSCOPY) to visualize the hemorrhoids. Examination of the entire rectum and lower colon with flexible sigmoidoscopy (another form of ENDOSCOPY) is also required in many circumstances to exclude

Hemorrhoids, often called *piles*, are a common affliction of the anal canal that can cause inflammation and discomfort.

other causes of bleeding. A complete BLOOD COUNT is usually performed to evaluate the patient for ANEMIA.

COMPLICATIONS

THROMBOSIS of an external hemorrhoid is the development of a blood clot in the hemorrhoid. It is very painful and causes a firm mass and swelling in the perianal area.

Prolapsed hemorrhoids are internal hemorrhoids that protrude from the anus. They can easily become irritated and cause soiling of anal secretions which, in turn, causes discomfort and perianal ITCHING.

TREATMENT

SELF TREATMENT:

Patients may obtain relief with warm baths (sitz baths), which soothe and cleanse the perianal area. (See also Prevention below.)

MEDICAL TREATMENT:

Dietary changes and fiber supplements are instituted to control bowel habits. Anal suppositories with or without cortisone may ameliorate symptoms.

SURGICAL TREATMENT:

- HEMORRHOID BANDING
- HEMORRHOID REMOVAL
- Infrared or electrocoagulation of hemorrhoids

PREVENTION

The development and progression of hemorrhoids can be avoided or impeded by avoiding CONSTIPATION and straining with bowel movements. A high-fiber diet is best for long-term control of bowel habits, but many patients require fiber supplements to control the consistency of bowel movements.

HEPATITIS

Hepatitis is an infectious or inflammatory condition of the liver. It most often is an acute self-limited event, although patients may be ill for weeks. Some forms of hepatitis may linger chronically and occasionally progress to substantial scarring or cirrhosis of the liver.

CAUSES

Hepatitis may be caused by a variety of viruses including, hepatitis A, hepatitis B, hepatitis C, hepatitis delta, cytomegalovirus, and Epstein-Barr. A parasite, *Toxoplasma*, can also cause infectious hepatitis. Not all viral hepatitis has a demonstrable virus and unknown viruses responsible for hepatitis remain to be discovered.

Most viral hepatitis is transmitted silently from person to person. Hepatitis B, C, and delta may be transmitted by blood products or the sharing of needles in illicit use of injectable drugs. Hepatitis B can be transmitted sexually.

A wide variety of prescription and over-the-counter medications can also cause hepatitis. This form of hepatitis is self-limited when discovered early and does not usually progress to a chronic state.

Alcohol, when used excessively and chronically, can cause hepatitis. Toxins such as carbon tetrachloride and food poisoning from certain rare mushrooms may also result in acute hepatitis.

SYMPTOMS

- Malaise
- Loss of appetite (see APPETITE, LOSS OF)
- FEVER
- Nausea and occasionally VOMITING
- Upper right ABDOMINAL PAIN or ache
- Yellowing of the eyes and skin (jaundice)
- Dark urine (see URINE, ABNORMAL APPEARANCE)
- Diffused ITCHING

> Most of the forms of hepatitis are self-limited, and the patient recovers completely. Some, however, can result in a more chronic condition and complications.

DIAGNOSIS

A diagnosis of hepatitis may be suspected in a patient with jaundice (yellowing of the skin and eyes) when other appropriate symptoms are present. The diagnosis is corroborated with blood tests that measure the activity of liver enzymes and bilirubin. BLOOD TESTS to measure exposure to hepatitis A, B, C, and delta; cytomegalovirus; Epstein-Barr virus; and *Toxoplasma* are available and will confirm the cause of infectious hepatitis in most instances.

If the diagnosis is unclear, ULTRASOUND or COMPUTED TOMOGRAPHY of the liver may be performed. On rare occasion, in cases without clear cause, a liver BIOPSY may be needed.

COMPLICATIONS

Most hepatitis is a self-limited condition, and after a period of several weeks, the patient fully recovers. On very rare occasion, viral hepatitis can be quite severe, even resulting in liver failure with coma.

Some forms of hepatitis (hepatitis B, C, and delta) can progress to a chronic condition that causes continued inflammation of the liver for months or years and may eventually even result in cirrhosis of the liver or LIVER CANCER. Follow-up with a physician and periodic evaluation of liver enzyme BLOOD TESTS will help in recognition and treatment of these complications.

TREATMENT

SELF TREATMENT:

- The need for prolonged bed rest in hepatitis is no longer considered essential; the patient should undertake only activity that does not cause undue fatigue.
- Nutrition is important, and the diet should be liberal; patients frequently will have a poor appetite and may find sweets and carbohydrates more palatable.
- Alcohol should be strictly avoided.
- The use of over-the-counter or prescription medication should be discussed with a physician.

MEDICAL TREATMENT:
- There is no nonexperimental treatment for acute viral hepatitis. Like other viral diseases, it is usually a self-limited illness that the patient's own immune system overcomes.
- Treatment with injectable interferon-alpha may be used in chronic hepatitis (more than six months of illness) caused by hepatitis B or C.
- Withdrawal of offending drugs, toxins, or alcohol is usually all that is required when these agents are the cause of hepatitis.

SURGICAL TREATMENT:

Liver transplantation has been used in cases of unremitting liver failure in patients who become desperately ill.

PREVENTION

Public health measures and modern sanitation have severely curtailed outbreaks of hepatitis in the United States and the industrialized world. Routine screening for hepatitis B and C in donated blood has virtually eliminated the risk of transfusion-related hepatitis. Hepatitis can still be spread within groups of illicit drug users who share needles, however. Hepatitis B can be spread sexually, and partners of patients should take precautions with protected sex.

Vaccines against hepatitis B are available and recommended for most children and groups of adults at higher risk for acquiring hepatitis B, including
- Medical professionals
- Patients on hemodialysis
- Patients with hemophilia or thalassemia requiring transfusion
- Morticians
- Homosexually active men
- Intimate contacts of persons with active hepatitis B

In the rare event that a patient is exposed to blood from a patient with active hepatitis B, injectable hepatitis B immune globulin may reduce the risk of acquiring hepatitis B. Immune gamma globulin is recommended for close household contacts of persons with hepatitis A.

HERNIA

Hernias can theoretically occur almost anywhere in the body, but the abdominal wall is the most common site.

A hernia is a defect in the abdominal wall that allows internal structures to protrude through the wall. The most common type of hernia, inguinal hernia, occurs in the groin, but a hernia can occur anywhere in the abdominal wall. A hernia in the naval (umbilical) or above it (epigastric) is also very common. A hernia can also occur at the site of a previous surgical incision.

CAUSES

Inguinal, umbilical, and epigastric hernias occur at a weak site in the abdominal wall that formed as the abdomen developed. Children who develop a hernia early in life are probably born with the defect. Adults who develop a hernia later in life are most likely born with a minimal defect that enlarges as tissues age and weaken. Increased pressure in the abdomen from lifting and straining may contribute to the development and enlargement of a hernia.

Healed abdominal incisions are never as strong as the normal abdomen tissues, and a hernia may develop in the wound. An incisional hernia is more likely to occur in patients with

- ABDOMINAL SWELLING
- Wound infection
- Obesity
- Critical illness
- Malnourishment

All of these factors are thought to interfere with normal wound healing.

SYMPTOMS

A hernia most often appears as a mass that causes only mild discomfort. If the hernia becomes trapped, or incarcerated, in the defect, it may cause significant, unremitting pain, especially if the blood supply to the contents of the hernia has been cut off—a so-called *strangulated* hernia. These complications require prompt medical attention.

DIAGNOSIS

The PHYSICAL EXAMINATION alone is used to diagnose a hernia in almost all cases. In rare cases, COMPUTED TOMOGRAPHY or ULTRASOUND may be used.

COMPLICATIONS

- An incarcerated hernia is one in which the mass cannot be pushed back into the abdomen.
- A strangulated hernia occurs when the blood supply to the contents of the hernia is compromised. If the blood supply is cut off for too long, gangrene can result.

TREATMENT

SELF TREATMENT:

None. Some patients use trusses to hold their hernia in place and claim that they improve comfort, but there is no evidence that a truss is beneficial.

MEDICAL TREATMENT:

None.

SURGICAL TREATMENT:

HERNIA REPAIR, either open or laparascopic, is the only treatment. Small hernias that are not progressing and are not causing serious symptoms may be observed without treatment, holding surgery in reserve for any problems that might develop.

PREVENTION

None.

HERNIATED DISK

A herniated disk, sometimes known as a slipped disk, is usually the result of an injury and can cause debilitating pain.

A herniated disk is a rupture or bulging of the intervertebral disks (soft tissue spacers) located between the bones of the spine. When the bulging causes pressure or irritation of the nerve roots that provide the sensation and motor power of the legs, there may be NUMBNESS, TINGLING, weakness, and radiating pain in the affected leg or arm.

CAUSES

A herniated disk is most often caused by a combination of wear and tear changes in the disk that allow a portion of the disk to press on the nerve roots that run out of the spine. When this process is present, an inciting event—a fall, a heavy lifting episode, or a twisting injury—may be a contributing factor.

Repetitive spinal injuries, exposure to vibration in the workplace, obesity, and smoking have been demonstrated to increase the risk of a disk herniation.

SYMPTOMS

Patients with a disk herniation frequently notice
- A radiating pain from the buttock and thigh area into the calf or foot
- NUMBNESS or tingling in the same area
- Muscle weakness or fatigue in the affected limb

Much less frequently, a herniated disk in the neck can cause these symptoms in an arm.

DIAGNOSIS

The diagnosis of a herniated disk is made by a combination of specific symptoms and objective evidence of motor weakness, reflex loss, and decreased sensation noted during the PHYSICAL EXAMINATION. Plain X rays (RADIOGRAPHY) are not usually helpful; special radiologic studies such as MAGNETIC RESONANCE IMAGING, COMPUTED TOMOGRAPHY, and myelography (a form of RADIOGRAPHY) may be needed to confirm the diagnosis in patients whose symptoms are worsening. Electrical testing is occasionally useful in identifying the specific nerve root that is irritated.

COMPLICATIONS

While the vast majority of patients with disk herniation recover with patience and nonsurgical treatment, changes in bowel or bladder function or progressive extremity weakness should be evaluated as soon as possible, as these may lead to permanent nerve deficits.

TREATMENT

SELF TREATMENT:
- Depending on the severity of symptoms, a decrease in activity is usually in order.
- Minor pain can be treated with over-the-counter analgesics and anti-inflammatories such as aspirin, acetaminophen, or ibuprofen.

MEDICAL TREATMENT:
More severe pain can be managed by prescription oral analgesics and anti-inflammatories, such as an acetaminophen and codeine combination, or by epidural anti-inflammatory injections.

SURGICAL TREATMENT:
Diskectomy (see LUMBAR DISK REMOVAL).

PREVENTION

The chance of a disk herniation can be reduced by avoiding the risk factors such as
- Vibrations in the workplace
- Obesity
- Smoking
- Improper lifting techniques

However, as degenerative changes of the disk occur in everyone with time, there is no preventative tactic that can completely eliminate the risk.

HODGKIN DISEASE

Although the disease sounds ominous and treatment can be difficult, 80 percent of patients with Hodgkin disease can be cured.

Hodgkin disease is a type of lymphoma. Lymphomas are cancers that arise from the lymph system, a network of small nodes and vessels that help to fight infections by filtering lymph fluid. Small lymph nodes may sometimes normally be felt in the neck or groin. In Hodgkin disease, lymph nodes become enlarged due to the presence of a tumor. Lymph nodes in the neck region are often involved.

CAUSES

The cause of Hodgkin disease is unknown. Some researchers believe that Epstein-Barr virus, the virus that causes mononucleosis, may be involved in the development of Hodgkin disease.

Immunosuppressant drugs used after transplantation surgery (see KIDNEY TRANSPLANT) may also be a factor in rare cases.

SYMPTOMS

Symptoms include
- Persistent swelling of a lymph node or nodes
- FEVER
- Night sweats (see SWEATING, EXCESSIVE)
- Unintended WEIGHT LOSS
- Generalized body ITCHING

DIAGNOSIS

Diagnosis is made by surgically removing an involved lymph node and examining it under the microscope. Once the diagnosis is made, other tests, such as bone marrow BIOPSY and COMPUTED TOMOGRAPHY of the chest and abdomen, are used to evaluate the extent of the disease and plan treatment strategies.

COMPLICATIONS

Without treatment, the immune system becomes progressively impaired, resulting in serious infections that can become life threatening.

Treatment

SELF TREATMENT:

None.

MEDICAL TREATMENT:

The use of chemotherapy and radiation therapy is determined by the stage of disease. One or the other or a combination of the two are options. With modern therapy, about 80 percent of patients with Hodgkin disease can be cured of their malignancy.

SURGICAL TREATMENT:

Spleen removal, also called splenectomy, is sometimes performed if the spleen—part of the lymphatic system—becomes dangerously enlarged, unresponsive to other therapies, and a potential source of complications.

Prevention

Any persistently swollen lymph node greater than one centimeter in diameter (the size of a marble) should be evaluated by a physician. Early detection is the key to successful treatment.

HYPERLIPIDEMIA

The elevated level of lipids in the blood is a major risk factor for cardiovascular disease and one of the precursors to potentially life-threatening atherosclerosis.

Hyperlipidemia involves elevated blood levels of fats such as cholesterol and triglycerides. These high levels are associated with the formation of fat deposits on the inner surface of blood vessels (see ATHEROSCLEROSIS).

A related problem is abnormally low high-density lipoprotein (HDL) cholesterol—the so-called "good" part of total cholesterol—which is believed to help remove fat deposits from the lining of the blood vessel walls.

CAUSES

Risk factors for hyperlipidemia include
- Obesity
- High-fat diet
- Lack of exercise
- Family history of the condition

Other conditions that can contribute to the problem include
- Thyroid disorders (HYPOTHYROIDISM)
- DIABETES
- Certain kidney and liver disorders

SYMPTOMS

The disease is relatively silent as far as what the patient can notice on his or her own. Only rarely do fatty skin deposits appear around the eyes or the ankle tendon above the heel. Other symptoms are related to the complications of ATHEROSCLEROSIS.

DIAGNOSIS

The characteristic fatty skin deposits may be detected by PHYSICAL EXAMINATION, but a BLOOD TEST of fasting lipid levels, including total cholesterol, triglycerides, and HDL cholesterol are necessary to make the diagnosis. Since random variation is significant, most physicians require two or three measurements over time to label a patient as having a problem.

COMPLICATIONS

The main danger of hyperlipidemia is its association with the formation of fatty deposits on the walls of blood vessels (ATHEROSCLEROSIS), which can lead to HEART ATTACK or STROKE.

Extremely high levels of triglycerides in the blood can cause PANCREATITIS.

TREATMENT

SELF TREATMENT:

- A diet low in cholesterol and fat (especially saturated fat)
- Regular exercise
- Maintenance of a healthy weight

MEDICAL TREATMENT:

Cholestyramine, lovastatin, gemfibrozil, and niacin are examples of drugs commonly used to lower blood lipid levels. These have the most impact on patients with existing ATHEROSCLEROSIS.

Patients with multiple risk factors for ATHEROSCLEROSIS may also receive significant benefits from these drugs, depending on their lipid levels, after all dietary efforts have been pursued. Drug therapy for others is generally reserved only in rare instances.

SURGICAL TREATMENT:

A procedure to divert fats from the body into the bowel (called an *ileal bypass*) can be quite effective in severe cases.

PREVENTION

The same measures listed under Self Treatment above may help avert hyperlipidemia.

HYPERTENSION

Hypertension is abnormally high blood pressure. It is, unfortunately, very common in the United States, but because it usually causes no noticeable symptoms, the condition is only diagnosed by regular BLOOD PRESSURE TESTING.

CAUSES

In most cases, the cause of the high blood pressure is not clear. Multiple factors probably play a role, including family history and salt intake. Blacks and men are more commonly affected. Other factors include
- Emotional stress
- Obesity
- Excessive alcohol intake
- Smoking
- A sedentary lifestyle

In rare cases, hypertension results from specific diseases; adrenal gland tumors, kidney diseases, and congenital abnormalities of the aorta, (the largest vessel coming out of the heart) can be the cause.

SYMPTOMS

Most patients with hypertension are without any symptoms. Some may experience HEADACHES, DIZZINESS, or nosebleeds, but these symptoms usually have other causes.

Unfortunately, the first symptoms of hypertension are usually from a complication. That's why periodic BLOOD PRESSURE TESTING is valuable.

DIAGNOSIS

Healthy people may have temporarily elevated blood pressure (for example, when they are under stress). Hypertension is diagnosed, however, when an individual has persistently elevated blood pressure—that is, elevated pressure measured on two or three occasions.

Although the cutoff is somewhat arbitrary, the usual definition of "abnormally high" is blood pressure greater than 140/90 mm Hg. Some patients' blood pressure is so variable that a 24-hour ambulatory blood pressure monitor or frequent home BLOOD PRESSURE TESTING may be needed.

> Hypertension is sometimes known as the silent killer because it causes no noticeable symptoms, but it can be deadly.

COMPLICATIONS

Hypertension promotes ATHEROSCLEROSIS, KIDNEY FAILURE, CONGESTIVE HEART FAILURE, and STROKE. Any symptoms related to these complications can be a clue to hypertension, too, including

- BREATHING DIFFICULTY
- ANGINA
- Claudication (pain during activity, relieved by rest)
- Swelling (see ANKLE SWELLING)
- NUMBNESS or weakness on one side of the body

TREATMENT

SELF TREATMENT:

Measures that may aid in lowering blood pressure include

- Limiting sodium intake
- Avoiding excessive alcohol
- Weight loss (if appropriate)
- Exercise (if hypertension is reasonably controlled)
- Relaxation techniques for stress reduction

MEDICAL TREATMENT:

If lifestyle changes don't improve hypertension enough or if the blood pressure is seriously elevated at the time of diagnosis, many types of medication can be used, including

- Diuretics such as hydrochlorothiazide
- Beta-blockers such as atenolol, metoprolol, and propranolol
- Calcium channel blockers such as nifedipine, diltiazem, verapamil, and amlodipine
- ACE inhibitors such as captopril and enalapril
- Alpha-blockers such as prazosin and terazosin

SURGICAL TREATMENT:

For the rare cases in which kidney or adrenal gland disorders are the cause, surgery may be necessary on those organs.

PREVENTION

Regular exercise, avoiding excess weight, moderation of salt intake, and limiting alcohol to no more than two drinks a day may help prevent hypertension.

HYPERTHYROIDISM

Thyroid hormone affects the entire body, and a wide variety of problems can be related to the excess amount of hormone produced in this disorder.

Hyperthyroidism is a disorder caused by excessive levels of thyroid hormone. Generally, excessive levels are caused by an overactive thyroid gland either acting on its own or being overstimulated by the pituitary gland.

CAUSES

- In some cases, excess thyroid hormone can be caused by an autoimmune disease in which antibodies attack thyroid tissue and lead to an overproduction of the hormone.
- Infections may occasionally cause an overstimulation of the thyroid gland, temporarily leading to excessive amounts of thyroid hormone in the bloodstream.
- Genetics seem to play a factor, because thyroid diseases tend to run in families and are more common in women.

SYMPTOMS

Excess thyroid levels can develop quite slowly or very quickly; the symptoms, therefore, may develop insidiously or rapidly. Symptoms include
- ANXIETY and restlessness
- Rapid heartbeat (see ARRHYTHMIA)
- TREMBLING of the fingers
- Intolerance to heat
- WEIGHT LOSS despite an increased appetite
- FATIGUE
- Weakness of the muscles, particularly the shoulders and thighs
- MENSTRUAL IRREGULARITIES

The thyroid gland may be noticeably swollen (a condition known as *goiter*), and when the autoimmune disease called *Grave disease* is the cause of excess thyroid stimulation, deposits behind the eyes may also develop, causing a bulging of the eyeballs.

DIAGNOSIS

The PHYSICAL EXAMINATION may lead to the initial suspicion of hyperthyroidism and BLOOD TESTS confirming high levels of hormone or suppressed levels of the pituitary hormone will confirm the diagnosis. A thyroid scan (a form of NUCLEAR MEDICINE) or ULTRASOUND may also be used to examine the thyroid gland.

COMPLICATIONS

- Excess thyroid hormone can lead to overstimulation of the heart muscle and may rarely cause a HEART ATTACK.
- Long-term hyperthyroidism may also lead to softening of the bones (OSTEOPOROSIS).
- The deposits behind the eyes, if allowed to progress, can lead to VISION DISTURBANCES.

TREATMENT

SELF TREATMENT:

None.

MEDICAL TREATMENT:

Radioactive iodine, which collects in the thyroid gland, can be used to destroy enough of the thyroid gland so that it produces less thyroid hormone.

Other medications that may interfere with the production of thyroid hormone and can be used for treatment include propylthiouracil and methimazole.

SURGICAL TREATMENT:

In some cases, very large thyroid glands or portions of the thyroid gland may be removed to control thyroid hormone production with both surgery (THYROIDECTOMY) and radioactive iodine.

Removing too much is not uncommon, causing the gland to produce too little thyroid hormone (HYPOTHYROIDISM), but this condition is relatively easily treated with the appropriate amount of thyroid hormone medication.

PREVENTION

None.

HYPOTHYROIDISM

Thyroid hormone affects the entire body, and a wide variety of problems can be related to the reduced amount of hormone produced in this disorder.

Hypothyroidism is a disorder caused by the thyroid gland's failure to make an adequate amount of thyroid hormone. Because the hormone is integral to the regulation of metabolism, this disorder has widespread effects on the body's functions.

CAUSES

- Hypothyroidism is frequently the end stage of an autoimmune disorder in which the body's immune system has attacked the thyroid gland tissue over a period of years.
- Also common is the understimulation of the thyroid gland by hormones from the pituitary gland, which helps regulate thyroid hormone production.
- Rarely, some viral infections may cause a temporary excess and then a temporary inadequacy of thyroid hormone.
- Genetics seems to play a role; hypothyroidism can run in families.
- Lack of dietary iodine can cause a decrease in thyroid function, but such a deficiency is very uncommon today.

SYMPTOMS

Symptoms of hypothyroidism include
- FATIGUE
- Intolerance to cold
- Unexplained WEIGHT GAIN
- A hoarse voice
- Puffiness around the eyes
- Dry skin
- Hair loss
- Slowing of mental function (see MEMORY PROBLEMS)
- CONSTIPATION
- MENSTRUAL IRREGULARITIES, particularly abnormally heavy, prolonged periods

DIAGNOSIS

The diagnosis is usually suspected from the symptoms and a PHYSICAL EXAMINATION, and it is confirmed by a BLOOD TEST of blood level of thyroid hormone.

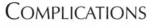

COMPLICATIONS

If hypothyroidism is left untreated, it can progress to coma and even death. If left untreated during infancy, it can result in permanent mental retardation and cretinism.

TREATMENT

SELF TREATMENT:

None.

MEDICAL TREATMENT:

Hypothyroidism is usually treated with thyroid hormone (thyroxine).

SURGICAL TREATMENT:

Without adequate iodine, the thyroid gland enlarges. If the thyroid gland is large enough to interfere with breathing or swallowing, THYROIDECTOMY may be required.

PREVENTION

Most people in the United States now have an adequate amount of iodine in the diet—most of it from iodized salt. Before this became a widespread practice, insufficient dietary intake of iodine was a cause of hypothyroidism.

IMPOTENCE

Impotence is a very common condition. Almost all men experience it at some point in their lives, although it is usually temporary.

Impotence is the inability to achieve or maintain an erection satisfactory for intercourse. Erection depends on many factors including the proper functioning of the
- Circulatory system
- Endocrine system
- Nervous system

The penis is mostly made up of spongy erectile tissue that fills with blood to become erect. This event requires each of these systems to work together in ways that are still not fully understood.

CAUSES

The causes of impotence are as varied as the systems involved in proper erectile functioning. The most common causes are psychological. Performance anxiety is a common cause, even in stable, loving relationships. Other common psychological factors that can lead to impotence include
- General anxiety
- Stress
- DEPRESSION

Loss of function can be caused by disorders involving the actual erectile mechanisms. Risk factors for this type of impotence include
- DIABETES
- Vascular disease (ATHEROSCLEROSIS)
- Smoking
- High blood cholesterol levels (HYPERLIPIDEMIA)

Hormonal imbalances and the side effects of certain medications such as beta-blockers (propranolol) and antihistamines can also cause impotence. Rarely, nerve damage from surgery in the area, STROKE, or MULTIPLE SCLEROSIS can be the cause.

DIAGNOSIS

Diagnosis of impotence includes determining the cause. An individual's MEDICAL HISTORY is a vital clue. A BLOOD TEST to determine circulating hormone levels and a general PHYSICAL EXAMINATION can also be useful.

TREATMENT

SELF TREATMENT:

See Prevention below.

MEDICAL TREATMENT:

- Medication that is suspected of causing the problem can be withdrawn.
- Hormone medication, such as bromocriptine and testosterone, is used as treatment for men with hormone imbalances.
- In men for whom the difficulty cannot be resolved, self-injection of vasoactive agents into the penis can provide temporary erection.
- A special vacuum device placed over the penis can also help engorge the penis to allow a temporary erection.

SURGICAL TREATMENT:

For permanent cases of impotence, penile implantation is an option.

PREVENTION

- Avoidance of smoking
- Control of blood cholesterol levels through diet and exercise
- Avoidance of alcohol and depressant drugs which can interfere with proper functioning

INCONTINENCE

Incontinence is a condition that becomes more common with age. For various anatomic reasons, it is more often seen in women than it is in men.

Incontinence is the involuntary loss of urine from the bladder. The severity can range from minor leakage to near complete loss of all bladder control. The most common forms are either *urgency incontinence*, in which urine is lost because of a sudden urge to urinate, and *stress incontinence*, in which any sudden strain such as a cough or sneeze causes a loss of some urine.

CAUSES

Stress incontinence can be caused by the weakening of the muscles of the pelvic floor. These muscles, which are responsible for closing off the opening to the bladder and holding the urine in, can become weaker and looser with age, especially in women after childbirth. Menopause also contributes to the condition because of the effects of decreased hormonal levels on the mucous membranes lining the urethra.

Sometimes another disorder is the cause of stress incontinence; cystocele and urethrocele are common culprits.

Urge incontinence can be caused by intrinsic bladder problems such as BLADDER INFECTION.

Damage to the nervous system, such as that caused by STROKE, can also lead to incontinence.

DIAGNOSIS

To determine the type and cause of incontinence, a PHYSICAL EXAMINATION and a complete MEDICAL HISTORY are useful. A catheter is sometimes used to determine the adequacy of bladder emptying. A CULTURE to detect the presence of any infection may also be performed.

COMPLICATIONS

Leaked urine can cause skin irritation, but this is not a very serious problem. The biggest problem caused by incontinence is the social stigma that accompanies it. Incontinence or fear of it can lead to a gradual withdrawal from social situations and activities.

TREATMENT

SELF TREATMENT:

- Moderation of excessive fluid intake can decrease episodes.
- Completely emptying the bladder as much as possible with each urination can help.
- Kegel exercises (repeated contraction of the muscles of the pelvic floor) can strengthen the muscles and lead to better bladder control.

MEDICAL TREATMENT:

- Anticholinergic drugs such as oxybutynin and hyoscyamine can help with incontinence by acting on certain nerve pathways and decreasing the frequency of urination.
- Biofeedback, using electrical equipment, can help increase awareness and control of muscles involved in control of the bladder.

SURGICAL TREATMENT:

Bladder suspension is a surgical technique that can repair the muscles of the pelvic floor and prevent leakage from stress incontinence.

PREVENTION

Hormone replacement therapy may prevent incontinence in some postmenopausal women whose incontinence relates to changes in the urethra's lining.

INFLUENZA

Influenza (commonly known as the flu) viruses have been an important cause of respiratory tract infections for centuries. The virus can cause worldwide outbreaks (pandemics), local outbreaks (epidemics), or sporadic cases (endemic). The different strains of the virus have the unique ability to change their outer coat, resulting in more severe infections in individuals not previously exposed. Global pandemics generally occur every 20 to 30 years.

CAUSES

The cause of influenza is a virus that frequently changes its genetic material. Although there are three viruses—A, B, and C—types A and B account for the vast majority of all cases.

SYMPTOMS

Influenza is characterized by
- FEVER (often very high)
- COUGH
- HEADACHE
- Muscle aches
- Weakness and FATIGUE

A characteristic finding that helps distinguish influenza from the common cold is that patients with influenza often have severe FATIGUE requiring bed rest. The FEVER and FATIGUE usually last three to four days, but the COUGH, weakness, and muscle aches may persist for weeks. Influenza may be indistinguishable from other viral infections in young children.

DIAGNOSIS

The diagnosis of influenza is generally made on the basis of the clinical symptoms. However, there are tests that can confirm the diagnosis.
- A CULTURE of oral secretions can identify the virus, but this takes several days.
- Recently, a rapid diagnostic test was developed that can give doctors the diagnosis in 24 hours.
- There are also BLOOD TESTS available, but they require confirmation two to four weeks later and are rarely helpful clinically.

> Influenza is a seasonal illness that occurs during the winter months. It is uncommon before November 15th or after March 15th.

COMPLICATIONS

Influenza is usually a self-limited disease, but complications can occur. Although influenza rarely causes PNEUMONIA, when it does, the mortality is high. The virus can also damage the heart muscle (MYOCARDITIS) and cause disease in the nervous system. Influenza B is an important cause of Reye syndrome, which can be fatal in children.

TREATMENT

SELF TREATMENT:

Individuals with influenza infection should adhere to the following basic care guidelines:

- Drink plenty of fluids
- Get plenty of rest
- Take acetaminophen to reduce FEVER and aches

Fluid intake is especially important to prevent DEHYDRATION. Aspirin should be avoided, particularly in children; aspirin use during viral infection is associated with Reye syndrome, an often fatal condition.

MEDICAL TREATMENT:

There are two antiviral medications that are effective against influenza. Amantadine is effective for both the treatment and prevention of influenza, but is associated with nervous system side effects, especially in the elderly. Rimantadine, a recently approved medication, is less toxic but more costly. Both of these medications must be administered within 48 hours of symptoms for maximum efficacy.

SURGICAL TREATMENT:

None.

PREVENTION

The most effective method of preventing influenza is vaccination. A new influenza vaccine is developed every fall to immunize people against the most commonly encountered strains in the community. Patients who are allergic to eggs should not receive the vaccine. For patients who do not get vaccinated, amantadine and rimantadine can be given to prevent infection. Treatment with either medicine is about 70 percent effective in preventing the illness.

INTESTINAL OBSTRUCTION

Intestinal obstruction occurs when the normal movement of intestinal contents through the digestive tract is interrupted. Intestinal obstruction usually refers to a lesion that mechanically blocks the intestine, but movement of intestinal contents can also be impeded when the normal contractions (motility) of the bowel are impaired.

CAUSES

Intestinal obstruction can be caused by
- Scars from previous operations (most commonly)
- Tumor (see COLORECTAL CANCER)
- Incarcerated HERNIA
- Twisting of the bowel (called *volvulus*)
- Telescoping of the bowel into itself
- Intra-abdominal abscesses pressing on the bowel
- Inflammatory diseases of the intestines

Bowel obstruction can sometimes result from impacted fecal material, parasites, foods that cannot be completely digested, and occasionally, large GALLSTONES.

SYMPTOMS

The symptoms of intestinal obstruction depend on the level of the obstruction. Obstruction high in the gastrointestinal tract causes nausea and VOMITING early. The food is undigested or only partially digested. Lower obstruction is manifest by crampy ABDOMINAL PAIN and ABDOMINAL SWELLING. Nausea and VOMITING are later symptoms.

Although patients with complete intestinal obstruction may have bowel movements early, as the contents of the bowel beyond the obstruction are eliminated, they are usually unable to pass stool and flatus. Patients with partially obstructed intestines will continue to pass small amounts.

DIAGNOSIS

The diagnosis of obstruction is based largely on the history of the illness and the PHYSICAL EXAMINATION. It is confirmed by abdominal X rays (RADIOGRAPHY), which show distended intestinal loops filled with fluid and gas.

Laboratory tests, including complete BLOOD COUNT and other BLOOD TESTS, are performed to assess kidney function and the amount of fluid lost into the obstructed bowel.

> Intestinal obstruction may occur anywhere in the gastrointestinal tract, from the esophagus to the anus.

COMPLICATIONS

The most serious complication from a bowel obstruction occurs when obstruction compromises blood supply to the involved intestine resulting in bowel death (gangrene) and perforation. Patients can develop infection of the abdominal cavity (peritonitis). This is a potentially life-threatening complication.

Patients can also suffer from severe DEHYDRATION and may develop KIDNEY FAILURE.

TREATMENT

SELF TREATMENT:

None.

MEDICAL TREATMENT:

Fluid and electrolyte imbalances must be corrected with intravenous fluids before the obstruction can be addressed.

The obstruction may resolve spontaneously if it

- Occurs shortly after another operation
- Is the result of an inflammatory disease of the bowel such as CROHN DISEASE or DIVERTICULAR DISEASE
- Is a partial, rather than a complete, obstruction

In other cases, the patient may be treated initially with a nasogastric tube placed on suction.

SURGICAL TREATMENT:

If the cause of obstruction is an incarcerated HERNIA, prompt HERNIA REPAIR may be required. If the bowel is found to have a compromised blood supply during HERNIA REPAIR, the bowel must be removed.

Patients with other causes of intestinal obstruction may require exploratory surgery to find the problem. The obstruction may be relieved by cutting or destroying adhesions, or by removing or bypassing a severely scarred portion of intestine or intestine involved with tumor. Bowel with compromised blood supply also must be removed.

PREVENTION

None.

IRRITABLE BOWEL SYNDROME

Irritable bowel syndrome is a very common affliction. It is often a frequently recurring condition. For reasons that are not clear, it affects women much more often than men.

In general, irritable bowel syndrome (IBS) is an increased sensitivity of the large intestine—and possibly the small intestine as well—to certain stimuli such as food, stress, and hormones. In IBS, nerve impulses to the intestine generate higher and more prolonged pressure within the bowel wall, resulting in changes of bowel habits, ABDOMINAL PAIN, and bloating.

IBS has many synonyms, including *spastic colon* and *mucous colitis*. *Colitis* is not a good term, though, because it is actually a different condition, one that involves inflammation. There is no visible or microscopic inflammation or damage associated with IBS.

CAUSES

The cause of IBS is unclear. Some studies indicate that the pressure generated within the colon in patients with IBS is higher than in other healthy individuals. The colon relaxes more slowly in IBS, and patients also seem to have a lower pain threshold within the intestine—even small increases in the amount of gas or stool can cause substantial discomfort.

SYMPTOMS

- Sense of incomplete evacuation of bowel movements
- ABDOMINAL SWELLING and gas
- ABDOMINAL PAIN
- Sense of CONSTIPATION, at times even alternating with DIARRHEA
- Rectal discharge of mucus

These symptoms are frequently improved, at least temporarily, after a bowel movement.

DIAGNOSIS

There is no specific test that will diagnose this condition; it remains largely a diagnosis of exclusion. It can be diagnosed if the typical symptoms are present and the results of a PHYSICAL EXAMINATION are normal. Other tests, if done, are usually used to exclude other conditions.

COMPLICATIONS

Although the symptoms can be quite distressing to the patient, this condition does not progress into a situation in which significant complications develop. RECTAL BLEEDING, WEIGHT LOSS, persistent DIARRHEA, or other unremitting symptoms, however, should guide the patient to seek medical advice.

TREATMENT

SELF TREATMENT:
- Exercising regularly
- Eating a diet rich in fiber (whole-grain breads, bran, vegetables)
- Avoiding fats and fried food
- Avoiding laxatives
- Limiting dairy products (IBS is often associated with lactose intolerance)

MEDICAL TREATMENT:
- Fiber supplements, such as methylcellulose or psyllium
- Antispasmodic or antimotility agents such as dicyclomine or hyoscyamine.
- Rarely, antidepressants such as amitriptyline

SURGICAL TREATMENT:
None.

PREVENTION

There is no specific prevention strategy, although a high-fiber, low-fat diet may reduce the severity of symptoms. For those with lactose intolerance, avoiding dairy products is also helpful.

KIDNEY FAILURE

The kidneys are the body's waste-treatment facility, filtering excess water and metabolic wastes from the blood to make urine. Kidney failure can have devastating effects.

Kidney failure describes the loss of the kidney's ability to eliminate excess water and bodily wastes from the bloodstream. This can happen over a period of hours (as in BLOOD POISONING or the very low blood pressure of shock), over a period of days (as in the toxic effects of medication such as gentamicin, anticancer drugs, and amphotericin B), or over a period of years (as in DIABETES, uncontrolled HYPERTENSION, excessive use of pain killers, or ATHEROSCLEROSIS).

CAUSES

High blood pressure (HYPERTENSION) and DIABETES are the most common causes of kidney failure. Other less common factors that can damage the kidneys and lead to kidney failure include

- Prolonged low blood pressure (shock)
- Persistent urinary obstruction from KIDNEY STONES, BLADDER STONES, or enlarged prostate (PROSTATE, ENLARGED)
- Infection
- Hereditary diseases
- Massive muscle damage or certain forms of LEUKEMIA, which can release protein in the blood that "plugs up" the kidneys
- CONGESTIVE HEART FAILURE, in which the heart cannot pump enough blood through the kidneys to make them effective
- Autoimmune diseases, such as systemic LUPUS ERYTHEMATOSUS

Some commonly used drugs can precipitate kidney failure, especially in the elderly. Nonsteroidal anti-inflammatory drugs such as ibuprofen and indomethacin are the main culprits, but they rarely lead to severe kidney failure.

SYMPTOMS

Early in kidney failure there are usually no symptoms at all. In advanced cases, though, the usual symptoms include

- Weakness
- Lethargy and FATIGUE
- Swollen or puffy extremities (ANKLE SWELLING)
- Nausea

In some cases, decreased urinary output and blood in the urine may be noted.

DIAGNOSIS

A PHYSICAL EXAMINATION may show edema (swelling) and enlarged kidneys in some cases, but the diagnosis of kidney failure primarily depends on

- BLOOD TESTS for creatinine and blood urea nitrogen
- URINALYSIS to detect inflammation of the kidneys or any metabolic abnormalities
- ULTRASOUND of the kidneys to reveal their size and the presence of any obstruction

COMPLICATIONS

- HYPERTENSION can result from kidney failure.
- CONGESTIVE HEART FAILURE can be precipitated by the kidney's inability to eliminate excess fluid and salt.
- Potassium buildup, acid buildup, and pericarditis are potentially life-threatening complications.
- Calcium imbalances can lead to OSTEOPOROSIS.

TREATMENT

SELF TREATMENT:
A carefully selected and prescribed diet can be helpful in slowing the progression of kidney failure. Usually, the diet is a low-sodium, low-potassium, low-protein diet.

MEDICAL TREATMENT:
Treatment is aimed at the underlying condition, such as HYPERTENSION. Tight control of DIABETES is also important. Early in kidney failure, ACE inhibitors such as captopril and enalapril may slow the progression of failure in some cases.

SURGICAL TREATMENT:
- Dialysis
- KIDNEY TRANSPLANT

PREVENTION

- Control of HYPERTENSION
- Tight control of DIABETES
- Early relief of urinary obstructions such as BLADDER STONES and KIDNEY STONES

KIDNEY STONES

For reasons that are not entirely understood, middle-aged men and people with recurrent urinary tract infections are more susceptible to the development of kidney stones.

Kidney stones are deposits of mineral or organic substances from urine that form in the kidneys. The stones can be very tiny or as large as a walnut.

CAUSES

Stones can form because of metabolic abnormalities that change the chemistry of the urine. This abnormality can simply be a constant predisposition, or it can be a definitive metabolic problem. Examples of predisposing problems include CROHN DISEASE and an overactive parathyroid gland.

Bacterial infections of the urine can also contribute to stone formation.

SYMPTOMS

The symptoms of kidney stones are usually unmistakable. The stones cause severe, colicky, flank pain. Occasionally, they can also cause blood in the urine, which can turn urine bright red or the color of tea, depending on the amount of blood (see URINE, ABNORMAL APPEARANCE).

DIAGNOSIS

Apart from consideration of the typical symptoms, diagnosis can involve
- BLOOD TESTS to check kidney function
- URINALYSIS
- CULTURE
- Intravenous pyelogram (RADIOGRAPHY)
- ULTRASOUND

COMPLICATIONS

Without proper treatment or with delayed treatment, a stone can cause an obstruction in the kidney or the urinary tract. An obstruction can lead to loss of kidney function (KIDNEY FAILURE). Another danger is a complicating infection, manifested by worsening pain and a FEVER.

TREATMENT

SELF TREATMENT:

See Prevention below.

MEDICAL TREATMENT:

- Some kidney stones will dissolve with medication, but most will not.
- Sometimes antispasmodic medications can encourage passage of the stone.

SURGICAL TREATMENT:

Extracorporeal shock-wave lithotripsy (ULTRASONIC LITHOTRIPSY) is a technique in which the patient is placed in a bath and tiny shock waves are pulsed through the water and the body to break up the stones. Once the stones are pulverized, they can pass through the urinary tract.

Another surgical option is kidney stone removal, which can be performed open (traditional surgery) or with a special flexible scope threaded up the ureter or inserted directly in the side (see ENDOSCOPY).

PREVENTION

- Adequate fluid intake (at least eight eight-ounce glasses of fluid per day) may help discourage stone formation.
- Dietary changes to decrease intake of calcium, uric acid, and oxalates (depending on the type of stone) may help prevent recurrences.
- Diuretic medication (such as hydrochlorothiazide), medication to lower uric acid levels (such as allopurinol), or other drugs that affect salts and change the acid balance of the urine may help prevent recurrence in some patients.

LARYNGEAL CANCER

Laryngeal cancer is a tumor of the larynx, or voice box. The disease most commonly affects middle-aged or older men who have a history of smoking and excessive alcohol consumption.

CAUSES

Laryngeal cancer is most consistently associated with smoking and heavy alcohol intake. Other possible factors include
- Chronic laryngitis
- Chronic gastric reflux (heartburn)
- Exposure to nitrogen mustard, asbestos, and ionizing radiation

SYMPTOMS

Hoarseness of the voice is the most common symptom. Heavy smokers are often hoarse anyway, which can lead to a masking of the telltale initial symptom and delay diagnosis and treatment. Any change in voice that does not resolve in a few weeks warrants a laryngeal examination.

WEIGHT LOSS without reduced caloric intake may also be one of the initial symptoms.

Cancers of the supraglottic larynx (the area above the vocal cords) do not produce early symptoms and signs, and it is not uncommon to see enlargement of the lymph nodes—a sign that the cancer may have spread to the lymph system—as the first sign. Early subtle symptoms include alteration of one's tolerance for hot and cold foods and scratchy sensations when swallowing.

DIAGNOSIS

The typical symptoms (hoarseness or change in voice associated with WEIGHT LOSS) in a person with a significant history of alcohol intake and smoking raises the index of suspicion for laryngeal cancer. Flexible laryngeal ENDOSCOPY can be done to inspect the area, while direct laryngoscopy (another form of ENDOSCOPY) is reserved for BIOPSY. COMPUTED TOMOGRAPHY is performed to evaluate the extent and stage of the disease.

> The peak incidence of this disease occurs in men in their 60s, although the disease is certainly not limited to this age group.

COMPLICATIONS

Upper airway obstruction can develop due to soft-tissue swelling around the tumor. Patients can develop shortness of breath and the sensation of inability to breathe (BREATHING DIFFICULTY). Speech and SWALLOWING DIFFICULTIES are often related to the cancer, but sometimes to the side effects of treatment as well.

TREATMENT

SELF TREATMENT:
Tobacco smoking and alcohol use should be discontinued immediately.

MEDICAL TREATMENT:
Early stage disease is highly curable by radiation therapy or surgery. Advanced stage disease is usually treated with a combination of chemotherapy, radiation, and surgery.

SURGICAL TREATMENT:
Supraglottic laryngectomy, hemilaryngectomy, and total laryngectomy are considered—surgeries to remove various parts of the larynx—based on the stage of cancer. The ability to speak can sometimes be preserved in early cases.

PREVENTION

Abstinence from alcohol and smoking is important. Ongoing clinical trials will determine if retinoic acid (a vitamin A-like compound) has a role in the prevention of second primary cancers.

LEUKEMIA

Leukemia is a cancer of the bone marrow causing an abnormal proliferation of white blood cells. Leukemia can be divided into acute and chronic forms. In acute leukemia, immature white blood cells proliferate. In chronic leukemia, mature white blood cells proliferate.

CAUSES

The cause of leukemia is unknown. Risk factors for developing leukemia include
- Radiation exposure
- Chemotherapy, especially for HODGKIN DISEASE, lymphoma (LYMPHOMA, NON-HODGKIN), multiple myeloma, or OVARIAN CANCER
- Chemical exposure such as exposure to the solvent benzene

SYMPTOMS

The symptoms of leukemia are very diverse. They can include
- FATIGUE
- Pallor (see ANEMIA)
- Easy bruising (BRUISING, UNEXPLAINED) or easy bleeding
- Shortness of breath (BREATHING DIFFICULTY)
- FEVERS
- Recurrent infections
- WEIGHT LOSS
- Loss of appetite (APPETITE, LOSS OF) or feeling full soon after eating

DIAGNOSIS

Diagnosis of leukemia is suspected by an abnormal complete BLOOD COUNT. To confirm the diagnosis, a bone marrow BIOPSY must be performed. Chromosomes are also analyzed at that time.

PHYSICAL EXAMINATION may show fast heart rate, pallor, bruises (BRUISING, UNEXPLAINED), RASH, and enlarged spleen, liver, or lymph nodes. There may also be evidence of infection.

High-dose chemotherapy with bone marrow transplantation can cure some types of leukemia, but the acute forms of leukemia are difficult to treat and are often fatal.

COMPLICATIONS

Complications include
* Bleeding—most patients diagnosed with leukemia are at risk of bleeding or bruising (BRUISING, UNEXPLAINED) due to low platelet counts.
* Infection—although there are numerous white blood cells available, they do not function normally. Patients are susceptible to bacterial, viral, and fungal infections.
* The transformation of chronic forms of leukemia into acute forms of leukemia or lymphoma (LYMPHOMA, NON-HODGKIN)—these are difficult to treat and are usually fatal.

TREATMENT

SELF TREATMENT:
None.

MEDICAL TREATMENT:
* Chemotherapy is given to treat leukemia. (The type of medication and duration of treatment depends on the form of leukemia.)
* Transfusions of platelets and red blood cells are given as needed.
* Prevention of infection with vaccines and antibiotics is crucial.
* High-dose chemotherapy with bone marrow transplantation is given for many types of leukemia with a goal of curing the disease.

SURGICAL TREATMENT:
With some types of leukemia, splenectomy (SPLEEN REMOVAL) may be helpful, but in general, there is no surgical intervention available for leukemia.

PREVENTION

Avoidance of unnecessary exposure to radiation and chemicals that can cause the disease is the only preventive strategy.

LIVER CANCER

Although relatively rare in the United States, liver cancer is one of the most common fatal malignancies in the world, causing more than one million deaths a year. It is most common in Africa and Asia.

The prognosis for this cancer is usually quite poor, with progression to death usually in 6 to 12 months.

CAUSES

Risk factors for the disease include long-standing HEPATITIS B infection, cirrohosis of the liver, and alcoholism.

SYMPTOMS

Liver cancer can cause ABDOMINAL PAIN, ABDOMINAL SWELLING, jaundice, FATIGUE, internal bleeding (possibly RECTAL BLEEDING), and generalized ITCHING.

DIAGNOSIS

COMPUTED TOMOGRAPHY and ULTRASOUND of the abdomen can detect even small liver cancers. A BLOOD TEST for a substance called *alpha-fetoprotein* may be helpful. Ultimately the diagnosis is made by BIOPSY of the liver.

COMPLICATIONS

Complications are most commonly seen in relation to chronic liver disease or cirrhosis of the liver.

TREATMENT

SELF TREATMENT:
A well-balanced diet should be maintained.

MEDICAL TREATMENT:
Chemotherapy does not appear to offer any advantage in the treatment of this cancer.

SURGICAL TREATMENT:
Resection of this tumor offers the only reliable cure for this cancer. Liver transplantation is curative in few patients.

PREVENTION

Abstinence from alcohol consumption and the screening and prevention of chronic HEPATITIS B infections can go a long way in the prevention of this cancer.

LUNG CANCER

Lung cancer is an overgrowth of cells originating in the lung. This cell growth proceeds outside the body's normal control mechanisms. It commonly spreads to the lymph nodes, bone, liver, brain, and adrenal glands.

CAUSES

Tobacco smoking is the most common cause of lung cancer, but it is not the only cause. An increased risk of lung cancer is also seen after occupational exposure to

- Asbestos
- Chromium
- Nickel
- Radon
- Hydrocarbons
- Arsenic
- Ether

There may also be a genetic predisposition to developing lung cancer, but this has not been shown definitively.

SYMPTOMS

Symptoms of lung cancer include
- BREATHING DIFFICULTY
- CHEST PAIN or pressure
- FATIGUE
- WEIGHT LOSS
- Loss of appetite (APPETITE, LOSS OF)
- Bloody sputum

DIAGNOSIS

Diagnostic tests include
- Chest X ray (RADIOGRAPHY)
- COMPUTED TOMOGRAPHY of the chest to locate the tumor precisely and to check for the spread of the disease to the lymph nodes, liver, and adrenal glands
- BIOPSY of the tumor to determine the exact type of cancer is done with either bronchoscopy (a form of ENDOSCOPY) or COMPUTED TOMOGRAPHY (guided fine needle aspiration). A surgical procedure is rarely needed for BIOPSY.
- Sputum testing, for evidence of cancer (CYTOLOGY)

Lung cancer is the most common form of cancer, and 80 to 90 percent of newly diagnosed cases are caused by tobacco smoking.

- BLOOD TESTS to evaluate liver function, calcium level, and electrolytes
- Bone scan (NUCLEAR MEDICINE) and COMPUTED TOMOGRAPHY of the head and neck to determine the extent of the disease

COMPLICATIONS

Possible complications of lung cancer include
- PNEUMONIA
- High blood calcium levels
- Hoarseness
- SWALLOWING DIFFICULTIES
- Arm pain
- Facial swelling
- Fluid collection around the lung

Other complications related to tumor spread to other organs can occur.

TREATMENT

SELF TREATMENT:

Many people feel an improvement in their BREATHING DIFFICULTY and COUGH after they stop smoking, although it may have no effect on the tumor itself.

MEDICAL TREATMENT:

Some types of lung cancer are responsive to chemotherapy given in either oral or intravenous form. Most types of lung cancer, though, have either minimal or no response to chemotherapy. These tumors often benefit from radiation therapy.

SURGICAL TREATMENT:

Small tumors that have not spread are best treated by surgical removal (LUNG RESECTION). The size and location of the tumor determine the surgical procedure and amount of lung tissue removed.

PREVENTION

Tobacco smoking and occupational exposures should be avoided.

LUPUS ERYTHEMATOSUS

Lupus erythematosus is an inflammatory disease of the small blood vessels in various organs of the body, especially the joints, the kidneys, the lungs, the brain, and the skin.

Depending upon the site of the inflammation, the process can be damaging or of only temporary concern. The joint disease in lupus, for instance, is usually nondestructive; whereas the kidney disease, brain disease, and lung disease in lupus can cause life-threatening organ destruction.

CAUSES

No cause is known. As in RHEUMATOID ARTHRITIS, there may be extrinsic, or environmental, factors, but none has been recognized. Some forms of lupus occur in response to medication; drugs such as procainamide (used for cardiac ARRHYTHMIAS), or phenytoin (used in the treatment of epilepsy) can precipitate lupus. Once these drugs are discontinued, however, the lupus process tends to correct itself.

Intrinsic factors involved in lupus are less well defined than they are in RHEUMATOID ARTHRITIS, but genetic features may be important. No specific genetic abnormality has thus far been determined, however.

SYMPTOMS

Symptoms depend upon the organs that are involved. In the skin, the usual symptoms include a RASH that causes a reddened, slightly thickened skin. The reaction is usually nondestructive and involves the areas on the nose and the cheekbones. Some patients experience a destructive skin RASH, which is called *discoid lupus*. This RASH occurs on the face and sun-exposed areas of the body, the scalp (where hair loss can take place), and in the ear canals.

Joint inflammatons resemble the symptoms of RHEUMATOID ARTHRITIS. Multiple joints can be inflamed, but unlike RHEUMATOID ARTHRITIS, long-term damage is not likely.

Brain involvement is revealed by seizures, mental confusion, MEMORY PROBLEMS, and in rare cases, coma. Restriction of lung expansion leads to BREATHING DIFFICULTY.

Lupus erythematosus affects women ten times more often than it affects men, and it can afflict people of any age.

DIAGNOSIS

The diagnosis of lupus can be difficult at times because the disease takes many different forms; its manifestations vary widely. However, a diagnosis of lupus is usually made when all three of the following conditions are true:

- Inflammation of several of the signature organs (mentioned above)
- Positive results on certain laboratory tests (mentioned below)
- Absence of other causes of the inflammation

The laboratory tests that are involved are BLOOD TESTS for the antinuclear antibody (ANA) and its subsets. The presence of ANA is very characteristic of this disease, but it can also appear, with a weaker reaction, in several other conditions.

COMPLICATIONS

The list of complications is extraordinarily large in lupus because so many organ systems can be involved. (See Symptoms above.)

TREATMENT

SELF TREATMENT:

The patient's help in managing the disease is critical. Drug compliance is particularly important. The patient needs to take medications, even at times when it seems as though they have little effect.

The patient must be alert to the disease's progression in critical areas of the body. Regular visits for examination and tests are required to monitor the inflammatory process.

Many patients with lupus are extremely sensitive to the sun. Direct exposure to certain ultraviolet rays cannot only cause a sunburn, but can increase and accelerate the symptoms of the lupus process itself. Thus, all patients with lupus should avoid direct exposure to the sun, wear long sleeves and a hat when going out in the daytime, and apply sunscreen with a sun protection factor (SPF) of 15 or higher on sun-exposed areas of the body.

MEDICAL TREATMENT:

Routine tests to monitor the disease include

- BLOOD COUNTS (in part to check for ANEMIA)
- URINALYSIS to detect protein in the urine or red cells (a sign of kidney involvement)
- BLOOD TESTS to monitor whether liver or kidney damage is occurring either as a result of the disease or sometimes as a consequence of the treatment and to determine the activity level of the disease process

The need for medications to control inflammation are governed by two considerations. The first consideration is the activity of the disease. More activity requires larger doses and more potent drugs. The second consideration is knowledge of the particular organs that are under attack. If joints are involved with lupus, only mild treatment may be required, since damage is not likely to occur, even on a long-term basis. On the other hand, if the kidneys are involved, more aggressive therapy must be applied early.

Unfortunately, aggressive therapy can have significant side effects. For example, corticosteroid drugs, such as prednisone, in high doses can cause

- WEIGHT GAIN, especially around the face and trunk
- Thinning of the bones (OSTEOPOROSIS)
- DIABETES
- CATARACTS

Other drugs include hydroxychloroquine, which has a good safety record but requires eye checks one or more times a year, and cyclophosphamide, which is given intravenously each month in cases of severe kidney, brain, or lung disease.

SURGICAL TREATMENT:

Surgical treatment is not ordinarily considered in the treatment of lupus; however, a KIDNEY TRANSPLANT may be performed if kidney function has become obliterated by lupus, particularly if dialysis treatment is not well tolerated.

PREVENTION

None.

LYMPHOMA, NON-HODGKIN

Lymphomas are cancers that arise from the lymph system, a network of small nodes (especially in the neck, groin, and armpits) and vessels that help to fight infections. Lymphoma is divided into two major categories: HODGKIN DISEASE and non-Hodgkin lymphoma.

In lymphoma, lymph nodes become enlarged due to the presence of a tumor. Any area where there is lymphoid tissue, including the chest and abdomen, may be involved.

CAUSES

The cause of lymphomas is unknown, but some viral infections may be a contributing factor. Immunosuppressant drugs used after transplant surgery (see KIDNEY TRANSPLANT) to prevent organ rejection may also increase the risk of lymphoma.

SYMPTOMS

Symptoms of lymphoma include
- Persistent swelling of a lymph node or nodes
- FEVER
- Night sweats (SWEATING, EXCESSIVE)
- Unintended WEIGHT LOSS

DIAGNOSIS

The diagnosis can be suspected from the symptoms, but is made definitively only by surgical BIOPSY of an involved lymph node. The examination of the sample of lymphatic tissue permits a determination of the type and stage of lymphoma present (non-Hodgkin lymphomas are categorized as low grade, intermediate grade, or high grade).

Once the diagnosis is made, other tests such as COMPUTED TOMOGRAPHY of various areas are used to evaluate the extent of the disease.

BLOOD COUNT and chest X rays (RADIOGRAPHY) may also be useful.

COMPLICATIONS

Without treatment, the immune system becomes progressively more and more impaired, resulting in serious infections that can be life threatening.

TREATMENT

SELF TREATMENT:
None.

MEDICAL TREATMENT:
Treatment depends on both the grade (low grade versus intermediate or high grade) and the degree to which the tumor has spread and involved other areas and other organs. Treatments presently used for the management of non-Hodgkin lymphomas are
- Chemotherapy
- Radiation therapy
- Bone marrow transplantation

SURGICAL TREATMENT:
None.

PREVENTION

Any lymph node greater than one centimeter in diameter (the size of a small marble) should be evaluated by a physician.

MIGRAINE HEADACHE

Migraine headaches are an extremely frequent benign headache syndrome; they are sometimes called *vascular headaches*. Migraines can cause intense pain and other symptoms. They are often presaged by a phenomenon known as an *aura*.

CAUSES

The cause of migraines is unknown; however, there seems to be some hereditary connection, as a family history of the condition is not uncommon.

There do appear to be triggers for certain individuals. Some patients develop a headache related to physical exertion—for example, while lifting weights or during sexual climax. Certain drugs and substances in food and drink may also play a role for some individuals.

SYMPTOMS

Not all migraines are preceded by preliminary symptoms, or auras, but if they are, the symptoms associated with an impending migraine usually involve some kind of VISION DISTURBANCE such as

- Bright or dark spots (sometimes resembling champagne bubbles)
- Tunnel vision
- Zigzag lines (called *fortification spectra*)

The aura is followed by an intense crescendo of a HEADACHE, frequently behind one eye or on one side of the head. The pain may be pounding, throbbing, viselike, or stabbing; frequently it feels like the head is going to explode from pressure. Other symptoms that can accompany the headache of a migraine, include

- Sensitivity to light
- Nausea
- VOMITING

DIAGNOSIS

The diagnosis of migraine can usually be made from the symptoms and a PHYSICAL EXAMINATION that reveals no neurologic problems.

Migraines are more common in women, although there is a counterpart in men: the cluster headache.

Many individuals experience the head pain predominantly on one side, but if they have not had at least one instance involving the opposite side, there may be cause for concern. In cases of unilateral headache or those related to exertion, MAGNETIC RESONANCE IMAGING and ELECTROENCEPHALOGRAPHY may be indicated to rule out other possibilities.

COMPLICATIONS

There should be no lasting complications from a migraine, although some research indicates that patients who are prone to experience migraines may have an increased risk of STROKE.

TREATMENT

SELF TREATMENT:
Rest in a quiet, darkened room and an adequate fluid intake can help one weather a migraine. (See also Prevention below.)

MEDICAL TREATMENT:
Medications used to treat various aspects of migraine episodes include
- Ergotamine
- Isometheptene
- Butalbital
- Acetaminophen and codeine combination
- Butorphanol nasal spray
- Antinauseants such as prochlorperazine, chlorpromazine, or metoclopramide
- Certain nonsteroidal anti-inflammatory drugs such as ibuprofen
- Corticosteroids such as prednisone (limited use under strict supervision)
- Sumatriptan
(See also Prevention below.)

SURGICAL TREATMENT:
None.

PREVENTION

Prevention of migraines involves two approaches. The first is avoidance of potential triggers. Strategies include

- Regularizing intake of caffeine so as not to induce symptoms of caffeine withdrawal
- Avoiding food containing tyramine such as chocolate, ripe cheese, yogurt, nuts, sour cream, and onions
- Avoiding foods high in nitrates such as processed meats
- Avoiding certain food additives such as monosodium glutamate and aspartame
- Limiting or eliminating alcoholic beverages, especially red wine, champagne, and beer
- Avoiding overuse of pain-killing medication

The second preventive approach involves the use of medication to head off migraines. Medications used for prevention include

- Propranolol
- Antidepressant drugs such as amitriptyline or imipramine
- Verapamil
- Anticonvulsants such as carbamazepine, phenytoin, and divalproex
- Methysergide
- Cyproheptadine
- Lithium

MULTIPLE SCLEROSIS

Multiple sclerosis is an inflammatory disease of the central nervous system. It usually starts in young adulthood, and its course is chronic but highly variable. It attacks different portions of the nervous system to a varying and unpredictable extent in episodes that remit and recur over many years.

CAUSES

The cause of multiple sclerosis is not known, but viruses have been implicated.

SYMPTOMS

The initial manifestations of the disease may be very minor and not enough to be brought to medical attention. Symptoms include

- Weakness
- VISION DISTURBANCES such as decreased or double vision
- Incoordination
- Tingling
- NUMBNESS

The symptoms may spontaneously subside, but after a variable interval (up to ten years), there may be a recurrence of the same or new symptoms. As the disease progresses, the deficits become more significant and irreversible. Some more severe symptoms include

- FATIGUE, especially in the summer months
- INCONTINENCE
- Spasticity, especially of the legs
- Trigeminal neuralgia—bouts of facial pain

DIAGNOSIS

Diagnosis of the disease is generally suspected from the characteristic course and symptoms, the patient's MEDICAL HISTORY, and a PHYSICAL EXAMINATION that focuses on neurologic function.

The most important test used for diagnosis today is MAGNETIC RESONANCE IMAGING of the brain and brain stem, which can reveal the characteristic inflammatory lesions.

Multiple sclerosis is most prevalent in temperate climates. It is almost twice as common in women as it is in men, and twice as common in whites as in blacks.

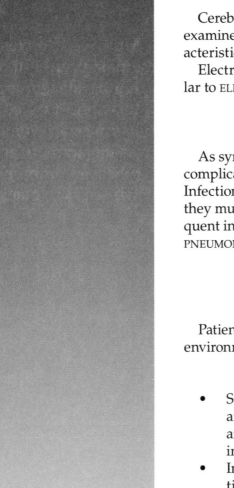

Cerebrospinal fluid obtained by a LUMBAR PUNCTURE can be examined for proteins and immunoglobulin G, which is characteristic of multiple sclerosis.

Electrophysiologic tests of the central nervous system similar to ELECTROENCEPHALOGRAPHY may also be useful.

COMPLICATIONS

As symptoms continue to cause irreversible damage, many complications can arise in a wide variety of body systems. Infections of any sort can cause exacerbations of the disease; they must be detected and treated promptly. The most frequent infections are kidney infection, BLADDER INFECTION, and PNEUMONIA.

TREATMENT

SELF TREATMENT:
Patients find it helpful to minimize their exposure to hot environments.

MEDICAL TREATMENT:
- Steroids such as prednisone and methylprednisolone are the mainstays of treatment. They function as anti-inflammatory agents and also suppress the immune system.
- Interferon-beta, a substance with antiviral properties that is produced by the body, is sometimes administered to decrease the frequency of relapses.
- Experimental treatments with plasmapheresis, immunomodulators, cytotoxics, copolymer-1, and other drugs are being studied, but none has proved to be beneficial.

SURGICAL TREATMENT:
None.

PREVENTION

None.

MYOCARDITIS

Myocarditis is the inflammation of the muscular walls of the heart (the thick middle layer of the heart wall is called the *myocardium*). Although the condition may subside when the underlying cause is treated, myocarditis—as with all conditions that affect the heart—can be dangerous, leading to CONGESTIVE HEART FAILURE.

CAUSES

Many times the cause of a specific case is uncertain, but the most commonly identified causes include
- Viral infection
- Lyme disease
- Rheumatic fever
- Parasitic infections
- Excessive alcohol intake (alcoholism)
- Ingestion of a toxic substance such as cobalt

SYMPTOMS

Often the condition will produce no symptoms, but the inflammation can impair the heart muscle enough to cause FATIGUE, BREATHING DIFFICULTY, and swelling of the extremities (see ANKLE SWELLING). Heart rhythm abnormalities (ARRHYTHMIAS) caused by myocarditis can also lead to palpitations, FAINTING OR FAINTNESS, or even cardiac arrest.

DIAGNOSIS

Careful PHYSICAL EXAMINATION of the heart, lungs, neck veins, and legs can help support a diagnosis of CONGESTIVE HEART FAILURE. ELECTROCARDIOGRAPHY may provide clues that suggest myocarditis. Special BLOOD TESTS looking for signs of viral infections may also be performed. An echocardiogram (ULTRASOUND) can document the degree of muscle impairment. Occasionally, a BIOPSY can be performed via a special catheter passed through the veins; the small amount of tissue obtained can document the inflammation and sometimes suggest the cause.

Myocarditis is often associated with some underlying disease, such as an infection. The degree of inflammation varies greatly and may cause few or no symptoms or progress to significant disability.

COMPLICATIONS

Myocarditis can lead to serious complications including
- CONGESTIVE HEART FAILURE leading to severe BREATH-ING DIFFICULTY
- ARRHYTHMIAS leading to FAINTING OR FAINTNESS
- Sudden cardiac death

TREATMENT

SELF TREATMENT:
Decreased physical activity may be important, particularly early in the course of myocarditis. A low-salt diet and avoidance of alcohol are also strongly recommended.

MEDICAL TREATMENT:
The general treatment of CONGESTIVE HEART FAILURE includes diuretics (such as furosemide), digoxin, and ACE inhibitors (enalapril and captopril).

Antibiotics for particular infections such as Lyme disease or parasitic infections may be used in some cases.

Drugs used to suppress the immune system such as prednisone may be warranted in selected patients.

SURGICAL TREATMENT:
In very severe cases, for appropriate patients, heart transplantation may be required.

PREVENTION

The risk of myocarditis can be reduced by
- Limiting alcohol consumption to moderate levels
- Seeking appropriate treatment for strep throat infections to avoid damage to the heart muscle
- Receiving a full series of childhood vaccinations

ORAL CANCER

Oral cavity cancer includes cancer of the various anatomic structures of the mouth such as the

- Lip
- Tongue
- Floor of the mouth
- Palate

Cancers of the mouth most commonly affect men older than 45 who have some history of having either chewed or smoked tobacco.

CAUSES

Cigarette smoking is the major cause. A clear relationship has been identified between the extent of tobacco exposure and the risk of oral cancer.

Additional risk factors include

- Vitamin A deficiency
- Alcohol abuse (alcoholism)
- Chronic irritants, such as poor dental hygiene
- Syphilis

SYMPTOMS

Common symptoms are based on anatomic location of the tumor, including

- Lip—ulcerative lesion of the lower lip or NUMBNESS of the skin of the chin
- Tongue—difficulty in speech and swallowing (SWAL-LOWING DIFFICULTIES) and greater likelihood of spreading to the lymph nodes
- Insides of the cheeks (buccal mucosa)—pain, difficulty chewing, and bleeding
- Floor of the mouth—pain
- The bone beneath the teeth (alveolar ridge)—pain exacerbated by chewing, loose teeth, and bleeding

A sore anywhere in the mouth that does not heal in a few weeks should be evaluated by a physician or dentist.

At one time, cancer of the mouth was often a disfiguring, if not deadly, disease. Now, cosmetic surgery techniques have minimized disfigurement and made rehabilitation easier.

DIAGNOSIS

PHYSICAL EXAMINATION of the oral cavity typically reveals the tumor, which is either ulcerative or exophytic (growing on the surface of the structure from which it originated). Cervical lymph nodes can usually be felt. COMPUTED TOMOGRAPHY of the area, including the base of the skull, is necessary for staging purposes. A BIOPSY is necessary to confirm the diagnosis.

COMPLICATIONS

Bleeding from the ulcer is a common complication. Difficulties in speech and SWALLOWING DIFFICULTIES are also common complications.

TREATMENT

SELF TREATMENT:
Discontinue smoking and alcohol intake.

MEDICAL TREATMENT:
For advanced disease, a combination of chemotherapy, radiation, and surgery is standard therapy and may offer a cure for early-stage tumors.

SURGICAL TREATMENT:
For early cancers, surgical resection is the treatment of choice. Reconstructive surgery is based on the extent of the primary tumor.

PREVENTION

Avoidance of smoking and alcohol abuse can significantly reduce risk. Ongoing clinical trials are evaluating retinoic acid (a vitamin A–like compound) as a preventive agent for second tumors.

OSTEOARTHRITIS

Osteoarthritis is a chronic arthritis involving damage to the cartilage cushion that caps the bones at a joint. Later, secondary changes occur in the adjacent bone itself. This process begins insidiously, usually in middle age, and increases in extent as the person gets older.

CAUSES

Cartilage breakdown can be the consequence of decreased formation of cartilage, increased breakdown of cartilage, or of both. Ultimately, the two bones in the joint rub directly against each other. Bone formation increases at points where the two bones of the joint meet, forming spurs.

There are two possible causes of osteoarthritis:
- Excess strain caused by repetitive trauma or a muscle imbalance around the joint
- A (often genetic) defect in the way cartilage is formed, allowing increased breakdown of cartilage or decreased formation of new cartilage

SYMPTOMS

Major symptoms of osteoarthritis are
- Pain of the affected joint or joints, which is made worse by activity and improved by rest
- Inflammation (although this is less common in osteoarthritis than in RHEUMATOID ARTHRITIS)
- A bony enlargement, which appears as nodules at the last row of joints in the hand (Heberden nodes), at the middle row of joints of the fingers (Bouchard nodes), and at the joint at the base of the thumb
- Pain in the hip (often felt in the groin)
- Pain in the knee

Limitation of motion results when pain is severe.

DIAGNOSIS

No specific findings mark early osteoarthritis. When the disease is beginning, nondescript pain can appear. X rays (RADIOGRAPHY) at this point are normal. Occasionally, swelling in the hands begins before a Heberden node develops. Laboratory tests are not diagnostic of osteoarthritis either.

Later in the disease's progression, the loss of cartilage can be detected on X-ray films (RADIOGRAPHY).

Although injury may cause the degenerative process of osteoarthritis at an early age, most cases do not develop until after the age of 55.

COMPLICATIONS

Natural progression of the illness can limit the function of the involved joint.

TREATMENT

SELF TREATMENT:

Good body mechanics maintain normal bone and joint structure. Walking with a proper gait under good muscle control is beneficial. Obesity plays a role in causing abnormal posture in the patient, which in turn creates a greater strain on the joints. In this aspect, maintaining a healthy weight can be considered beneficial.

MEDICAL TREATMENT:

Pain relief is accomplished by medications including acetaminophen and various nonsteroidal anti-inflammatory drugs such as ibuprofen.

Supportive techniques are available for individual joints that are damaged by osteoarthritis, including splints, canes, and orthoses. Orthotics are particularly helpful in patients with foot osteoarthritis.

SURGICAL TREATMENT:

Although surgery is not necessary in the early phases of osteoarthritis, it is a dramatic and successful treatment for bone that is totally damaged and for which medical treatment is no longer effective. Joint replacement, in which an artificial metal or plastic material replaces the damaged bone, can be performed. KNEE ARTHROPLASTY and HIP ARTHROPLASTY can be very successful in this regard. Sometimes a joint or vertebrae can be fused. The amount of motion that is lost may be negligible, and pain is eliminated.

PREVENTION

No successful prevention strategy is now available, although maintenance of good posture, good gait, and strong muscle development without obesity over the course of one's life ought to be helpful in retarding the progress of osteoarthritis.

OSTEOPOROSIS

Osteoporosis is a condition in which bone substance is lost from the bone found at the ends of long bones, the pelvis, and the ribs, or from the shaft of long bones in the arm or leg. Bone loss weakens the bone structure and makes it vulnerable to easy injury. Bone fracture, even with little or no provocation, can result from a minor fall.

CAUSES

Bone is a complex, dynamic tissue with an even balance between formation and removal. During periods of growth in childhood and in early adulthood, such remodeling is necessary to increase the size of the skeleton to reach its full maturity. After this time, density of the skeleton slowly decreases.

This thinning process continues over the course of a person's life span. In women, however, the thinning process is accelerated after menopause. If the skeleton is too small to begin with or if bone has been lost at a faster rate than normal because of illness, drugs such as prednisone and thyroid hormone, or alcohol use, bone damage can ensue.

SYMPTOMS

No symptoms are noted until the bone has become so weak that a bone fracture occurs even after a trivial insult. The vertebrae in the spine can be slowly compressed in height, leading to rounding of the upper back.

DIAGNOSIS

The diagnosis is made accidentally in many cases when a routine X ray (RADIOGRAPHY) is taken for other purposes. Bone density measurements (bone mineral density testing) can accomplish this objective, and by repeating them, the rate of bone loss over time can be determined.

COMPLICATIONS

Complications include bone fractures, especially hip fractures, and postural changes in the body, particularly rounding of the upper spine area.

Osteoporosis is more common in women than men, and for reasons that are not entirely understood, white and Asian women are more likely to develop the disease than are black women.

TREATMENT

SELF TREATMENT:

(See Prevention below.)

MEDICAL TREATMENT:

For small-sized women who are postmenopausal and who have not had estrogen replacement therapy, constant intake of calcium is stressed. In addition, a source of vitamin D should be provided either in milk or in a daily multivitamin preparation that contains 100 percent of the adult requirement for vitamin D. Estrogen replacement therapy is recommended for postmenopausal women if there are no contraindications to its use.

If osteoporosis has been shown and particularly if bone fractures have occurred, medications are available that may retard further thinning of the bone and possibly increase the amount of bone in the skeleton. These medications include

- Calcitonin
- Etidronate
- Alendronate

SURGICAL TREATMENT:

No treatment is indicated except for treatment if a bone fracture should occur.

PREVENTION

Prevention of the complications of osteoporosis is possible. All individuals should maintain a lifestyle that encourages exercise and adequate intake of calcium and vitamin D. Estrogen replacement for select postmenopausal women completes the usual preventive measures.

Calcium intake should be approximately 1,500 mg daily. This amount of calcium is found in a quart of milk. Those who are lactose intolerant can get calcium from calcium-fortified orange juice and vegetables such as spinach, which do not contain lactose. Calcium can also be made up by any number of commercial supplements that are available over the counter.

Regular physical activity, particularly in the early years of life, is a plus in maintaining a strong skeleton. Weight-bearing exercise such as walking or weight training are useful in maintaining a healthy skeleton.

OVARIAN CANCER

Cancer of the ovaries is the deadliest of the gynecologic cancers. It accounts for approximately 14,500 deaths per year compared with only around 5,000 each for UTERINE CANCER and CERVICAL CANCER.

CAUSES

The exact cause of ovarian cancer cannot be pinpointed, but risk factors for the disease include
* Advancing age (The group at highest risk is between 75 and 79 years of age.)
* Nulliparity (having never given birth to a live infant)
* Personal history of endometrial cancer, COLORECTAL CANCER, or BREAST CANCER
* Family history of ovarian cancer

There appears to be no risk associated with the use of fertility drugs.

A very small number of women (less than 0.05 percent) are at significantly increased risk because of hereditary ovarian cancer syndromes.

SYMPTOMS

Symptoms are not noticeable in the early stages of the disease. The first symptoms usually appear after the cancer is advanced. They include
* Increasing abdominal girth
* Early satiety
* Changes in bowel or bladder habits
* Pelvic pressure
* VAGINAL BLEEDING

DIAGNOSIS

The diagnostic approach to ovarian cancer involves a complete PHYSICAL EXAMINATION including pelvic examination. If an enlarged ovary is suspected, ULTRASOUND can be used to determine the size of the tumor and the rate of bloodflow to the area.

A BLOOD TEST for CA-125 may be helpful in the diagnosis of the disease in some cases, especially in postmenopausal women.

Unfortunately, no appropriate screening method exists for ovarian cancer, so the disease is rarely caught in the early stages.

COMPLICATIONS

Untreated ovarian cancer can lead to
- Internal bleeding
- Spread of the cancer to other parts of the body
- Continued WEIGHT LOSS

TREATMENT

SELF TREATMENT:
None.

MEDICAL TREATMENT:
After surgery, chemotherapy is required. The exact regimen depends on the type of tumor and the stage.

SURGICAL TREATMENT:
The first line of treatment for ovarian cancer is surgical removal. The extent of the operation depends on the stage and size of the tumor and on whether the woman would like to preserve her reproductive capabilities. In advanced cases, total hysterectomy with complete removal of the ovaries and fallopian tubes may be necessary, but some cases may only require removal of one ovary, leaving the rest of the reproductive system intact.

PREVENTION

Although there are no specific strategies to prevent ovarian cancer, there may be some protective factors, including
- Having more than one full-term pregnancy
- Using oral contraceptives for more than five years
- Breast-feeding

In women who have a hereditary ovarian cancer syndrome, the ovaries can be removed surgically to prevent the development of the disease. Prophylactic removal of the ovaries can be performed on women at risk who do not have the hereditary syndrome if they are undergoing abdominal surgery for another reason and do not desire children in the future. This preventive approach is not appropriate for women who do not have the hereditary syndrome and are not undergoing abdominal surgery for another reason.

OVARIAN CYSTS

An ovarian cyst is an abnormal growth consisting of various cell types within normal ovarian tissue.

CAUSES

Although some ovarian cysts may develop from gonadotropin stimulation or fertility medications, most cysts have no specific cause.

SYMPTOMS

Although many cysts of the ovary are asymptomatic, some produce symptoms such as

- Dull or pressure-like pain in the lower abdominal or pelvic region (see ABDOMINAL PAIN), which may be chronic
- Abnormal uterine bleeding, including spotting and MENSTRUAL IRREGULARITIES
- Acute severe lower abdominal or pelvic pain (see ABDOMINAL PAIN) if an ovarian cyst ruptures or torsion (twisting) occurs
- Dyspareunia (painful intercourse)
- Abdominal enlargement (ABDOMINAL SWELLING) with large ovarian cysts or ascites (fluid in the abdomen)
- Gastrointestinal symptoms
- Urinary tract obstruction (rarely)

DIAGNOSIS

Ovarian cysts may be detected during a pelvic exam either incidentally or when investigating suspicious symptoms that suggest the possibility of an ovarian cyst. However, to define the characteristics of an ovarian cyst more precisely, such as its size, location, and consistency, an ULTRASOUND may be required. This can be done either abdominally or vaginally.

In rare cases, COMPUTED TOMOGRAPHY or MAGNETIC RESONANCE IMAGING is useful for defining ovarian cysts. These two procedures may be useful in people suspected of having OVARIAN CANCER or those with ovarian cysts that cannot be seen adequately by ULTRASOUND, but at present there is no reliable imaging technique to screen for OVARIAN CANCER.

> Ovarian cysts are common, usually asymptomatic, and benign in the vast majority of cases.

COMPLICATIONS

Complications of ovarian cysts include
- Rupture or torsion (twisting) of the cyst, which may require immediate surgery
- Internal bleeding caused by cyst rupture
- Infection (rare)
- Malignant degeneration in which cancer develops in the cyst (very rare)

TREATMENT

SELF TREATMENT:

None.

MEDICAL TREATMENT:
- Nonsteroidal anti-inflammatory drugs such as ibuprofen may be used for mild to moderate pain.
- Narcotics may be required in cases of severe pain.
- Oral contraceptives may reduce development of new ovarian cysts in the future.

SURGICAL TREATMENT:

Indications for surgery include
- Persistent or enlarging ovarian cyst greater than six centimeters after four to six weeks of observation
- Cysts greater than eight to ten centimeters
- Postmenopausal cysts greater than five centimeters
- Cysts that occur before menstruation starts
- Complex characteristics on ULTRASOUND or pelvic examination
- Ascites (abdominal fluid collection)

The procedure of choice is an ovarian cystectomy or OVAR-IAN CYST REMOVAL. Oophorectomy (removal of the entire ovary) may be required in some cases.

PREVENTION

Ovarian cyst formation may be reduced with the use of oral contraceptives. In addition, oral contraceptives reduce the risk of epithelial OVARIAN CANCER.

PANCREATIC CANCER

The pancreas is an organ involved in endocrine functions such as the secretion of insulin, and exocrine functions such as the secretion of enzymes involved in digestion. It is located underneath the stomach and liver and adjacent to the duodenum (the first section of the small intestine).

CAUSES

The cause of this cancer remains unknown. The most established risk factor for the development of this cancer is cigarette smoking. Other less common risk factors are
- A high-fat diet
- DIABETES
- Chronic PANCREATITIS, generally related to high alcohol intake
- Contact with organic chemicals

SYMPTOMS

When the cancer originates in the head of the pancreas, which is the closest area to the duodenum, patients suffer from jaundice and generalized ITCHING. If, on the other hand, the tumor originates in the area of the tail of the pancreas, which is furthest from the duodenum, the tumor can grow to larger sizes before causing symptoms. This condition can result in the obstruction of bile excretion leading to the development of
- Jaundice
- Pale-colored stools (see STOOL, ABNORMAL APPEARANCE)
- Generalized ITCHING
- ABDOMINAL PAIN
- WEIGHT LOSS
- A palpable mass

Many patients with pancreatic cancer also have symptoms of cancer that has spread to other organs.

DIAGNOSIS

Cancer of the pancreas can be easily seen with COMPUTED TOMOGRAPHY or ULTRASOUND of the abdomen. The diagnosis needs to be confirmed by obtaining a BIOPSY.

Pancreatic cancer is the fourth leading cause of cancer death; only 15 percent of pancreatic tumors can be fully removed. Cessation of cigarette smoking can greatly reduce the incidence of this cancer.

COMPLICATIONS

Complications arise from the spread (metastasis) of the cancer to other organs or from the physical size of the tumor causing obstruction of the bile duct or other internal structures.

TREATMENT

SELF TREATMENT:
An overall healthy lifestyle with a well-balanced diet is essential to maintain general health during the treatment for pancreatic cancer.

MEDICAL TREATMENT:
Although treatment with chemotherapy has not been very encouraging, promising new chemotherapy agents are always being investigated.

Combinations of treatment with chemotherapy and radiation therapy may help control symptoms in some cases of advanced cancer.

SURGICAL TREATMENT:
Removal of the tumor offers the only chance for cure of this type of cancer. Unfortunately, only about 15 percent of patients can have their tumors fully removed. The rest have cancers that have grown too extensive to remove completely.

PREVENTION

The only well-established risk for the development of pancreatic cancer is cigarette smoking. Smoking cessation should, therefore, result in a decreased chance of developing this type of cancer.

PANCREATITIS

The pancreas aids in the digestive process by secreting various enzymes that break down nutrients directly into the intestine. The pancreas also secretes insulin into the bloodstream. Pancreatitis occurs when the pancreas is inflamed and these potent digestive enzymes leak out of the gland and self-digest tissues close to the pancreas gland.

CAUSES

The most common causes of pancreatitis are GALLSTONES and excessive alcohol intake. Passage of small GALLSTONES from the gallbladder into the ductal system of the liver may lead to blockage of the pancreatic duct, resulting in pancreatitis.

Alcohol may directly damage the pancreas in some patients. Although this type of pancreatitis is somewhat unpredictable, it usually relates to excessive and prolonged alcohol abuse.

Although rare, pancreatitis may also be caused by drugs such as azathioprine and hydrochlorothiazide, toxins (scorpion stings), blunt trauma to the abdomen, and metabolic conditions (severe HYPERLIPIDEMIA, elevated blood calcium).

SYMPTOMS

Pancreatitis may be acute, without prior symptoms, or chronic, if there are repeated episodes.

The symptoms of acute pancreatitis are sudden, severe mid-ABDOMINAL PAIN made worse with food, frequently radiating directly into the patient's back. VOMITING and FEVER are not unusual.

Chronic pancreatitis causes symptoms similar to acute pancreatitis with repeated episodes of mid-ABDOMINAL PAIN. Additional symptoms include DIARRHEA with foul, greasy stools and WEIGHT LOSS. The DIARRHEA is made worse with food, especially fats. At times, insulin release may be compromised, and elevated blood sugar may cause the symptoms of DIABETES.

DIAGNOSIS

A diagnosis of pancreatitis may be suspected in any case of severe or recurrent mid-ABDOMINAL PAIN. It is corroborated by BLOOD TESTS that measure levels of pancreatic enzymes, amy-

Because excessive alcohol consumption is a major cause of this condition, many cases of pancreatitis are preventable.

lase, and lipase. GALLSTONES as a cause of pancreatitis need to be ruled out with a gallbladder ULTRASOUND. In complicated or protracted cases, ULTRASOUND or COMPUTED TOMOGRAPHY of the pancreas may be performed.

COMPLICATIONS

Persistent pain beyond four or five days raises the possibility of inflammatory cysts within the pancreas. These cysts may become infected or bleed internally. If the pancreatitis is extensive or due to GALLSTONES, the main duct of the liver may become obstructed, resulting in jaundice. Rarely, and only with severe pancreatitis, the inflammatory substance released by the damaged pancreas may cause damage to the lungs, kidneys, and coagulation system. If the pancreatitis is chronic, some patients may develop chronic DIARRHEA, WEIGHT LOSS, and even DIABETES.

TREATMENT

SELF TREATMENT:
Patients with pancreatitis not due to GALLSTONES or a specific drug should avoid alcohol. Patients with chronic pancreatitis may benefit from less fat in the diet.

MEDICAL TREATMENT:
No direct medical therapy has been proved to be of obvious benefit. Patients with severe symptoms should be monitored in the hospital, and fasting or suctioning gastric secretions with a tube and introducing intravenous fluids and antibiotics may limit the course of pancreatitis.

SURGICAL TREATMENT:
If a GALLSTONE is blocking the common bile duct, removal of the stone may be attempted with ENDOSCOPY or surgery at an appropriate time (see GALLBLADDER REMOVAL). Open surgery is otherwise restricted to complications of pancreatitis.

PREVENTION

Limiting alcohol use eliminates this cause of pancreatitis. A low-fat diet to minimize HYPERLIPIDEMIA is also helpful.

PARKINSON DISEASE

Parkinson disease, named for the 19th century English physician James Parkinson, is a degenerative disease of the central nervous system. It is sometimes called *paralysis agitans*, especially when there is no readily apparent cause.

There are other syndromes and conditions that have similar features to those of Parkinson disease, but are not the same. These conditions are often refered to as *Parkinsonism* or *Parkinsonism plus* if they share some of the same aspects but are not the strictly defined disease. (See Diagnosis below.)

The part of the brain that the disease mainly affects is a structure called the *substantia nigra*, which is located deep in the area of the brain called the *brain stem*. The disease slowly destroys the nerve cells in this area of the brain and can go unnoticed for a long time; it is believed that by the time the symptoms of the disease begin to be noticeable, about 75 to 80 percent of the nerve cells in the substantia nigra have already degenerated.

The degeneration of the cells in the substantia nigra causes changes in other parts of the brain, as well, because the substantia nigra is responsible for producing a substance called *dopamine*—a neurotransmitter that is needed for the proper communication between nerve cells. The other parts of the brain begin to suffer from the deficiency of dopamine caused by the damage in the brain stem.

CAUSES

In most cases, the cause is unknown. However, some cases can be caused by
- Hereditary factors
- Brain injury from infection or carbon monoxide poisoning
- Tumors

SYMPTOMS

The symptoms of Parkinsonism are generally related to the nervous system's inability to control movement normally. Vol-

About 20 percent of patients who seem to have Parkinson disease actually have something different. Some of these other conditions are amenable to treatment, but most are not.

untary muscle movement becomes affected. Specific, characteristic symptoms include
- Tremor of the muscles while they are at rest (TREMBLING)
- Slowness of movements
- Rigidity
- Shuffling gait
- A tendency to fall

DIAGNOSIS

The diagnosis of Parkinson disease is a clinical one, based on the MEDICAL HISTORY and a thorough neurologic examination. Nonetheless, in up to 20 percent of cases, the physician may later change the diagnosis from Parkinson disease to Parkinsonism or Parkinsonism plus, based on either
- Other symptoms that develop and that do not fit the profile for true Parkinson disease
- The fact that the condition does not seem to respond to specific treatments that would have an effect in Parkinson disease

Physicians may order COMPUTED TOMOGRAPHY or MAGNETIC RESONANCE IMAGING of the brain to look for changes in the brain's anatomy.

COMPLICATIONS

Progression in severe cases can lead to MEMORY LOSS and immobility. Even before severe progression, hazardous falls can lead to injury, and the condition can precipitate associated problems such as DEPRESSION.

TREATMENT

SELF TREATMENT:
Staying active with regular exercise can help optimize functioning.

MEDICAL TREATMENT:
The major treatment strategies for Parkinson disease are directed toward supplying or increasing the amount of dopamine or dopamine-like substances in the brain. Recent basic science discoveries have resulted in some newer approaches that may prove useful.

Drugs being used include
- Deprenyl, a drug that provides some symptomatic relief and is also thought to slow down the development of the disease (It is not entirely clear yet that the disease can be slowed.)
- Carbidopa-levodopa, the mainstay of symptomatic treatment at all stages of the disease
- Bromocriptine and pergolide, which mimic the effect of dopamine in the brain (These can be used early or later in the disease, alone or as adjuncts to carbidopa-levodopa.)
- Trihexyphenidyl and benztropine, anticholinergic drugs that work by a different mechanism "downstream" of where dopamine works in the brain
- Amantadine, better known as an antiviral agent

Physical and occupational therapy are beneficial.

Treatment of associated conditions (such as DEPRESSION) or supportive services for dementia or general disability should not be neglected.

SURGICAL TREATMENT:

Several surgical options are being studied. In very advanced cases, small destructive lesions in the brain are carried out with small needles rather than with major surgery. This is effective in treating disabling tremor. Implantation of fetal tissue appears to have some promise but is still highly experimental.

PREVENTION

None.

PELVIC INFLAMMATORY DISEASE

One million women per year are treated for pelvic inflammatory disease in the United States, with 150,000 undergoing surgical procedures for complications of the disease.

Pelvic inflammatory disease (PID) is a profound infection of the fallopian tubes, ovaries, and pelvis in women who have unchecked or untreated sexually transmitted diseases such as gonorrhea or chlamydia. Typically, the infection starts in the fallopian tubes, but it can sometimes involve the ovaries. Advanced infection can be diffusely disseminated throughout the pelvis.

CAUSES

Pelvic inflammatory disease is usually caused by sexually transmitted diseases such as gonorrhea and chlamydia, although sometimes the infection occurs spontaneously in women who are not sexually active. Infection in these women occurs from the normal organisms that live in the vagina.

Risk factors for PID include
- New or multiple sex partners
- Low socioeconomic status
- Being unmarried
- A history of sexually transmitted diseases
- The lack of barrier contraceptive use
- The use of an intrauterine device (IUD)

SYMPTOMS

Typical symptoms of acute PID include
- Acute lower ABDOMINAL PAIN
- Pain on pelvic examination
- VAGINAL DISCHARGE
- FEVER higher than 100°F
- MENSTRUAL IRREGULARITIES

However, some cases of PID can be asymptomatic, and laboratory tests can usually help make the diagnosis when the symptoms are not as pronounced.

DIAGNOSIS

The diagnosis of PID is based on a thorough MEDICAL HISTORY and PHYSICAL EXAMINATION. Patients undergo a careful pelvic examination, and CULTURES of the cervix are performed. BLOOD TESTS including a complete BLOOD COUNT are also necessary to make the diagnosis, and on occasion, an ULTRASOUND may be useful. In some cases, surgery may be required to confirm the diagnosis.

COMPLICATIONS

Acute complications include diffuse pelvic infection, which if unchecked can be life threatening. As with any serious infection, if this disease is not treated quickly and aggressively, diffuse sepsis (BLOOD POISONING) may ensue and death could result. Death from acute PID, however, is rarely seen in developed countries.

There are two major long-term complications of PID, both of which impact upon future reproduction. The first is tubal factor infertility, and the second is an increased risk for ectopic pregnancy. Tubal factor infertility occurs in 20 to 60 percent of women who have PID. Ectopic pregnancy tends to increase by at least 15 percent for each episode of PID. Other less common complications of PID include chronic pelvic pain, pain with intercourse, and pelvic adhesions.

TREATMENT

SELF TREATMENT:
(See Prevention below.)

MEDICAL TREATMENT:
There are a variety of antibiotic regimens available for treating PID. Depending on the severity of the disease, either outpatient therapies or inpatient therapies with intravenous antibiotics might be indicated. A decision to hospitalize depends on the severity of the infection.

SURGICAL TREATMENT:
Surgical treatments, including laparoscopy (a form of ENDOSCOPY) and laparotomy (open abdominal surgery), may be indicated in women with life-threatening infection; however, most of the time, the diagnosis can be made without surgery, and medical treatment can be instituted.

PREVENTION

The key to prevention of this disease is avoiding sexual contact with partners infected with sexually transmitted diseases. Abstinence or monogamous relationships are safer. Women who are sexually active may significantly decrease the incidence of infection by using the male or female condom.

PERIODONTITIS

Periodontitis is a chronic inflammation of the supporting structures of the teeth that leads to the formation of pockets in the gingiva—the gum tissue—and bone loss in tooth sockets. Loosening of the teeth is a late warning sign that advanced bone loss has already occurred.

CAUSES

The primary cause of periodontitis is poor oral hygiene. The accumulation of plaque (deposits of bacteria) and calculus (the hardened form of plaque) can lead to the development of GINGIVITIS and then proceed to periodontitis. Tobacco smoking has been shown to be a factor in the development of periodontitis since this habit increases irritation of the gingival tissues. It can be definitively shown that any habit that creates chronic gingival irritation, such as smoking does, makes a person more susceptible to periodontitis.

SYMPTOMS

Periodontitis is often asymptomatic in its early stages. The loosening of teeth is usually a sign of advanced, long-standing periodontal disease. In certain instances, an acute periodontal abscess may develop and act as a warning sign. A periodontal abscess is a localized, painful swelling of the gingiva around the tooth. Occasionally, bad breath can accompany periodontitis.

DIAGNOSIS

The diagnosis of periodontal disease is made by measuring the periodontal pocket depths over time. Pockets that have increased to deeper than three millimeters must be evaluated for periodontal breakdown. Bleeding on probing is also recorded to assess the amount of inflammation present. A measurement of the plaque index is often used to determine the effectiveness of the patient's home oral efforts.

Many practitioners advocate the use of a DNA analysis to identify the microorganisms in cases of periodontitis that do not respond to conventional periodontal therapy. This allows the dental professional to prescribe an antibiotic or combination of antibiotics that are highly active against the specific microorganism.

> Unlike gingivitis, which is often the precursor to this condition, periodontitis is not reversible.

COMPLICATIONS

The primary complication of periodontitis is loss of teeth that occurs after loss of supporting bone. Many times the early symptom, loose teeth, is a sign that the disease is already advanced.

TREATMENT

SELF TREATMENT:

A patient with a diagnosis of periodontal disease must practice greatly improved oral hygiene, including brushing after every meal, daily flossing, and more frequent visits to the dentist's office for a thorough professional dental cleaning.

MEDICAL TREATMENT:

Periodontal disease is first treated with a procedure called *scaling and root planing*—a nonsurgical deep cleaning of the roots of the teeth. If periodontal pocketing persists after scaling and root planing, treatment could consist of surgical intervention.

SURGICAL TREATMENT:

If the patient's periodontitis does not favorably respond to conventional nonsurgical techniques, PERIODONTAL SURGERY may be required. The primary purposes of periodontal surgery are to eliminate periodontal pockets and to allow a direct view of the tooth roots to ensure that all debris has been removed.

PREVENTION

Periodontal disease can be prevented by practicing good oral hygiene, which includes brushing after every meal and flossing once daily. In addition, visits to the dentist at least twice a year for professional cleaning aid in the early detection and management of any periodontal problems. Tobacco use should be stopped.

PNEUMONIA

Pneumonia can strike previously healthy individuals, but most often, patients have an identifiable risk factor such as alcoholism, diabetes, chronic heart or lung disease, neuromuscular weakness, or HIV infection.

Pneumonia is an infection of the lower respiratory tract, particularly of the air sacs, or alveoli, at the ends of the bronchial tubes. Infected alveoli fill with pus and fluid and interfere with the delivery of inhaled oxygen to the bloodstream.

CAUSES

Pneumonia can be caused by a variety of infectious agents. Most of the time, it is caused by a virus, bacterium, or some bacterium-like organism. The most commonly responsible organisms include

- *Streptococcus pneumoniae* (pneumococcal pneumonia)
- *Mycoplasma pneumoniae*
- Viruses such as INFLUENZA

Pneumonia caused by the bacteria *Pneumocystis carinii* is rare, except in patients with AIDS.

SYMPTOMS

Bacterial pneumonia causes

- FEVER
- COUGH
- Excess mucus
- BREATHING DIFFICULTY
- CHEST PAIN

The symptoms get worse over the course of hours or days until they are severe enough for the patient to seek medical attention. Viral and mycoplasmal infections tend to cause less severe illness with more aches and pains.

DIAGNOSIS

Pneumonia is generally suspected after the MEDICAL HISTORY and the PHYSICAL EXAMINATION reveal FEVER and respiratory distress. The most useful diagnostic test is the X ray (RADIOGRAPHY), which can show the poorly aerated lung tissue and the area involved. Laboratory tests include

- Tests of blood oxygen level (see BLOOD TESTS)
- BLOOD COUNT
- Possibly CULTURE of blood or mucus

In particularly difficult cases, bronchoscopy (a form of ENDOSCOPY) may be needed to establish a definitive diagnosis.

COMPLICATIONS

Severe cases of pneumonia can lead to respiratory failure requiring mechanical ventilation. Lung tissue can be damaged, causing tissue death, internal bleeding, and possibly lung collapse. Infectious agents can spread to other specific organs, such as the brain, or throughout the bloodstream (see BLOOD POISONING).

TREATMENT

SELF TREATMENT:

General measures such as bed rest and adequate fluid intake are appropriate, but medical attention is necessary.

MEDICAL TREATMENT:

Bacterial pneumonia is primarily treated with antibiotics such as erythromycin, clarithromycin, and azithromycin. Frequently, more than one antibiotic is prescribed to cover all the likely organisms before the specific one is identified; often the organism is never identified, and the broad-spectrum antibiotics are used.

Viral infections are much less easily treated. General supportive therapy may be all that can be done, but some medications can be helpful against specific viruses. These include

- Amantadine
- Rimantadine
- Acyclovir
- Ganciclovir

SURGICAL TREATMENT:

None.

PREVENTION

Yearly INFLUENZA vaccination is the single most effective preventive strategy. Pneumococcal vaccine offers protection from pneumonia caused by *Streptococcus pneumoniae* (pneumococcal pneumonia). These vaccines are appropriate for people at high risk, including

- Those with chronic heart, lung, or kidney disease
- Those with DIABETES
- Those older than 65

PROSTATE CANCER

Prostate cancer is the second most common cancer in men, with more than 85,000 new cases diagnosed each year.

Prostate cancer is a growth of tumor cells within the prostate gland in men. This growth is stimulated by androgens (male sex hormones), especially testosterone.

CAUSES

The cause of prostate cancer is unknown. Several factors associated with an increased risk of prostate cancer include
- High-fat diet
- Cirrhosis of the liver
- Occupational exposure to rubber and cadmium
- Being married
- Certain demographics (high risk in Sweden and the United States; low risk in Asia), suggesting environmental factors
- A family history of the disease

SYMPTOMS

Often there are no symptoms at the time of diagnosis. Symptoms frequently indicate advanced disease and include
- Difficulty passing urine (URINATION, PAINFUL)
- Blood in the urine
- Frequent urination (URINATION, FREQUENT)
- Back pain (BACKACHE)
- Bone pain at any site

DIAGNOSIS

Routine blood work includes a complete BLOOD COUNT, kidney and liver function tests, and tests for calcium, phosphorous, and alkaline phosphatase levels (see BLOOD TESTS). A URINALYSIS and chest X ray (RADIOGRAPHY) are also performed. Acid phosphatase and prostate-specific antigen (PSA) are BLOOD TESTS for relatively specific markers for prostate cancer. They are also used to follow the disease course. A needle BIOPSY of any nodules found during rectal examination is used to make the diagnosis and help determine the stage of the cancer. A bone scan (see NUCLEAR MEDICINE) and COMPUTED TOMOGRAPHY of the abdomen and pelvis are needed to determine the extent of the disease.

COMPLICATIONS

Complications of prostate cancer can include
* Spread (metastasis) of the cancer into bone, which can cause pain or bone fractures
* Spinal cord compression, which can result from metastasis of the cancer to the spine and may be accompanied by weakness, NUMBNESS, INCONTI-NENCE, and a loss of bowel control (BOWEL CONTROL, LOSS OF)
* IMPOTENCE as a result of therapy
* ANEMIA, in advanced disease, with associated symptoms of FATIGUE, BREATHING DIFFICULTY, and pallor
* KIDNEY FAILURE from obstruction of urine outflow by the prostate

TREATMENT

SELF TREATMENT:

None.

MEDICAL TREATMENT:

Very early stage disease may be treated by observation alone. Tumors confined to the prostate can be treated with radiation therapy. Hormone therapy can be useful. Chemotherapy is only used in patients with recurrent advanced disease.

SURGICAL TREATMENT:

The disease can be treated with PROSTATE GLAND REMOVAL surgery. Removal of the testicles can also cause prostate cancer to shrink.

PREVENTION

There is no established means to prevent prostate cancer. Men 40 years of age and older should have an annual digital rectal examination to detect early stage disease; early detection improves prognosis.

PROSTATE, ENLARGED

The benign growth and enlargement of the prostate gland occurs in the majority of men older than 40 years of age.

During puberty, the prostate gland goes through a growth spurt until it becomes the mature adult size and remains at this size through most of adulthood. Then, for reasons that are not entirely understood, around the age of 45 or 50, the prostate can go through another growth spurt causing the symptoms of enlarged prostate.

CAUSES

No specific cause or risk factors have been identified for prostate enlargement in older men. Aging seems to be a contributing cause, and levels of male hormones are also a factor.

SYMPTOMS

When the gland enlarges, it can interfere with or obstruct the urinary tract, causing
- Diminished urinary stream pressure
- FREQUENT URINATION during the day and night
- Incomplete bladder emptying

DIAGNOSIS

An individual's MEDICAL HISTORY and a PHYSICAL EXAMINATION are usually sufficient to make a diagnosis. Additional tests may include cystoscopy (a form of ENDOSCOPY) and urodynamic testing of bladder function.

COMPLICATIONS

Urinary retention can lead to problems such as BLADDER INFECTION.

WARNING SIGNS:
- Infrequent urination
- Urination of small volumes
- Needing to strain to pass urine
- Urine leakage (INCONTINENCE)

TREATMENT

SELF TREATMENT:

None.

MEDICAL TREATMENT:

The drug finasteride can shrink the size of the prostate gland. The drugs terazosin and doxazosin can decrease the amount of urinary obstruction and relieve some of the symptoms.

SURGICAL TREATMENT:

There are several surgical options for the treatment of an enlarged prostate. All involve removing part of the gland to reduce its size (see PROSTATE GLAND REMOVAL).

- Transurethral resection of the prostate involves the use of a cystoscope to pass an instrument up the urethra to the gland. Part of the gland is then removed.
- Transurethral incision of the prostate involves the use of a cystoscope to cut the gland in a key location to improve urine flow.
- Simple prostatectomy is a traditional open surgical technique to remove the gland.
- Laser ablation of the prostate involves destroying part of the gland with lasers.

PREVENTION

None.

PSORIASIS

Two to three percent of the population have psoriasis, a chronic skin condition.

Psoriasis is a chronic affliction of the skin featuring red plaques with thick scales. Characteristically, it involves the scalp, elbows, knees, and sacral area of the lower back.

CAUSES

The cause is unknown, although a genetic component is likely in some patients.

SYMPTOMS

Most of the time, psoriasis causes minimal ITCHING, except when it is in the scalp and skin folds. The patient will readily recognize red inflammatory plaques with thick scale on the scalp, elbows, knees, sacral area, and other sites.

Psoriasis can involve the entire skin surface in some severe cases and often involves fingernails and toenails, causing discoloration and pitting of the nails. Although it may involve the face in some cases, most of the time the face is spared.

Another kind of psoriasis occurs after an infected throat or upper respiratory tract infection. This condition occurs with the sudden onset of crops of salmon-pink or red half-inch-wide papules and small plaques with scale all over the body, especially the torso. This is called *guttate* (meaning teardrop-like) psoriasis.

DIAGNOSIS

The clinical presentation is usually highly suggestive to a trained professional, and further testing may be unnecessary. Where confirmation is needed, a skin BIOPSY can be performed for a tissue diagnosis.

COMPLICATIONS

Normal-appearing skin in a patient with psoriasis is not really normal. If the skin is scraped or cut, psoriasis may form at the site of injury.

Persons with psoriasis may also have RHEUMATOID ARTHRITIS.

In some patients, psoriasis invokes a significant amount of emotional turmoil, including feelings of dependency, anger, DEPRESSION, resentment, passive-aggressive behavior, and low self-esteem.

TREATMENT

SELF TREATMENT:
Trauma to the skin should be avoided. The skin should be kept well lubricated with topical emollients. Mild soaps should be used, and the patient should not overbathe.

MEDICAL TREATMENT:
Many medications can be used in the treatment of psoriasis, including
- Topical steroid creams and ointments
- Topical tar preparations
- Topical vitamin D
- Topical anthralin
- Short-wave ultraviolet light
- Long-wave ultraviolet light after the oral administration of 8-methoxypsoralen (a photosensitizer)
- Oral administration of vitamin A analogues
- Oral or intramuscular methotrexate
- Oral cyclosporine A, a powerful immunosuppressive agent
- Oral administration of sulfasalazine, an agent used for inflammatory bowel disease
- Oral administration of hydroxyurea

SURGICAL TREATMENT:
None.

PREVENTION

None.

PULMONARY EMBOLISM

More than half a million people experience pulmonary embolism each year. Early, appropriate treatment makes a major difference, because untreated, pulmonary embolism can have a mortality rate as high as 30 percent.

When a blood clot travels into the lung, it is called a pulmonary embolism. The clot may interfere with blood flow through a portion of the lung so that oxygen from the air spaces cannot be delivered to the blood by that portion of the lung. That area of the lung may even die (infarct). Pulmonary embolism is an extremely dangerous complication of other disorders of the circulatory system.

CAUSES

Clots can come from many portions of the body because all the blood from the legs, arms, and abdominal and pelvic organs drains into the right side of the heart and is pumped into the lungs.

The most common sites for clots to form are the deep veins of the legs (especially the thigh and groin region). Less often the clot may come from the veins draining the kidneys or the larger veins leading up to the right side of the heart.

Risk factors for these clots are varied, but they usually involve

- Prolonged immobility
- Damage to veins
- Drugs or cancers that increase the clotting of the blood in general

SYMPTOMS

The most common symptom is sudden shortness of breath (BREATHING DIFFICULTY). It may be associated with

- Sweating (SWEATING, EXCESSIVE)
- COUGH
- CHEST PAIN
- Coughing up blood
- FAINTING or FAINTNESS
- Signs of a clot in the leg (THROMBOSIS)
- Fast pulse
- FEVER

Almost always, the risk factors for THROMBOSIS will be apparent, including

- Immobility such as that after surgery or a STROKE
- Vein damage from hip, knee, or pelvic surgery or trauma

- An overactive coagulation system from smoking, estrogen therapy, a genetic predisposition, or cancer

DIAGNOSIS

The presence of risk factors and compatible symptoms raises the suspicion of pulmonary embolism.

ELECTROCARDIOGRAPHY or chest X ray (RADIOGRAPHY) may provide additional clues. Measurement of oxygen level in the blood (arterial blood gas) is usually done as a next step (see BLOOD TESTS).

Other new tests of coagulation may be helpful, but usually a NUCLEAR MEDICINE scan of the lungs is required to confirm the diagnosis. If this is not definitive, an angiogram (RADIOGRAPHY) may be necessary to see the clot, or serial blood flow studies of the leg, which involve ULTRASOUND to examine the dynamics of blood in vessels, may be done to assess the risk of recurrent clot formation.

COMPLICATIONS

Cyanosis, a bluish coloring of the skin associated with dangerously low oxygen levels in the blood, may be seen in more severe pulmonary emboli. Even with treatment, pulmonary embolism can lead to

- Dangerously low blood pressure
- HEART ATTACK
- Death

TREATMENT

SELF TREATMENT:
(See Prevention below.)

MEDICAL TREATMENT:
- Heparin is the main initial treatment. (New forms of this drug may even be more effective and safer.)
- Clot-dissolving drugs like tissue plasminogen activator (TPA), streptokinase, and urokinase may be used for more life-threatening emboli.
- Oxygen is generally given to raise blood levels.

Longer-term prevention of recurrence is accomplished with warfarin or heparin.

SURGICAL TREATMENT:

On rare occasion, for a life-threatening massive clot to the lungs, immediate surgical removal may be attempted.

For patients who cannot be on anticoagulants like heparin or for whom the medication fails to work, the large vein in the abdomen that drains the blood from both legs and the pelvis (the vena cava) may be interrupted with a filter of some type. The filter can trap subsequent clots to help prevent a life-threatening recurrence. Nowadays these filters can be placed without major surgery by special catheters threaded through the veins with X ray (RADIOGRAPHY) guidance.

PREVENTION

Special compression stockings—some with inflatable compartments to keep blood from flowing too slowly and clotting—can be placed on the legs before and after high-risk times for clots to form, such as with hip or knee surgery, or during other times of immobility, such as after a STROKE. Low-dose anticoagulants are also given at these times to decrease the chance of THROMBOSIS.

Other strategies to help prevent clots or recurrences include

- Not smoking
- Maintaining an active lifestyle
- Maintaining a healthy weight
- Rapid rehabilitation after surgery
- Frequent leg movement on long trips by car, plane, or train

RHEUMATOID ARTHRITIS

Rheumatoid arthritis is an inflammation of the membrane lining the joint; this membrane is called the *synovium*. An inflammation called *synovitis* results in thickening of the membrane and the formation of extra fluid within the joint. As a consequence, the joints, tendons, or bursas—all of which have a synovial lining—become swollen and painful and experience a reduced range of motion.

Multiple joints are usually involved in a symmetrical fashion; that is, both wrists, both thumbs, both middle fingers, and so on.

CAUSES

No cause has been recognized for this disease, but two factors are likely contributors: 1) extrinsic or environmental factors, and 2) intrinsic or genetic factors.

Although no specific extrinsic or environmental factors have yet been recognized, viruses or toxic factors in the environment could play a role in the development of the disease. Rheumatoid arthritis did not seem to exist before the industrial era several centuries ago, implying that toxic factors due to industry may be involved. At this point, however, these are only speculations.

More knowledge is available about intrinsic factors. These are some well-studied genetic abnormalities of the immune system involving a specific part of the human genetic code. Research in this area continues, but has not yet yielded any practical treatments.

SYMPTOMS

Rheumatoid arthritis usually involves morning stiffness lasting 15 minutes or more and an associated swelling of the joints. The patient begins to feel better late in the day, but then fatigue may set in.

Not only are the joints involved, but sometimes inflammation exists in other areas such as

- The whites of the eye
- The lungs—where increased fibrous scar tissue can form
- Near the elbows—where nodules can appear
- The blood vessels

Although often associated with aging, rheumatoid arthritis can affect people of any age. Climate conditions are not important. Women have a slightly greater frequency of the disease than men.

DIAGNOSIS

The diagnosis of rheumatoid arthritis is usually made by observation of the symptoms: the persistent swelling of multiple joints that does not disappear in 6 to 12 weeks. If the symptoms do disappear in that time, other conditions that may mimic rheumatoid arthritis, including LUPUS ERYTHEMATOSUS or some viral disease, may be involved.

Laboratory tests are helpful in diagnosis. BLOOD TESTS are used to search for an elevation in the sedimentation rate which reflects the inflammatory process that underlies the disease, a slight ANEMIA, and rheumatoid factor. The rheumatoid factor test is positive in about 80 percent of the patients with rheumatoid arthritis.

COMPLICATIONS

In the joints, complications include damage by destruction of the cartilage and bone that underlies the cartilage. Natural cartilage and bone tissue are replaced by the inflamed synovium. Such joints become unstable and lack sufficient motion, interfering with function. Hand function or the ability to walk normally can be impaired. In some cases these complications can be life threatening. If bone erosion takes place high in the spine, the top joint in the neck becomes unstable and pressure can be exerted against the spinal cord with serious consequences such as paralysis.

In rare instances, rheumatoid arthritis can cause blood vessel inflammation that leads to damage in organs, peripheral nerves, or the skin—sometimes leading to gangrene in the tips of the fingers or in the intestines. Lung disease, seen in a small number of patients, is the result of an increase in fibrous tissue that impairs the lungs' ability to oxygenate the blood.

A few patients have a decreased white blood cell count and are vulnerable to infections. Lastly, some patients develop an inflammation of the glands that produce saliva and tears. When this happens, they experience dryness of the mouth and eyes. This complication is called *Sjögren syndrome*—a problem that can also exist independently of rheumatoid arthritis.

TREATMENT

SELF TREATMENT:

The patient's response to the illness is critical. Education about the disease helps the patient develop a realistic approach to his or her own particular case. Rest periods are beneficial. Exercise is encouraged but should be moderated to suit the degree of illness. Compliance with medication intake is important.

MEDICAL TREATMENT:

Physical therapy is important. It can be accomplished through structured programs under the care of a physical therapist, and once the patient is educated, the program can be maintained on his or her own.

Drug treatment is geared to the amount and type of drugs needed to control the inflammation. Almost all patients benefit from nonsteroidal anti-inflammatory drugs such as ibuprofen and naproxen. Some joints can be treated by injection of corticosteroids such as triamcinolone directly into the joint.

Long-term therapy with medications such as methotrexate, sulfasalazine, azathioprine, cyclophosphamide, hydroxychloroquine, and gold salts can prevent acceleration of tissue damage.

SURGICAL TREATMENT:

Surgical treatment is reserved for two circumstances:

- The removal of inflamed synovial tissue from joints or tendons to avoid damage to these structures
- Replacement of the total joint, particularly the knee (KNEE ARTHROPLASTY) and the hip (HIP ARTHROPLASTY)

In contrast to patients with OSTEOARTHRITIS, the bone structure of patients with rheumatoid arthritis is usually weaker. As a consequence, they may have less successful results. Even so, the results can be truly dramatic in selected patients.

PREVENTION

No known preventive techniques are available.

SHINGLES

> Shingles can be viewed as a recurrence of chicken pox virus in adults, usually the elderly, but it affects the skin in a different way from the chicken pox of childhood.

Shingles is a skin eruption that is usually localized within one or two areas of the skin. When a shingles eruption begins in adult life, it is thought that the dormant chicken pox virus becomes active again and escapes the person's immune system, which has kept the chicken pox virus dormant for many years. Common areas of involvement are linear segments of the trunk that follow the skin lines, along the arms or legs, over a linear area of the scalp, and around the eyes or nose.

CAUSES

Shingles is caused by activation of the dormant chicken pox virus (varicella) and its escape of the person's immune surveillance.

SYMPTOMS

Often before anything is seen on the skin, the patient will experience a localized area of skin that is painful, burning, or ITCHING. This is often in a linear distribution. Then, a day or two later, small clusters of small water blisters erupt on the skin, which is usually red and inflamed. These blisters pop and leave open sores (erosions) that eventually form thick, crusty scabs. The scabs may persist for 7 to 14 days before they fall off, leaving pink or white spots in a localized linear distribution.

There may be associated burning, ITCHING, and pain throughout the course of the active eruption. This pain may persist for a long time even after the skin lesions have completely healed.

DIAGNOSIS

The PHYSICAL EXAMINATION and the telltale symptoms usually provide enough clues to make the diagnosis of shingles. The physician can confirm this diagnosis in the office with a Tzanck Smear. In this test, the physician unroofs a blister or early crust, gently scrapes the blister roof and base, makes a thick smear on a slide, and examines it under the microscope. Alternatively, the physician can make a thick smear of blister and blister base fluids on a slide and send it for direct immunofluorescence at a laboratory, which can positively identify the chicken pox virus. Or, the physician can take the same fluid for viral CULTURE; the chicken pox virus, however, is notoriously difficult to CULTURE.

COMPLICATIONS

Secondary infection of the open erosions is common. Severe pain and continuous pain after the skin eruption has abated is another frequent complication.

When the eruption involves the eye, there may be injury and scarring of the eye as a severe complication.

In patients with weakened immune systems, shingles may become a widespread systemic infection rather than just a localized infection of the skin.

TREATMENT

SELF TREATMENT:
- Aluminum acetate solution on cool, wet compresses
- Antibacterial ointment on open erosions
- Chlorpheniramine or diphenhydramine antihistamines for ITCHING
- Aspirin for pain

MEDICAL TREATMENT:
If the patient is seen early, an antiviral drug such as acyclovir or valacyclovir can inhibit the virus and shorten the course of the eruption.

SURGICAL TREATMENT:
None.

PREVENTION

A new vaccine to prevent chicken pox entirely is being offered for children, but it is not helpful for adults who have already had chicken pox.

SKIN CANCER

> Most skin cancers occur on the head, neck, and hands— the sun-exposed areas of the body.

The four essential types of skin cancer are
- Melanoma, a pigmented skin tumor that is quite serious and may be life-threatening
- Basal cell carcinoma, the most common skin tumor, which is locally invasive and destructive (it destroys tissue in the immediate area), but it usually does not spread or result in death
- Squamous cell carcinoma, which is three times more rare than a basal cell carcinoma but behaves in a similar manner
- Bowen disease, a cousin of the squamous cell carcinoma that is more superficial, involving only the outermost layer of the skin

The typical basal cell carcinoma is an elevated round-oval, pearl-like bump with some red coloration due to fine red blood vessels going across or into it. Sometimes several small bumps form a circle. They bleed easily and sometimes ulcerate. The squamous cell carcinoma is less well-defined, has uneven, poorly visualized borders, and may be a scaly, crusted, red elevation with a rough surface. Bowen disease usually is a red or pink plaque-like elevation with very clear borders. Basal cell carcinoma and squamous cell carcinoma tend to occur on sun-exposed sites of the skin.

CAUSES

The cause of cancer is unknown. It is thought, however, that squamous cell carcinoma and basal cell carcinoma are related to an accumulation of sunlight over a lifetime. People with light complexions have these tumors more often than people with dark complexions.

Malignant melanoma is believed to be associated with numerous severe sunburns during childhood, adolescence, or young adulthood. It, too, occurs more commonly in lightly pigmented people, especially those with blue or green eyes, freckles, and almost white skin. A tendency to develop melanoma seems to run in families.

SYMPTOMS

- Skin lesions with persistent ulceration or bleeding
- Persistent skin lesion that changes size, shape, or color (SKIN CHANGES)

DIAGNOSIS

A BIOPSY should be done on any suspicious skin lesions. When evaluating pigmented skin lesions, the physician usually looks for good and bad signs. Bad signs include

- Uneven pigmentation or coloration of the lesion
- Irregular borders
- Asymmetry
- Marked elevation
- Large size (bigger than a pencil eraser)

TREATMENT

SELF TREATMENT:

None.

MEDICAL TREATMENT:

Skin cancer requires surgical treatment.

SURGICAL TREATMENT:

All of the skin cancers described above can be treated by means of excision and removal of the tumor. Surgical removal results in a better than 90 percent cure rate for nonpigmented tumors (basal cell carcinoma, squamous cell carcinoma, and Bowen disease). Alternative methods for destroying the cancer include using liquid-nitrogen freezing (cryosurgery) or scraping with a curette and burning the tissue with electric cautery (electrodesiccation and curettage).

The treatment of melanoma depends upon the thickness of the tumor and the depth of invasion when examined with the microscope. When the tumor is thin and superficial, excision may be all that is necessary. Deeper lesions may require an examination of the lymph nodes draining the skin area and chemotherapy (see MALIGNANT MELANOMA REMOVAL).

PREVENTION

Prolonged sun exposure increases the risk of skin cancer, so limiting exposure to the sun is the best prevention, particularly for those with fair complexions. Most skin cancers occur on the head, neck, and hands, so clothing (wide-brimmed hats, long sleeves) and use of sun block with a sun protection factor of 15 offers adequate protection.

STOMACH CANCER

Although stomach cancer was the leader among cancer deaths worldwide until 1988, its incidence has decreased dramatically in the last three decades, most likely due to changes in dietary habits.

Most stomach tumors occur in the lower third of the stomach, arising from cells in the lining of the stomach. A second tumor occurs in up to 20 percent of patients. The cancer is isolated to the stomach in only about 10 percent of cases. By the time it causes symptoms and is diagnosed, the cancer has usually spread to the adjacent tissues and lymph nodes.

CAUSES

Stomach cancer is associated with consumption of smoked or salty foods. There is an increased incidence of gastric cancer in

- Smokers
- Japanese and Chilean people (possibly related to dietary habits)
- Asbestos workers
- People with lower socioeconomic status
- Patients who have undergone stomach resection for the treatment of peptic ulcer disease—as many as three decades after the operation
- People infected with *Helicobacter pylori*, a bacteria known to cause gastritis

SYMPTOMS

Most patients have symptoms similar to those of ULCER disease, such as

- Anorexia (APPETITE, LOSS OF)
- Stomach fullness
- Abdominal discomfort worsened by some foods and improved by antacids.

Patients may also experience painless gastrointestinal bleeding with black tarry stools. Less commonly, patients may experience symptoms related to the advanced nature of their tumor, such as early satiety and WEIGHT LOSS.

DIAGNOSIS

The diagnosis of stomach cancer is most commonly made by performing a stomach ENDOSCOPY with BIOPSY of a suspicious lesion. Barium-enhanced X rays (RADIOGRAPHY) of the upper gastrointestinal tract may also lead to the discovery of the disease. COMPUTED TOMOGRAPHY of the abdomen is later performed to determine the extent of the cancer at diagnosis.

COMPLICATIONS

Complications include
- Bleeding from the tumor, leading to ANEMIA
- Rupture of the tumor, resulting in ACUTE ABDOMINAL PAIN
- Other complications in advanced cancer

TREATMENT

SELF TREATMENT:
Abstinence from tobacco and alcohol and maintenance of a well-balanced diet will help during treatment of this disease.

MEDICAL TREATMENT:
Treatment with antacids and ulcer medications such as cimetidine and ranitidine are most helpful in the control of pain.

At present there is no role for treatment with chemotherapy in early stomach cancer, but chemotherapy may be used to treat patients with advanced cancer. Its use may result in shrinkage of up to 50 percent of stomach cancer and may result in improved control of symptoms.

SURGICAL TREATMENT:
Total gastrectomy (removal of the entire stomach) offers the best chance of cure.

PREVENTION

Abstinence from tobacco and alcohol may help decrease the chance of stomach cancer.

Screening programs for gastric cancer have been instituted in Japan where this cancer is responsible for 40 percent of cancer deaths. Screening has resulted in improved survival.

STROKE

More than any other organ, the brain depends on an adequate supply of oxygen. If part of the brain is deprived of oxygen, it becomes damaged or dies—this is a stroke.

CAUSES

Some of the possible causes include
- HEART VALVE DISEASE, which can lead to the formation of blood clots that can break off and flow to the brain, where they block smaller arteries
- ATHEROSCLEROSIS, which can cause build-up of plaque along the walls of the arteries, potentially blocking flow because of narrowing of the artery or plaque breaking off and causing blockages farther downstream
- ARRHYTHMIAS or ATRIAL FIBRILLATION
- Polycythemia
- Weak spots in the blood vessels of the brain that rupture (ANEURYSM)
- HYPERTENSION—the single most important cause

The major risk factors for stroke are
- Age older than 60 years
- Smoking
- High blood pressure (HYPERTENSION)
- DIABETES
- ATRIAL FIBRILLATION
- Previous stroke or transient ischemic attack

SYMPTOMS

The symptoms of stroke can be very diverse. They include
- Weakness in one part of the body
- Drooping of the face
- Difficulty walking
- VISION DISTURBANCES, such as double vision
- NUMBNESS of the face or an extremity

If any of these symptoms are temporary and resolve in a matter of minutes or hours, it is a transient ischemic attack, which can be a warning sign of an impending stroke. The fact that they resolve should *not* reassure the patient into delaying medical evaluation.

DIAGNOSIS

A MEDICAL HISTORY and PHYSICAL EXAMINATION are performed. Other tests include
- COMPUTED TOMOGRAPHY of the brain
- MAGNETIC RESONANCE IMAGING of the brain
- ULTRASOUND to evaluate the blood flow
- ELECTROCARDIOGRAPHY
- BLOOD COUNT

COMPLICATIONS

A stroke is as life threatening as a HEART ATTACK and can cause permanent neurologic damage and death.

TREATMENT

SELF TREATMENT:
None.

MEDICAL TREATMENT:
The main course of treatment is the intravenous administration of powerful blood thinners such as heparin. This treatment is appropriate in only certain types of strokes; it can be harmful in others.

SURGICAL TREATMENT:
(See Prevention below.)

PREVENTION

Reducing risk factors includes
- Avoiding smoking
- Eating a diet low in fat, cholesterol, and sodium
- Maintaining a healthy weight
- Avoiding excessive alcohol intake
- Taking steps to control HYPERTENSION

After a stroke or a transient ischemic attack has occurred, therapies can reduce the risk of another. Antiplatelet drugs such as aspirin or ticlopidine, and anticoagulants such as heparin and warfarin can reduce the risk of blood clot.

CAROTID ENDARTECTOMY, a procedure used to open carotid arteries that have become occluded, can be helpful in a select group of medically stable patients at high risk of stroke.

TESTICULAR CANCER

Testicular cancer is a malignancy that arises in one of the testicles, the paired male reproductive organs that produce sperm and the hormone testosterone.

CAUSES

The cause of testicular cancer is unknown. There is a higher risk of testicular cancer, though, in men with a history of undescended testes (cryptorchidism), but the reason for this connection is unknown.

SYMPTOMS

Testicular cancer usually occurs as a painless swelling or firm nodule in one testicle. This may be accompanied by a dull aching in the scrotum. In about 10 percent of patients, pain in the testicle is present (TESTICLES, PAINFUL OR SWOLLEN).

Occasionally, symptoms may result from the metastatic spread of tumor to other locations, such as the lungs (LUNG CANCER).

DIAGNOSIS

ULTRASOUND examination of the testicle may assist the physician in determining whether a mass in the scrotum is within or outside of the testicle. In patients with a mass within the testicle, testicular cancer must be ruled out. Removal of the abnormal testicle (orchiectomy) through an incision in the groin is the only accepted method of diagnosing testicular cancer.

Once the diagnosis is made, other studies used to determine whether the cancer has spread beyond the testicle include

- BLOOD TESTS
- X rays (RADIOGRAPHY)
- COMPUTED TOMOGRAPHY

COMPLICATIONS

As with all cancers, metastasis of the cancer to other areas in the body is a danger.

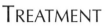

TREATMENT

SELF TREATMENT:

None.

MEDICAL TREATMENT:

Chemotherapy and radiation therapy are most helpful. Because of advances in therapy, 90 percent of patients can be cured of their cancer.

SURGICAL TREATMENT:

Two surgical treatments are used: orchiectomy (removal of the testicle) and retroperitoneal lymph node dissection (removal of lymph nodes in the pelvic region where testicular cancer may spread).

PREVENTION

All men between the ages of 15 and 35 can perform monthly testicular self-exams. The normal coiled, slightly tender structure (the epididymis), found at one pole of each testicle, should not be a cause for concern. Any nodule or abnormal thickening of a testicle should be evaluated by a physician.

THROMBOSIS

There is a delicate balance in the blood between too much and too little clot formation. Too little can lead to bleeding problems; too much can lead to thrombosis.

Thrombosis, or blood clotting, is an essential protective mechanism of the body to help with daily trauma. However, clots can also be problematic. The most common problem is when they form in the deep veins of the legs (called *thrombophlebitis*) and travel downstream, potentially obstructing a blood vessel in the lungs (PULMONARY EMBOLISM). Other problems include clots that form on top of cholesterol plaques in arteries (ATHEROSCLEROSIS), which can lead to HEART ATTACK, STROKE, or gangrene. Clots also form in the heart, in such circumstances as ATRIAL FIBRILLATION or HEART VALVE DISEASE, and can travel downstream to obstruct a blood vessel.

CAUSES

Inappropriate clots may form because of several major risk factors, including
- Vessel damage from ATHEROSCLEROSIS, hip or knee surgery, or trauma
- A slowing of blood flow from immobility on account of obesity, surgery, STROKE, or prolonged travel
- Overactivity of the clotting system because of familial disorders, smoking, cancer, or estrogen therapy

SYMPTOMS

Deep vein thrombosis only causes noticeable symptoms in about half of cases (swelling and leg pain). Once a clot breaks off and obstructs a downstream vessel, it usually causes symptoms (see STROKE; HEART ATTACK; PULMONARY EMBOLISM; and gangrene). Sometimes clots form in an area that is more apparent, such as in HEMORRHOIDS or in VARICOSE VEINS on the surface of the leg (superficial thrombophlebitis). These are not dangerous because of their location but are more often painful and recognized as a tender lump in a vein.

DIAGNOSIS

The diagnosis is based on clues from the MEDICAL HISTORY and PHYSICAL EXAMINATION. Usually, a blood flow study such as an ULTRASOUND is done to check the veins of the leg for signs of clotting. This can be definitive and therapy can be started. If it is inconclusive, then venography (RADIOGRAPHY) is performed, injecting contrast dye into the vein to help visualize the clot.

COMPLICATIONS

Deep-vein thrombosis of the leg can break off and travel to the lung, causing a PULMONARY EMBOLISM. Thrombosis in an artery can cause a STROKE, HEART ATTACK, or gangrene.

TREATMENT

SELF TREATMENT:

Warm compresses and leg elevation may help a superficial thrombophlebitis of the leg.

MEDICAL TREATMENT:

Heparin is the main initial treatment. Clot-dissolving drugs like tissue plasminogen activator (TPA), and streptokinase may be used for more life-threatening thrombosis. The risk of recurrence can be decreased with warfarin or heparin.

Aspirin is used for patients at risk of thrombotic STROKE or HEART ATTACK to decrease the risk of thrombosis.

SURGICAL TREATMENT:

For patients who cannot be on anticoagulants like heparin or for whom the medication fails to work, the large vein in the abdomen (the vena cava) may be interrupted with a filter of some type. The filter can trap subsequent clots to help prevent a life-threatening recurrence. Nowadays these filters can be placed without major surgery by special catheters via the veins with X ray (RADIOGRAPHY) guidance.

A clot in the artery of the leg can sometimes be "fished out" with special plastic tubes (catheters).

Painful clots in HEMORRHOIDS may be removed with a scalpel.

PREVENTION

* Minimizing risk factors of immobility with early mobilization after surgery
* Special elastic or compression stockings on the legs
* Low doses of anticoagulant drugs such as aspirin, heparin, or warfarin in patients at significant risk
* Frequent leg movements on long trips to help keep the blood circulating
* Avoiding smoking
* Avoiding obesity

ULCER

Although ulcers can be temporarily healed by reducing gastric acid, permanent healing requires eradication of the bacteria *Helicobacter pylori.*

An ulcer is a sore that develops in the lining of the stomach or duodenum and visually resembles an excavated crater. The more generic term *peptic ulcer* does not indicate the ulcer's location, whereas *gastric ulcer* and *duodenal ulcer* clearly describe anatomic location and are the preferred terms.

CAUSES

At least 90 to 95 percent of duodenal ulcers and 70 percent of gastric ulcers are associated with the bacteria called *Helicobacter pylori.* Other less frequent causes of ulcers are

- Aspirin or nonsteroidal anti-inflammatory drugs such as ibuprofen
- Excessive amounts of gastric acid secreted in response to hormonal stimulation by an intra-abdominal tumor (Zollinger-Ellison syndrome)

SYMPTOMS

Localized discomfort, typically a dull ache rather than a severe pain, just below the end of the breast bone, usually occuring one to two hours after meals. The discomfort may be temporarily alleviated with food or antacids. It may occur in the middle of the night, and it is typically intermittent, with days or weeks separating episodes of distress.

DIAGNOSIS

At times, the diagnosis may be made by the physician based on typical symptoms without need for diagnostic testing. However, further tests might include

- BLOOD TESTS to detect exposure to *Helicobacter pylori*
- Gastroscopy (a form of ENDOSCOPY), allowing the physician to biopsy tissue (BIOPSY), assessing for the presence of *Helicobacter pylori*
- Barium X rays (RADIOGRAPHY) of the stomach and duodenum
- Breath tests, in which expired air from a patient is collected in a small bag after the patient consumes a pudding treated with minute amounts of radioactively labeled carbon, to diagnose *Helicobacter pylori* infection quickly (This test is under development and is not yet widely available.)

COMPLICATIONS

Complications are fairly rare. Ulcers may bleed internally, at times without prior symptoms. The bleeding may be noted as black, loose stool (STOOL, ABNORMAL APPEARANCE) or, more rarely, as VOMITING of dark, "coffee-ground" material or obvious blood.

If ulcers recur chronically, the outlet of the stomach and duodenum into the small intestine may become narrowed, causing obstruction. This results in the sensation of immediate fullness after meals, episodes of VOMITING or regurgitation, and at times VOMITING of undigested food, many hours after a meal.

Ulcers may also perforate into the abdominal cavity or adjacent organs, resulting in severe, intractable ABDOMINAL PAIN and FEVER; peritonitis, and even BLOOD POISONING.

TREATMENT

SELF TREATMENT:

Dietary adjustments do not have a major impact on ulcer disease. The previously held belief that milk, cream, and bland foods are beneficial has not held up to medical scrutiny. Patients should avoid foods that upset their stomach, and each individual may have different food sensitivities. A regular meal schedule (avoiding long periods of not eating) should be followed, simply because food within the stomach buffers stomach acid. Coffee and tea (both caffeinated and decaffeinated) and alcohol should be avoided. Tobacco should be totally avoided.

MEDICAL TREATMENT:

Oral antacids (many available over the counter) can help alleviate symptoms.

Antibiotics to eradicate *Helicobacter pylori* include
- Metronidazole
- Amoxicillin
- Tetracycline
- Azithromycin
- Bismuth products (these are used in combination with antibiotics to eradicate *Helicobacter pylori;* use of bismuth alone is not effective)
- Pepto-Bismol

Histamine$_2$-receptor antagonists that suppress stomach acid production include
- Cimetidine
- Ranitidine
- Famotidine
- Nizatidine

Proton pump inhibitors that suppress stomach acid production include
- Omeprazole
- Lansoprazole

Other effective agents include
- Sucralfate
- Misoprostol

SURGICAL TREATMENT:

Surgery (peptic ulcer surgery) is primarily reserved for the complications of ulcer and is very rarely done today for symptoms not responding to medical treatment. Surgical procedures include
- Vagotomy and pyloroplasty
- Highly selective vagotomy
- Antrectomy with Billroth I or II anastomosis

PREVENTION

No good preventive measures are available. Since this is in large part a bacterial infection, improvement in general sanitation has decreased the incidence of ulcer in underdeveloped countries. Researchers are working on possible vaccines against *Helicobacter pylori,* which may be useful in areas of the nonindustrialized world where the infection seems to start at an early age.

ULCERATIVE COLITIS

Ulcerative colitis is an inflammatory condition that causes ulceration of the inner lining of the large intestine. When only the lower part of the large intestine is involved, it is called *ulcerative proctitis;* when the entire colon is involved, it is called *ulcerative colitis.* Unlike CROHN DISEASE, it does not involve the small intestine.

CAUSES

As in CROHN DISEASE, the specific cause of ulcerative colitis is not known. Most recent research suggests that the body's immune system is reacting against some substance in the digestive tract that induces the body's own defenses to produce an inflammatory response. It remains quite unclear as to what this foreign substance is, though.

SYMPTOMS

- Loose, frequently bloody stools (STOOL, ABNORMAL APPEARANCE)
- Urgency to have a bowel movement
- Sense of incomplete evacuation
- Crampy ABDOMINAL PAIN
- Skin RASH or painful lumps in the skin
- Joint pain or pain in the lower back

DIAGNOSIS

In addition to a thorough PHYSICAL EXAMINATION, barium X rays (RADIOGRAPHY) of the lower bowel or sigmoidoscopy or colonoscopy (forms of ENDOSCOPY) are needed to diagnose ulcerative colitis. A BLOOD TEST to detect antineutrophilic cytoplasmic antibody is being used by researchers in an attempt to learn more about various subtypes of ulcerative colitis.

COMPLICATIONS

On rare occasion, the ulcerative colitis may become severe and not respond to medical therapy, resulting in fulminant colitis. Patients with this condition are quite ill with
- FEVER
- Intractable DIARRHEA
- RECTAL BLEEDING
- ABDOMINAL SWELLING

Although any age group can be affected by ulcerative colitis, it tends to begin between the ages of 15 and 40.

A few patients may develop large, nonhealing sores on the skin (pyoderma gangrenosum) or inflammation of the bile ducts of the liver (sclerosing cholangitis) (see CHOLECYSTITIS AND CHOLANGITIS).

Some people with chronic ulcerative colitis have an increased risk of developing COLORECTAL CANCER. This risk is primarily restricted to those patients with involvement of the entire colon who have had the disease for more than 10 years.

TREATMENT

SELF TREATMENT:

Good nutrition is essential. Although specific foods play no role in causing ulcerative colitis, soft, bland foods may be better tolerated and cause less discomfort when the disease is active. A unique association between discontinuing smoking and flare-ups of ulcerative colitis has been noted in several studies. The general health risks of smoking, however, greatly outweigh any potential benefit.

MEDICAL TREATMENT:

Medications that can be helpful in the condition include
- Sulfasalazine
- Mesalamine (pill and enema formulations)
- Olsalazine
- Corticosteroids, such as prednisone and methyl-prednisolone
- 6-mercaptopurine
- Azathioprine

SURGICAL TREATMENT:

Surgery is usually reserved for those patients with unremitting symptoms unresponsive to medical treatment, or in instances of fulminant colitis. Unlike CROHN DISEASE, where surgery is not curative, removal of the entire colon will cure ulcerative colitis (see ILEOSTOMY).

PREVENTION

Very long-term use of such medications as sulfasalazine or mesalamine may keep the disease in remission, preventing relapses.

UTERINE CANCER

Endometrial carcinoma, cancer of the lining of the uterus, is the fourth most common malignancy in women in the United States, behind BREAST CANCER, bowel cancer (COLORECTAL CANCER), and LUNG CANCER. Overall, about two to three percent of women will develop endometrial cancer.

CAUSES

There are several risk factors for the development of endometrial cancer, including
- A history of infertility and MENSTRUAL IRREGULARITIES
- Late natural menopause
- Obesity
- Estrogen replacement therapy without progestins
- DIABETES

SYMPTOMS

Approximately 90 percent of women with endometrial carcinoma will have VAGINAL BLEEDING as their only symptom. Fortunately, most women recognize the importance of this symptom and seek medical consultation within three months.

DIAGNOSIS

PHYSICAL EXAMINATION seldom reveals any evidence of endometrial carcinoma, although obesity and HYPERTENSION are commonly associated constitutional factors. Endometrial BIOPSY is the accepted first step in evaluating a woman with abnormal uterine bleeding (VAGINAL BLEEDING; MENSTRUAL IRREGULARITIES) or suspected endometrial problems.

A PAP SMEAR is an unreliable diagnostic test in the evaluation of uterine cancer, since only 30 to 50 percent of women with endometrial cancer will have an abnormal PAP SMEAR. (Its main role is detecting CERVICAL CANCER.)

Hysteroscopy (a form of ENDOSCOPY) and DILATION AND CURETTAGE should be reserved for situations in which an office endometrial BIOPSY cannot be performed, bleeding recurs after a negative BIOPSY, or the specimen obtained is inadequate to explain the bleeding.

Transvaginal ULTRASOUND may be a useful adjunct to endometrial BIOPSY for evaluating abnormal uterine bleeding (VAGINAL BLEEDING; MENSTRUAL IRREGULARITIES) and for selecting women for additional testing.

The overall five-year survival rate for women with endometrial cancer is 73 percent.

COMPLICATIONS

Some women experience pelvic pressure or discomfort indicative of uterine enlargement or disease spread. Bleeding may not have occurred because of cervical stenosis (in which the cervix blocks the blood from passing out of the uterus) and may be associated with the collection of blood within the uterine cavity and a worse prognosis.

TREATMENT

SELF TREATMENT:

None.

MEDICAL TREATMENT:

Medical therapy is secondary to surgical treatment. Postoperative radiation therapy may result in improved survival. Women with metastatic (spread) disease may benefit from hormonal therapy or chemotherapy.

SURGICAL TREATMENT:

The surgical procedure would minimally include
- Sampling of peritoneal fluid for evaluation (CYTOLOGY)
- Exploration of the abdomen and pelvis with BIOPSY or excision of any suspicious lesions
- Total HYSTERECTOMY
- Removal of both fallopian tubes and ovaries
- Sampling of lymph nodes in the pelvis and alongside the abdominal aorta

PREVENTION

Screening for endometrial cancer should currently not be undertaken because of the lack of an appropriate, cost-effective, and acceptable test that reduces mortality. Abnormal perimenopausal and postmenopausal uterine bleeding (VAGINAL BLEEDING; MENSTRUAL IRREGULARITIES) should always be taken seriously and properly investigated.

VAGINITIS

Vaginitis is an inflammation of the vagina that can cause bothersome symptoms. Vaginitis is a common problem that, although annoying, does not pose major health problems if treated promptly.

CAUSES

Vaginitis is usually a result of some infectious agent, although other irritants can cause inflammation as well. Frequent causes of vaginitis include
- *Candida* organisms (a yeast infection)
- *Trichomonas* organisms
- Bacterial vaginosis
- Lack of estrogen in postmenopausal women
- A foreign body, such as a lost tampon, in the vagina

SYMPTOMS

The symptoms of vaginitis include
- Vaginal ITCHING and burning
- VAGINAL DISCHARGE
- Foul odor

DIAGNOSIS

The symptoms themselves can usually point to the diagnosis of vaginitis. Important information for the physician to know in the patient's MEDICAL HISTORY includes
- The character of the VAGINAL DISCHARGE, especially whether it is itchy or odorous
- Any new sexual partners, since some causes of vaginitis are sexually transmitted
- Use of douches, since they can cause a chemical reaction
- Recent treatment with antibiotics
- Any new medications, such as oral contraceptives
- Any medical problems, such as DIABETES

To diagnose the cause of vaginitis, a PHYSICAL EXAMINATION of the vulva, or entrance to the vagina, and the vagina will be done. A sample of the VAGINAL DISCHARGE is obtained and examined under a microscope.

If the cause of the vaginitis is sexually transmitted, CULTURES for CHLAMYDIA and gonorrhea and a BLOOD TEST for syphilis and human immunodeficiency virus (HIV) are sometimes warranted.

Vaginitis is an inflammation that can usually be treated with antibiotics or vaginal creams.

COMPLICATIONS

Infections need to be treated promptly to avoid progression. Unattended vaginitis could potentially progress to wider infection, PELVIC INFLAMMATORY DISEASE, and infertility.

TREATMENT

SELF TREATMENT:

If the patient has had documented yeast infections in the past and experiences the classic recurrent symptoms (ITCHING and thick, white, odorous VAGINAL DISCHARGE), self treatment with over-the-counter clotrimazole may be appropriate.

MEDICAL TREATMENT:

- For vaginitis caused by candidal organisms, treatment is usually a vaginal cream or suppository. An oral medication (fluconazole) is also available.
- For a trichomonal vaginitis, an oral antibiotic (metronidazole) is prescribed. It is important that both sexual partners receive treatment simultaneously, or the infection can recur.
- For bacterial vaginosis, treatment is usually an oral antibiotic (metronidazole) or vaginal cream. Sometimes this infection can be sexually transmitted and the partner or partners needs treatment also.

SURGICAL TREATMENT:

None.

PREVENTION

Strategies to help prevention of vaginitis include
- Taking showers rather than baths
- Wearing cotton panties or pantyhose with a cotton crotch rather than nylon
- Wiping from front to back after urination or bowel movements
- Avoiding frequent douching
- Limiting sweets and increasing yogurt intake
- Maintaining a healthy body weight
- Limiting the number of sexual partners and employing safe-sex techniques

VARICOSE VEINS

Varicose veins are dilated curving veins usually on the legs. Veins return blood to the heart and lungs to be reoxygenated and then to be recirculated to the rest of the body via the arteries.

The pressure in veins is much lower than in the arteries, so blood's return trip via the veins is more difficult, especially since it's uphill most of the time from the legs when standing or sitting. The veins normally have one-way valves that help blood flow back toward the heart, but in varicose veins, the valves often fail, allowing blood to pool and contributing to the swelling problem.

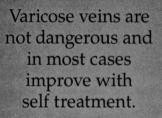

Varicose veins are not dangerous and in most cases improve with self treatment.

CAUSES

Although hereditary factors play a major role for many people, other causes include
- Prolonged standing or sitting
- Obesity
- Lack of exercise
- Age
- Pregnancy
- Anything that causes long-term obstructions of the veins

Women are more often affected than men.

SYMPTOMS

The symptoms are
- Swollen, knotted, visible veins
- Swelling in the legs (ANKLE SWELLING)
- In long-standing cases, SKIN CHANGES such as discoloration, ITCHING, skin ulcers, and other skin breakdown problems

DIAGNOSIS

The diagnosis is apparent from seeing the veins on the legs. Blood flow studies (ULTRASOUND) may be used to document problems in the deeper veins under the muscles of the legs that are not visible on the surface.

COMPLICATIONS

- The skin breakdown (SKIN CHANGES) can lead to infections and ulceration.
- A clot may form in the vein and cause a tender swollen lump (a superficial thrombophlebitis). This is not dangerous.

TREATMENT

SELF TREATMENT:
- Tight belts or stockings that constrict the legs at the top should be avoided; they can make the obstruction to the vein flow worse.
- Elastic stockings specifically made for leg swelling should be worn. Care should be taken if the skin becomes dry or begins to break down.
- Elevation of the legs whenever possible during the day and at night helps, especially if the legs are raised a few inches above the level of the heart.

MEDICAL TREATMENT:
Diuretics such as hydrochlorothiazide may be used if necessary for severe swelling, but the self-treatment measures are preferred.

SURGICAL TREATMENT:
Sclerotherapy (injection of chemicals that shrink the vein) and surgical removal (VARICOSE VEIN REMOVAL) are reserved for the most bothersome cases.

PREVENTION

Persons with varicose veins should avoid obesity and prolonged standing or sitting and should adhere to a regimen of regular exercise.

TESTS & SURGERIES

ALLERGY TESTING

When patients have symptoms that may be a result of an allergic reaction, allergy testing can help identify the item that triggered the reaction (the item is called an *allergen*). However, because people can have positive reactions to allergy tests but not experience noticeable symptoms when exposed to the substance, the results of such testing must be interpreted carefully.

Allergy tests are most helpful for evaluating symptoms of hay fever. They play a smaller role in investigating causes of reactions such as ASTHMA and hives. Their use in evaluating food allergies is more uncertain, and they are probably unwarranted in the general evaluation of nonspecific symptoms such as FATIGUE.

There are a number of ways to test for allergies. The most certain way is to challenge and rechallenge a person to the item to which they are supposed to be allergic. That is, expose the person, look for a reaction, and repeat the same procedure again later to be certain. However, given the time and confounding factors, this approach is not always practical. The two most common methods for allergy testing are

- Skin tests in which the skin's reaction to a potential allergen is monitored
- Radioallergosorbent tests (RAST) or other BLOOD TESTS in which the laboratory searches for specific immunologic substances in the blood

PREPARATION

Because they modify the body's reaction to allergens, antihistamines and prednisone should be discontinued before various types of skin tests.

ANESTHESIA

None.

PROCEDURE

For skin testing
- A drop of purified allergen is placed on the skin.
- A small prick with a needle is made at the site to allow the allergen to come in contact with the immune system.

- If a hive forms within minutes, the test is positive
  and complete, but if the result is negative or unclear,
  a small amount of the allergen may be injected
  directly into the skin with a needle to be sure the
  test is not positive.

When skin testing some types of allergens, especially metals such as nickel, the material may be taped against the skin for a few days rather than injected.

For RAST and other BLOOD TESTS, blood is drawn from a vein and analyzed in special laboratories for specific antibodies to certain allergens. This method is particularly useful for fungal reactions and when investigating certain rare occupational exposures that cause lung symptoms. RAST is easy and widely available, but it is expensive and fraught with false-positive results.

HOSPITAL RECOVERY

Patients are observed for at least 15 minutes after skin testing so that any generalized reaction (see below) can be treated promptly.

AT-HOME RECOVERY

None.

COMPLICATIONS AND RISKS

In rare cases, skin tests may cause more than a local reaction on the skin. Examples of more drastic reactions include
- Wheezing
- Low blood pressure
- Diffuse hives (RASH)
- BREATHING DIFFICULTY or SWALLOWING DIFFICULTIES
  from swelling of the throat

Severe local reactions can be treated with topical hydrocortisone.

For RAST, the main "risks" are incurring the expense of further testing due to false-positive results.

ANEURYSM, REMOVAL OF

Aneurysms can be life threatening, and if they rupture, the results are often catastrophic. Prompt repair of unstable aneurysms is crucial.

An ANEURYSM is a bulging out or ballooning of a blood vessel. There are two main dangers associated with an ANEURYSM: 1) Clots can form within the ballooned out area; and 2) The weakness of the wall can cause the vessel to rupture.

ANEURYSMS most often develop in the aorta, the body's largest blood vessel, in the chest portion leading from the heart or in the abdominal portion before the aorta divides into branches that provide blood to the legs. When an aortic ANEURYSM is threatening to rupture and the risk of surgery is warranted, a thoracic or vascular surgeon will repair or remove it. In some cases an interventional radiologist may also be able to repair an ANEURYSM using special devices passed through the blood vessels.

Cerebral ANEURYSMS of the brain blood vessels are usually repaired by a neurosurgeon. An ANEURYSM can also occur in the heart muscle and require repair.

ALTERNATIVE TREATMENTS

Not all ANEURYSMS need to be operated on. If the ANEURYSM is relatively small and not causing any problems, it can be monitored for expansion over a period of years using ULTRASOUND. Some blood pressure-lowering medicines, such as metoprolol and propranolol, can help slow or stabilize progressive expansion.

PREOPERATIVE PREPARATION

COMPUTED TOMOGRAPHY, ULTRASOUND, and angiograms (RADIOGRAPHY) are all used to define the extent and size of the ANEURYSM. Because the surgery is more stressful to the heart than most other operations and most people with ANEURYSMS have some degree of heart disease, special tests of the heart, such as a CARDIAC STRESS TEST, are also often performed.

Overnight fasting is required with general anesthesia.

ANESTHESIA

General anesthesia is necessary, and a heart-lung machine may also be needed.

Newer techniques that involve placement of special devices called *stents* inside an ANEURYSM can be performed under local anesthesia.

PROCEDURE

For aortic ANEURYSMS in the chest or abdomen
- An incision is made in the chest or abdomen along the midline.
- The ANEURYSM is located and the vessel is clamped off above and below the ANEURYSM site.
- The diseased section is removed and replaced with a synthetic pipe that is sized and sewn into place.
- The incision is then closed with sutures.

For some patients, a new technique may be possible using special grafts (stents) that can be placed inside the ANEURYSM and secured into place using plastic tubes (catheters) guided through the blood vessels and manipulated with the help of X rays (RADIOGRAPHY).

HOSPITAL RECOVERY

- The hospital stay is usually about seven to ten days, often with the first day in the intensive care unit.
- If the chest cavity was opened for surgery, chest tubes (drainage tubes that run under the rib cage to collection containers) are usually needed.
- A catheter in the bladder to drain urine for a day or two is common.

AT-HOME RECOVERY

- Activity can be gradually increased with full recovery in about four to six weeks.
- Synthetic grafts can become infected, so prophylactic antibiotics may be recommended before any subsequent procedures.

COMPLICATIONS AND RISKS

- Excessive bleeding
- Loss of blood flow to nearby branch arteries leading to damage of the areas they feed—for example, the spinal nerves (causing paralysis), the intestines (causing gangrene of the bowel), and the kidneys (causing kidney damage or KIDNEY FAILURE)
- Infection of the wound or graft

ANGIOPLASTY

Angioplasty, a relatively new technique in the treatment of vascular diseases, is now one of the most frequently performed cardiovascular procedures in the United States.

Angioplasty is used to shape the inside of a blood vessel to improve blood flow past blockages (see ATHEROSCLEROSIS). Various techniques to open up blockages in arteries using devices on long plastic tubes have been developed, but the most commonly used device is a narrow, inflatable, one- to two-inch-long balloon attached to a long plastic tube called a catheter.

The catheter is usually inserted through a hole punctured through the skin into the arteries in the groin and is then passed up to the target vessel until the balloon is placed alongside a blockage. It is then inflated to force an increase in the interior space of the vessel.

Besides balloons, other related devices include rotating small blades, drill-like devices, and lasers. The target vessels are usually partially occluded arteries to the heart (causing ANGINA) or large vessels in the leg (causing claudication—pain in the legs during activity that is relieved by rest).

ALTERNATIVE TREATMENTS

Angioplasty is best used when surgery (such as CORONARY ARTERY BYPASS GRAFT SURGERY) is otherwise necessary and when medications are not enough. Medications for ANGINA (one indication for angioplasty) include nitroglycerin, calcium channel blockers (diltiazem), and beta-blockers (metoprolol, atenolol). Medications for claudication usually provide a modest benefit.

PREOPERATIVE PREPARATION

A CARDIAC STRESS TEST and angiogram X ray (RADIOGRAPHY) are helpful in selecting the right patients for angioplasty and planning the procedure.

ANESTHESIA

Local anesthesia is all that is needed, but a surgical team and general anesthesia are usually available on standby.

PROCEDURE

- The balloon catheter is inserted into an artery in the thigh or occasionally in the upper arm.

- The catheter is guided with the help of RADIOGRAPHY to the site of the blockage.
- The balloon is inflated and deflated repeatedly to expand the opening of the blocked artery.
- X rays (RADIOGRAPHY), pressure readings, and ULTRASOUND images may be used to evaluate the vessel before and after the procedure.
- The catheter is withdrawn, and the opening to the entry artery is compressed or repaired.

HOSPITAL RECOVERY

- One to two days in the hospital may be required to allow the insertion site to start healing safely.
- The heart is monitored closely for the first 24 hours with continuous ELECTROCARDIOGRAPHY.
- Intravenous blood thinners, such as heparin and aspirin, may be used to reduce the chance of a clot forming where the lining of the artery is disrupted.

AT-HOME RECOVERY

For the first week or two, patients should generally avoid vigorous exercise involving bending at the insertion site.

COMPLICATIONS AND RISKS

Bleeding at the insertion site after the catheter is removed is the most common complication. The bleeding can be under the skin and may show up as an enlarging lump or as increasing pain in the area.

More serious but rare complications include

- Allergic reactions to the X ray contrast material, or dye, that is used to make the artery more visible during the procedure (see RADIOGRAPHY)
- Tearing, perforating, or completely occluding the target artery, possibly leading to HEART ATTACK and even death (very rare)

A few percent of patients may need emergency bypass surgery to help deal with these complications. (See CORONARY ARTERY BYPASS GRAFT SURGERY.)

BIOPSY

Because biopsy is usually the definitive test for certain diseases, and because many different tests can be run on a biopsy sample, the test is extremely helpful in diagnosis.

A biopsy is a procedure in which a small sample of tissue is taken from a particular part of the body so that it can be prepared and examined under a microscope. More advanced tests may also be done on this tissue sample, such as CULTURES for viruses or other germs. Often biopsies are used to check for cancer, but many other uses exist.

PREPARATION

Most biopsies don't require any preparation. If a sample is to be taken from the linings of the lungs or the gastrointestinal tract, fasting can minimize any risk of vomiting.

ANESTHESIA

Almost all biopsies are done with local anesthesia. Rarely, general anesthesia might be necessary if the biopsy is to be taken from a difficult area (for example, a brain biopsy).

PROCEDURE

The exact procedure varies with each biopsy location. Special scopes through which small samples can be removed are commonly used for biopsies of the gastrointestinal tract and lung (see ENDOSCOPY). Special catheters passed through the veins or arteries can be used in a biopsy of the heart (CARDIAC CATHETERIZATION). COMPUTED TOMOGRAPHY or ULTRASOUND can guide certain biopsies of internal organs using special needles passed through the skin directly to the organ.

RECOVERY

In most cases, biopsies are performed on an outpatient basis, and patients are released the same day. Observation can range from a few minutes for skin biopsy to hours or overnight for biopsy of an internal organ.

COMPLICATIONS AND RISKS

A biopsy is a relatively simple and safe procedure. Bleeding or infection are always a possibility but are rare. Some organs can be perforated during a biopsy and may require surgery; this complication is also rare.

BLADDER REMOVAL

Surgical removal of the bladder involves removing the bladder and creating a so-called urinary diversion, in which a segment of bowel is used to connect the ureters to a stoma—an opening to the outside of the abdomen. This urinary diversion allows urine to drain out into a collecting pouch on the outside of the body.

The surgery is performed by a urologist or general surgeon in a hospital setting.

ALTERNATIVE TREATMENTS

In some patients, a combination of radiation therapy and chemotherapy can replace surgery.

PREOPERATIVE PREPARATION

Cystoscopy (a form of ENDOSCOPY) and a BIOPSY of the tumor are usually necessary to confirm the diagnosis and determine the extent of the cancer.

The surgery requires a complete bowel preparation involving antibiotics and enemas to clean out the colon and decrease the chance of infection after surgery.

Overnight fasting is required with general anesthesia.

ANESTHESIA

General anesthesia.

PROCEDURE

- An incision is made in the lower portion of the abdomen over the bladder.
- The ureters from the kidneys to the bladder are identified and cut.
- The bladder is removed. Frequently, the prostate (in men) or uterus and ovaries (in women) are removed during this same procedure, as well.
- A conduit is fashioned from a section of the small intestine.
- The conduit is connected to the ureters on one end and the skin on the other.

> Surgical removal of the bladder is usually performed only in the case of invasive bladder cancer.

- A stoma, or opening in the skin, is created for the collecting device, which can be fitted tightly with an appliance to hold it in place.
- The incision is closed with sutures.

HOSPITAL RECOVERY

- The hospital stay is usually about 10 to 14 days, often with the first day spent in the intensive care unit.
- An intravenous line remains in place for about seven days until bowel function returns.

AT-HOME RECOVERY

- Strenuous activity must be restricted for about six weeks.
- A nurse may visit the patient in the home or while he or she is still in the hospital to teach the patient self-care techniques for the stoma site.
- Minor postoperative pain may require oral pain medication such as acetaminophen and codeine combination.

COMPLICATIONS AND RISKS

- Delayed return of bowel function, signaled by an inability to eat and keep down food
- Leakage from one of the urine connections, signaled by FEVER and excessive drainage from the surgical wound

BLOOD COUNT

Red blood cells carry oxygen to all parts of the body using the protein hemoglobin. White blood cells help fight infections. Smaller bits of tissue called platelets help seal leaks in blood vessels and aid in the formation of blood clots. Blood counts are the measurement of all three of these items in the blood.

PREPARATION

No special preparation is required for a blood count. Fasting, for example, is not required for a blood count as it is for some other BLOOD TESTS.

PROCEDURE

Blood is usually drawn from a vein in the middle of the arm, but other sites can be used in special circumstances. The procedure is usually as follows:

- A tourniquet is applied to the upper arm for a short period to enlarge the vein, making it easier to see and get blood from.
- The vein site is swabbed with alcohol or iodine to prevent infection.
- A sterile needle punctures the vein (a procedure called *venipuncture*) and suction draws out the required amount of blood.
- A dressing (bandage) is then applied. It can usually be removed in a few hours.

COMPLICATIONS AND RISKS

A bruise at the site of the venipuncture is the most common complication. An infection at the site is possible but extremely rare.

One of the most common laboratory blood tests, a blood count can help make the diagnosis of anemia or assess the body's response to an infection or its ability to fight one.

BLOOD PRESSURE TEST

Most people can learn to take their own blood pressure measurements, but it is necessary to do it carefully to get the most accurate results.

Blood pressure is one of the "vital signs." Chronic high blood pressure (HYPERTENSION) can contribute to many diseases, and because it causes no symptoms, monitoring it with this test is crucial.

PREPARATION

The patient should be sitting quietly for a few minutes, comfortably resting the arm to be measured at chest height.

PROCEDURE

- A blood pressure cuff is wrapped around the upper arm.
- The pressure is raised in the cuff with a pump until it is well above the patient's blood pressure, so that no flow is getting under the cuff.
- Very slowly, the pressure is released, and using a stethoscope, the person performing the test listens for the sound of blood flowing through the artery.
- When the pulse can be heard, the pressure of the cuff is recorded. This first number (the *systolic* pressure) is the peak pressure of the blood with each heartbeat.
- The pressure in the cuff continues to go down until the sound of the pulse momentarily disappears again, and the pressure of the cuff is recorded again. This is the second number (the *diastolic* pressure). It represents the lowest the blood pressure gets between heartbeats.
- The two measurements are normally written together: for example, *120/80*.

RECOVERY

The only recovery consists of waiting the minute or two for the blood flow in the arm to return to normal. (It is not uncommon for the lower arm and hand to have the sensation of "pins and needles" for a few moments.)

COMPLICATIONS AND RISKS

None.

BLOOD TESTS

Much can be learned from the chemistry of the blood, and there are many different laboratory tests that can be performed on a single sample. With the exception of different amounts of blood needed for different tests, the procedure for blood tests varies little as far as the patient is concerned.

Common tests include liver and kidney function, blood mineral balance, blood cholesterol levels, and blood sugar levels.

Screening tests for blood cholesterol and blood sugar levels are often performed on certain age groups and populations identified as being at risk for certain diseases (such as ATHEROSCLEROSIS or DIABETES) and are a reasonable and effective way to prevent some health problems.

Blood tests are performed for many reasons. They can be used to screen for disease in apparently healthy people, to help make a diagnosis, or to monitor the progress of a disease or treatment.

PREPARATION

Fasting for three or more hours may be necessary for some specific blood tests. Ask your doctor beforehand.

PROCEDURE

Blood is usually drawn from a vein in the middle of the arm, but other sites can be used in special circumstances. The procedure is usually as follows:

- A tourniquet is applied to the upper arm for a short period to enlarge the vein, making it easier to see and get blood from.
- The vein site is swabbed with alcohol or iodine to prevent infection.
- A sterile needle punctures the vein (a procedure called *venipuncture*) and suction draws out the required amount of blood.
- A dressing (bandage) is then applied. It can usually be removed in a few hours.

COMPLICATIONS AND RISKS

A bruise at the site is the most common complication. An infection at the site is possible but extremely rare.

False alarm test results can also be considered a common "complication" of using blood tests to screen healthy people. Approximately 50 percent of healthy people who have a 20-item blood panel performed will have at least one false-positive test result.

CARDIAC CATHETERIZATION

The definitive test for atherosclerosis of the heart is cardiac catheterization with coronary angiography. It is used to plan most heart surgeries.

A catheter is a long plastic tube that can be inserted into a vein or artery and can be manipulated with the help of RADIOGRAPHY. In a cardiac catheterization, catheters are passed up to the heart. Dye can be injected into the coronary arteries and into heart chambers in order to film the blood flow into and out of the chambers with RADIOGRAPHY.

Pressure measurements can also be made that help check heart valve function (see HEART VALVE DISEASE). The X-ray films of the arteries help identify any blockages that could interfere with blood flow to the heart muscle (as a result of ATHEROSCLEROSIS, for example).

PREPARATION

For individuals with a known allergy to the contrast dye, special preparation with medicines is useful in reducing allergic reactions. A cardiac catheterization is performed in patients who have fasted at least four to six hours, unless it's an emergency.

ANESTHESIA

Local anesthetic is used at the site where the catheter is inserted.

PROCEDURE

- A vein, artery, or one of each in the arm or leg is chosen as the entry point.
- The vessel is penetrated with a needle, or a small surgical incision is performed (a "cut down") to isolate the vessel.
- Guide wires are used to thread catheters up to the heart and to change to differently shaped catheters for different tasks.
- Pressure readings are recorded.
- A blood thinner such as heparin is given to minimize the chance of blood clots forming on or in the catheters.
- Dye may be injected by hand with a syringe, or a higher-volume pump may be used to take certain pictures.

- When the procedure is done, the catheters are removed and pressure is carefully applied to allow the entrance site to seal. If a "cut down" was necessary, the artery or vein is sewn and the skin sutured closed.

HOSPITAL RECOVERY

- Usually, patients may walk cautiously after six hours if the leg was the entry point, although overnight bed rest is common.
- An intravenous line with fluids is maintained initially.
- Patients may be released the next day, although some hospitals may let patients go home in the evening after a morning procedure.

AT-HOME RECOVERY

Avoidance of stressful activity that could affect the puncture site is reasonable for a few days.

COMPLICATIONS AND RISKS

- An allergic reaction to the dye is one of the most common complications, occurring in a few percent of patients.
- Less common but even more severe complications include blood clots forming on the catheters and breaking off and going downstream, possibly leading to a STROKE, HEART ATTACK, or gangrene, depending on where the clot travels.
- Heart rhythm abnormalities (ARRHYTHMIAS) may be seen during dye injections or when catheters touch the inside of the heart.
- The artery that serves as the entry site may be damaged and need additional special repair.
- Approximately 1 in 1,000 patients could have a life-threatening complication progressing to death.

CARDIAC STRESS TEST

This test, sometimes called a treadmill test, involves monitoring the subject's heart as it is put through the paces of moderate to strenuous exercise. In some cases, when strenuous exercise cannot be performed, the state of exertion can be simulated by using certain drugs.

A physician with some additional training in the area or a specially trained nurse or exercise physiologist usually performs a cardiac stress test. Advanced cardiac life-support equipment and a physician trained in its use need to be nearby in case any cardiac problems arise because of the extreme exertion.

PREPARATION

Depending on the type of stress test, certain medications may be suspended before the test. Theophylline and caffeine are avoided for stress tests in which certain drugs are used to affect the heart. Beta-blockers such as atenolol or metoprolol may be suspended before other types of stress tests because of their affect on the circulatory system.

The patient should avoid a large meal prior to the test. Baseline ELECTROCARDIOGRAPHY is checked before the stress is started so that the tester has a point of comparision with which to judge later readings.

PROCEDURE

There are two major categories of cardiac stress tests. The oldest and usually the best method is to use exercise to stress the heart while ELECTROCARDIOGRAPHY and BLOOD PRESSURE TESTING are monitored for changes. The exercise is usually on a treadmill, although stationary bicycles are sometimes used. NUCLEAR MEDICINE or ULTRASOUND techniques may be used during the procedure to assess other aspects of the heart's function.

The second approach uses drugs instead of exercise to stimulate the heart. The patient usually lays down quietly for this type of "stress," and it is most helpful in patients who cannot otherwise achieve the adequate cardiac stress levels through exercise. (This technique is useful for patients with disabilities, for example.)

Many types of stress testing are available nowadays to check blood flow to the heart and overall circulatory function.

RECOVERY

After the stress, the patient is monitored for a minimum of five to six minutes or until the physician feels it is safe to stop. For some NUCLEAR MEDICINE techniques, the patient may have to be scanned for 20 to 30 minutes and return late in the day for a repeat scan.

COMPLICATIONS AND RISKS

Generally, the risks associated with this test are low, and if a patient is so vulnerable to exercise-related stress that a complication does occur, it's better that it happens during the test in a monitored setting with health professionals rather than out on the street or at home.

Complications include
- Changes in heart rhythm (ARRHYTHMIA)
- Low blood pressure
- FAINTING OR FAINTNESS
- HEART ATTACK (rare)
- Cardiac arrest (extremely rare)

The overall risk of life-threatening complication is near 1 in 10,000. However, some patients should have their cardiac stress test deferred. Such patients include those with
- HEART VALVE DISEASE
- Uncontrolled ANGINA
- Uncontrolled high blood pressure (HYPERTENSION)
- Uncontrolled CONGESTIVE HEART FAILURE

CAROTID ENDARTECTOMY

The carotid arteries run through the neck on either side of the Adam's apple up to the brain and are the major source of blood flow to the brain. ATHEROSCLEROSIS can cause enough plaque build-up to interfere with blood flow to the brain or to serve as a site for clot formation, which can lead to either transient ischemic attack or STROKE. In carotid endartectomy, a vascular surgeon, cardiothoracic surgeon, or neurosurgeon opens the carotid artery and cleans out the plaque material in the area that is most problematic.

PREOPERATIVE PREPARATION

Aspirin, which is commonly used to treat transient ischemic attack, may be withheld temporarily before surgery to avoid bleeding complications.

Because approximately 70 percent of the people with ATHEROSCLEROSIS of the carotid artery also have it in their heart, some type of cardiac evaluation, such as ELECTROCARDIOGRAPHY, CARDIAC STRESS TESTING, or CARDIAC CATHETERIZATION, may be warranted, depending on the patient's other risk factors.

ULTRASOUND of the carotid artery and cerebral angiography (RADIOGRAPHY) are usually performed before the surgery is even considered to identify the problem and select the best candidate to benefit from surgical correction.

Overnight fasting is required with general anesthesia.

ANESTHESIA

General anesthesia is the most common, but local anesthesia with an intravenous sedative is an option in some cases.

PROCEDURE

- An incision is made along the neck under the jaw to identify the area of the carotid artery to be opened.
- Clamps are placed on the artery above and below the area of plaque build-up.
- Care is taken to not dislodge any plaque that could travel downstream and cause a STROKE.
- The artery is opened.
- The atherosclerotic debris is carefully removed.
- The artery is sewn closed, and the clamps are removed.
- The skin is sutured closed.

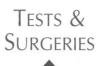

Monitoring by ELECTROENCEPHALOGRAPHY is sometimes done during the procedure in order to detect any complications during the time the patient is under general anesthesia.

HOSPITAL RECOVERY

Patients are usually kept in the hospital for three or four days. Aspirin or other blood thinners such as heparin may be used to decrease the risk of complications and improve blood flow.

AT-HOME RECOVERY

Patients can generally return to work in a few weeks. Wound care, such as cautious cleaning and inspection for signs of infection, is appropriate.

COMPLICATIONS AND RISKS

Carotid endartectomy and the preoperative angiography (RADIOGRAPHY) both carry a significant risk of STROKE. Complication rates vary from one to ten percent or more depending on the hospital and the surgeon. (Generally, hospitals that perform many carotid endartectomies have lower complication rates.)

Because of this significant risk, patients are very carefully selected so that the benefits clearly outweigh the risks. In recent years, the surgery has been reserved for patients who experience significant transient ischemic attacks associated with tight blockages in the carotid arteries. However, it may also modestly benefit patients with tight blockages not causing symptoms if performed at a hospital with a low complication rate.

Besides the risk of stroke, possible complications include excessive bleeding and infection at the wound sight.

CARPAL TUNNEL RELEASE

Surgical carpal tunnel release is recommended for patients who have not obtained relief of symptoms with conservative treatment.

Carpal tunnel release is a surgical procedure to relieve continuous or episodic pressure on the median nerve. Entrapment or compression of the median nerve and its blood supply cause CARPAL TUNNEL SYNDROME.

ALTERNATIVE TREATMENTS

Anti-inflammatory medication, such as ibuprofen or naproxen, given orally or steroids given by injection directly into the area may be helpful. A splint to keep the wrist in a neutral position, worn either full time or at night, may also relieve the symptoms.

PREOPERATIVE PREPARATION

In general, routine diagnostic tests such as ELECTROCARDIO-GRAPHY and BLOOD TESTS may be performed to make an assessment of general health. Specific preparation will depend on the type of setting (hospital, surgical center, or office surgery) in which the procedure will take place.

Overnight fasting is required for general anesthesia.

ANESTHESIA

Adequate anesthesia for a carpal tunnel release can be provided by general anesthesia, regional anesthesia (a nerve block of the arm only), or local anesthesia (a nerve block in the area of the carpal tunnel only).

PROCEDURE

Carpal tunnel release can be done either as an open procedure through a small incision overlying the underside of the wrist, or as an endoscopic procedure through small stab incisions to allow access for instruments and a lighted magnifying endoscope (see ENDOSCOPY).

Regardless of the method employed, the goal of the operation is to release the pressure from the transverse carpal ligament that constricts the space where the median nerve runs next to the tendons of the wrist and finger flexor muscles.

- In the open procedure, the incision is made and the transverse carpal ligament is exposed; in the endoscopic procedure, the instruments are put in place through small stab incisions.
- The ligament is carefully divided, releasing the pressure on the median nerve.
- The incisions in the skin are closed, leaving the cut ligament to heal on its own in the released position.

HOSPITAL RECOVERY

Carpal tunnel release is generally done as an outpatient procedure, so no hospital stay is necessary beyond the time it takes for anesthesia to wear off.

AT-HOME RECOVERY

- The affected arm and hand should remain elevated for 24 to 48 hours after the surgery to decrease swelling.
- The wrist may be placed in a splint or brace to limit the motion of the wrist joint.
- Oral pain medicine, such as an acetaminophen and codeine combination, is generally adequate for pain relief, and may be needed for 10 to 14 days after the operation.
- A period of restricted activity should be expected, and patients are generally advised to limit lifting, carrying, and other wrist movement activities for several weeks.

COMPLICATIONS AND RISKS

As with any surgery, there is a low risk of surgical wound infection; this would be noticed as increased redness, pain, swelling, and drainage from the wound and possibly a low-grade FEVER.

The operation itself may cause some irritation of the median nerve or flexor tendons; increasing NUMBNESS, tingling, or weakness should be evaluated by a physician.

CATARACT REMOVAL

In most cases today, cataract surgery includes removal of the cataract and replacement with a new plastic lens implant. The implanted lens corrects most of the need for glasses after surgery, but glasses may still be needed for reading or far vision.

A CATARACT is an opacity in the clear lens of the eye. The lens is positioned directly behind the colored portion of the eye known as the iris and is important for focusing a clear image on the back of the eye. When a CATARACT forms, visual function may be impaired. If the patient and eye surgeon (the ophthalmologist) agree that cataract surgery is necessary, plans for the operation can be made. The procedure is usually done on an outpatient basis, and the results are extremely successful in the vast majority of cases.

ALTERNATIVE TREATMENTS

Some CATARACTS can change the need for glasses due to a change in the optical properties of the lens. In these cases, adjusting the glasses by increasing the nearsighted correction or reducing the farsighted correction can improve sight.

Some CATARACTS are small and affect visual function because of their central location. In this case, self-administered pupil-dilating eyedrops can allow a patient to see around the cataract and improve eyesight.

If these measures are inadequate to control the problem, cataract surgery may be required.

PREOPERATIVE PREPARATION

Before the operation, the surgeon or a technician will measure the patient for the appropriate implant power. Everyone requires an implant power specific to his or her own eye. The goal is to avoid large differences in spectacle requirements between the two eyes. The power can be adjusted to reduce or eliminate any nearsightedness or farsightedness that may have been present before.

Other preoperative tests can include BLOOD TESTS, ELECTRO-CARDIOGRAPHY (for patients older than 40 years of age), and more sophisticated tests if the patient has complex medical problems.

In general, patients are asked not to eat or drink after midnight the night before surgery if the operation is planned for the morning. A light breakfast may be allowed if the surgery is to be performed in the afternoon. If a patient is on blood pressure or other heart medicine, this should be taken as usual on the morning of surgery. The patient should consult with the eye surgeon and medical doctor about adjusting anti-coagulants, or blood thinning medication, such as heparin, warfarin, and aspirin. Patients with DIABETES may be instructed to modify their medication on the day of surgery, when the diet is being altered.

ANESTHESIA

In most cases, local anesthesia is used for the surgery. The patient is sedated with medication administered through an intravenous line. The eye surgeon or anesthesiologist then injects local anesthetic around the eye, which blocks movement of the eye and lid, numbs the pain fibers, and blurs the vision in the eye. If the patient is unable to lie still for the operation, general anesthesia may be necessary. Some patients may be deemed good candidates for topical anesthesia, in which the surgery is performed with anesthetic eyedrops only and without sedation or general anesthesia.

PROCEDURE

Although there are several techniques available for removing a cataract, the most common today is a procedure called *phacoemulsification*, which takes only 30 to 45 minutes.

- The pupil is dilated widely with eyedrops before the patient is brought to the operating room.
- After anesthetic administration, the skin around the eye is cleansed with special soap, and drapes are positioned so that only the eye to be treated is exposed.
- A device is inserted to separate the eyelids and hold the eye open.
- A small incision (approximately ⅛ inch) is made in the upper portion of the eye at the edge of the iris.
- The phacoemulsification unit (a device the size of a marking pen with a small tapered tip) is introduced through the incision.
- The device breaks up and sucks out the clouded interior of the lens.
- The implant is placed inside the "skin" of the old lens in the space where the cataract was.
- The incision is closed with one stitch, or it may be self-sealing and require no stitches.

Antibiotics and cortisonelike medication may then be administered by injection or by placing a special drug-soaked dissolvable contact lens over the eye.

HOSPITAL RECOVERY

The surgery is done on an outpatient basis, which means that following the operation and some relaxation time, the patient, accompanied by a friend or relative, is allowed to go home.

AT-HOME RECOVERY

Postoperative discomfort is usually minimal. The patient will be examined by the surgeon the next day and will be given instructions on the use of eyedrop medications. The next follow-up visit occurs within one week of the surgery, and later appointments occur at longer intervals.

Because of the small incision technique, recovery time is rapid and restrictions are minimal. Activities of daily living are all permissible. Care should be taken to avoid falling, injury to the eye, or exposure to irritating materials around the eye. Swimming with the head under water should be avoided for approximately two weeks.

COMPLICATIONS AND RISKS

Problems occur only rarely, with the worst complications being the most rare. Complications include
- Loss of vision in the eye due to infection or bleeding
- Retinal detachment
- Reversible swelling of the retina
- GLAUCOMA
- Swelling of the front of the eye (the cornea)

In some cases, the tissue behind the implant may become hazy and require laser treatment to restore clarity. Finally, the best prediction of implant power may, on rare occasion, be poorly suited to the patient when actually implanted, requiring lens implant exchange or a contact lens.

WARNING SIGNS:
- Severe pain and redness that seem to be worsening
- Decrease in vision after the first postoperative day
- Pus discharge from the eye

These problems should prompt a call to and examination by the surgeon.

COLOSTOMY

A colostomy involves the creation of an opening between the abdominal wall and large bowel. The patient has bowel movements through the opening (or stoma) and must wear an appliance that holds an impermeable plastic bag in place to collect the fecal material.

Colostomy is required for patients who have their rectum removed or who need to have the fecal stream diverted from the distal large intestine. The operation can be necessary to decompress the colon when there is an INTESTINAL OBSTRUCTION. It can be a temporary situation or permanent one, as when the rectum is removed because of a disease such as COLORECTAL CANCER.

ALTERNATIVE TREATMENTS

None.

PREOPERATIVE PREPARATION

A colostomy is sometimes performed during another procedure, usually removal of the rectum or an emergency operation on the colon for infection (see DIVERTICULAR DISEASE) when sewing the colon back together right away is too dangerous.

If scheduled ahead of time, the patient is taught preoperatively about the care and maintenance of the colostomy and a point on the abdominal wall suitable for the colostomy is marked before the operation so that it will be located in the optimal position.

Except when performed in an emergency, colostomy requires the usual preparation for surgery. BLOOD TESTS and ELECTROCARDIOGRAPHY, for example, are standard before almost any surgery.

Overnight fasting is required with general anesthesia.

ANESTHESIA

General anesthesia.

PROCEDURE

- An opening in the abdominal wall, usually in the left lower abdomen, is made.

> Having a colostomy can be traumatic, and a patient can require a period of adjustment, but the operation should not prevent a person from leading a normal life.

- When the colon is obstructed on the left side, the colostomy is made from a loop of colon in the right upper abdomen.
- The end (or sometimes a loop) of large intestine is brought out through the opening and sewn to the edges of the skin.
- The opening is covered with an appliance and a bag to collect the fecal contents.

HOSPITAL RECOVERY

Recovery depends on the primary operation—whether the colostomy was performed during a more extensive procedure such as removal of the rectum. Generally, the procedure requires three to seven days in the hospital.

AT-HOME RECOVERY

Recovery depends on the primary operation. Activity should be restricted for approximately three to six weeks.

COMPLICATIONS AND RISKS

- The end of the bowel may retract into the abdominal wall causing difficulty with fitting the appliance.
- Infections can occur along the side of the stoma.
- A HERNIA—the protrusion of internal structures through the opening—may occur alongside the stoma.
- An abnormally long portion of colon may protrude, or prolapse, through the opening.
- If the appliance does not fit adequately, leakage of fecal material can damage the skin around the stoma.

COMPUTED TOMOGRAPHY

Computed tomography, or CT, is an X-ray procedure that uses computer technology to make a series of X-ray images, or scans, of a body part—much like slices of bread—that can then be reconstructed by the computer and viewed from different angles.

A technician may run the machine, but a radiologist administers the contrast, if any, and interprets the results.

PREPARATION

Special preparation depends on the part of the body studied and whether contrast material, a type of dye that allows better visualization of the area studied, is to be administered. For patients allergic to contrast material, special preparation with medication such as diphenhydramine and prednisone may be required. If the bowel or kidneys are scanned, fasting may be required for three to four hours before the procedure.

PROCEDURE

- The patient lies on a table.
- If contrast material is needed, an intravenous line may be started to administer the material.
- The area of the body to be imaged is passed into the scanning area.

The procedure may take 15 minutes or as long as an hour, depending on the size of the area studied, whether X rays are obtained both before and after injection of contrast material, and the ability of the patient to cooperate by lying still.

RECOVERY

Computed tomography is generally performed on an outpatient basis, and patients need no recovery time.

COMPLICATIONS AND RISKS

There is essentially little risk to undergoing CT. The amount of radiation from most scans is comparable to the amount of radiation one is exposed to during a day at the beach.

Individuals allergic to contrast material can experience serious reactions, including hives, and loss of blood pressure.

Computed tomography allows physicians to visualize areas of the body that formerly could only be examined through open surgery.

CORONARY ARTERY BYPASS GRAFT SURGERY

The selection of patients for bypass surgery has been studied a great deal, yet some controversial areas remain. In properly selected patients, bypass surgery may increase the likelihood of a patient being alive five years later by 10 percent to 30 percent or more. It may also relieve disabling angina when medications are not enough.

When ATHEROSCLEROSIS interferes with the blood flow to the heart muscle because of blockages in the coronary arteries, one of the ways to improve blood flow to the heart is coronary artery bypass graft surgery. A vein, usually from the leg, or an artery from along the breastbone is used to reroute the blood and bypass the blockages.

ALTERNATIVE TREATMENTS

Medications such as nitroglycerin, atenolol, and diltiazem can relieve symptoms and, in some cases, even prolong life. ANGIOPLASTY may also be an option for some patients facing bypass surgery.

PREOPERATIVE PREPARATION

A CARDIAC STRESS TEST can be very helpful in selecting which patients may benefit the most from bypass surgery. A coronary angiogram (RADIOGRAPHY) and CARDIAC CATHETERIZATION is also critical in selecting patients and planning the actual bypass operation. The patient may need to avoid aspirin for approximately one week before surgery. Other tests routinely done before the operation include
- BLOOD TESTS of various kinds
- ELECTROCARDIOGRAPHY
- Chest X ray (RADIOGRAPHY)
Overnight fasting is required for general anesthesia.

ANESTHESIA

General anesthesia is administered and an artificial heart-lung bypass machine is used to sustain life during parts of surgery in which the bypass grafts are being sewn.

PROCEDURE

- The chest is opened by some of the surgical team while veins in the leg, or occasionally the arm, are removed carefully to be used for the "bypass." In addition, one or two arteries along each side of the breastbone (the internal mammary arteries) may be isolated for bypass use.
- The heart is stopped while the heart-lung machine sustains life.

- The one end of the bypass vessel is sewn carefully to the aorta, and the other end is sewn to the coronary artery beyond the blocked area. This may be repeated, if necessary, for other blockages.
- The heart is restarted and the chest is closed in multiple steps.

HOSPITAL RECOVERY

In some hospitals, uncomplicated bypass surgery now only requires three days in the hospital with close home-care follow-up. Most hospitals, though, keep patients five to ten days, depending on the progress of recovery. Monitoring in the intensive care unit for one to two days is commonly followed by monitoring with ELECTROCARDIOGRAPHY for a few additional days. Gradually chest tubes, intravenous lines, and other support systems are removed.

AT-HOME RECOVERY

Patients are usually allowed to drive after six weeks. Before that, they may return to work full- or part-time, depending on their doctor's recommendation. Even during the first few days home, patients should get dressed and go out for progressively longer walks.

COMPLICATIONS AND RISKS

The following are mild complications:
- A suppressed appetite and mild depression can be common shortly after bypass surgery, so getting back to routine activities as soon as possible is helpful.
- The most common problems are tenderness at incision sites (legs and breastbone); less often, infection at these sites can be an issue.

More serious complications—including STROKE, HEART ATTACK, need for emergency reoperation, and even death—are quite uncommon but vary with age and the individual. For middle-aged men, the risk of death may be less than one percent. For older patients, mortality can be five to ten percent in some higher-risk patients.

CULTURE

A culture is a test in which a sample from a patient's body is taken and tested for any germs that can be grown from it. When they are grown, or cultured, the bacteria, viruses, or other microorganisms can then be identified. The most appropriate antibiotic treatment can also be suggested by testing various drugs against the germ grown from a culture.

> A culture is a common test used to confirm the presence and identity of any infectious agents.

PREPARATION

Cultures are best done before someone is treated with antibiotics, since the drugs may inhibit the growth of bacteria and lead to false-negative results.

To prevent contamination with the normal bacteria that are always on the skin and in the mouth, rigorous skin preparation with antibacterial swabs precedes the sample taking.

ANESTHESIA

None, unless the culture is part of a BIOPSY procedure.

PROCEDURE

There are various ways to sample for germs:
- A throat swab takes a small sample from the back of the throat to test for streptococcal bacteria, the cause of strep throat.
- Blood samples can be drawn (see BLOOD TEST) to look for PNEUMONIA and BLOOD POISONING.
- Bone samples may be needed to document infection and select antibiotics in cases of osteomyelitis.
- Fluid accumulations around lungs, heart, joint spaces, or abdomen may be aspirated by needle.
- Urine, sputum, or stool may be cultured.

RECOVERY

Depending on the technique, little recovery time is needed.

COMPLICATIONS AND RISKS

If a needle is used for the sample, there is a remote possibility of excessive bleeding or infection. False-positive results are also a "risk" that can lead to unnecessary treatment.

CYTOLOGY

Cytology uses a small sample of cells spread on a microscope slide to look for changes that can be clues to cancer or infections. The samples are somewhat easier to obtain than a BIOPSY but may also be collected with needles and special scopes just like a BIOPSY. Some common examples of cytologic tests are the PAP SMEAR to look for cancer of the cervix and the sputum cytology to look for lung cancer or certain infections such as *Pneumocystis carinii* PNEUMONIA.

Cytology is a test closely related to a biopsy, but cytology requires fewer cells, and, therefore, less tissue needs to be collected.

PREPARATION

For samples taken from the stomach or lungs, fasting for a few hours may be required to minimize the risk of vomiting.

ANESTHESIA

Usually, no anesthesia is required, but local anesthesia can be used, depending on how the sample is collected.

PROCEDURE

The exact procedure varies with the sample to be taken. To collect a PAP SMEAR, a wooden spatula is used. Special scopes with brushes are commonly used for samples collected from the lungs or gastrointestinal tract.

Needles may be used to aspirate cells from some organs such as the thyroid gland or suspected tumors in the lung, breast, or abdomen. Sometimes, accumulations of fluid around the heart, lungs, or in the abdomen will be drained off and searched for cells to be studied.

RECOVERY

Taking a cytology specimen usually requires little or no observation. When a needle is used, a period of observation of up to 24 hours may be necessary.

COMPLICATIONS AND RISKS

Bleeding and infection at the site from which the sample was taken are possible, but rare, complications.

DILATION AND CURETTAGE

Dilation and curettage (D & C) is used for both diagnostic and therapeutic reasons. Some of the more common reasons include

- Diagnosis of endometrial abnormalities (such as UTERINE CANCER or hyperplasia), incomplete or missed abortion, or molar pregnancy (the presence of a degenerated ovum, or egg)
- Evaluation of the endometrial lining in cases of infertility
- The control or treatment of dysfunctional uterine bleeding

The procedure is usually performed in an outpatient surgery center or an operating room of a hospital by a gynecologist.

ALTERNATIVE TREATMENTS

Depending on the reason for the D & C, options may include hormonal therapy, hysteroscopy (a form of ENDOSCOPY), or endometrial sampling.

PREOPERATIVE PREPARATION

Depending on the type of anesthetic being used, overnight fasting may be required.

ANESTHESIA

A variety of anesthetic techniques can be used for a D & C, including local anesthetic such as a paracervical block, intravenous sedation, spinal or epidural anesthetic, or general anesthetic.

PROCEDURE

- The patient is positioned in stirrups similar to that for an office pelvic examination.
- A speculum is placed in the vagina and the cervix is located.
- A clamp is placed on the cervix after the vagina has been cleansed.
- The cervix is dilated to the appropriate size for viewing and instruments.

Dilation and curettage is the second most common gynecologic procedure and is used to diagnose cancer and other serious diseases as well as to treat dysfunctional uterine bleeding.

- Either a suction curettage (scraping) or sharp curettage is performed to clean out the uterine contents.
- If the procedure is being performed for diagnostic reasons, the material obtained is sent to pathology for a definitive diagnosis.

HOSPITAL RECOVERY

The D & C is an outpatient procedure and postoperative recovery may range from 15 minutes to a few hours, depending on the type of anesthetic used and how long it takes the patient to come out of it.

AT-HOME RECOVERY

Recovery at home is minimal. Patients should expect some minimal vaginal spotting for a few days after the procedure. Patients also need to refrain from intercourse for one to two weeks and avoid any vigorous activity immediately after the procedure.

COMPLICATIONS AND RISKS

At home, patients should look for any signs of infection. These may include
- Lower ABDOMINAL PAIN and tenderness (although cramping is normal)
- Temperature higher than 100.4°F
- Any foul-smelling VAGINAL DISCHARGE

ELECTROCARDIOGRAPHY

Electrocardiography is a very common test used to evaluate the health of the heart.

Commonly referred to as an EKG or ECG, electrocardiography uses a machine to measure and record (on paper or computer screen) the electrical activity of the heart. With each heartbeat, the heart has an electrical discharge spike that can be recorded using electrodes on the surface of the body. The shape and pattern of the spikes can help diagnose a wide variety of heart problems, including myocardial infarction (HEART ATTACK) and problems with the electrical system of the heart.

PREPARATION

The skin may be shaved where the electrode recording patches are placed on the chest, arms, and legs. Otherwise, the procedure requires no preparation.

ANESTHESIA

None.

PROCEDURE

- The patient lies down quietly.
- The recording electrodes are placed on specific sites on the chest wall, arms, and legs.
- The machine is started and a sample (usually three to four seconds) from each electrode site is recorded.

The EKG may be monitored continuously during some procedures and surgeries.

In an attempt to diagnose certain heart rhythm problems (ARRHYTHMIAS), portable EKG monitors (called *Holter monitors*) may be worn for 24 hours or more to give an extended picture of the heart's rhythm.

RECOVERY

None.

COMPLICATIONS AND RISKS

Occasionally, the adhesive or gel used at the electrode sites can cause some local skin irritation.

ELECTROENCEPHALOGRAPHY

Electroencephalography (EEG) is a test of brain function that records the electrical activity of the brain. This test is used to aid in the evaluation of patients with a variety of problems. A change in brain function, seizures, or a loss of consciousness are the most common reasons for this test, but it may be used for patients with HEADACHES, mental changes, weakness, or changes in sensation. The test is performed by a technologist and typically requires one to two hours.

Electroencephalography helps evaluate patients with a variety of brain disorders, from headaches to mental changes to seizures.

PREPARATION

No extensive preparation is needed, and patients should continue to take their medications unless specifically instructed otherwise. Because electrodes will be placed on the scalp, the hair should be clean, hair dressings should not be used, and hair pieces should not be worn on the day of the EEG. Because it is frequently desirable for the patient to sleep during a portion of the test, coffee or other caffeine-containing beverages should be avoided on the day of the test.

PROCEDURE

- The technologist asks some questions about the problem for which the test is being performed.
- Electrodes are attached all over the head with a special paste or glue.
- The patient is asked to lie quietly with the eyes closed.
- The technologist may ask the patient to hyperventilate for a few minutes and look at a flashing light or do some other simple stimulating activities.
- The electrodes are removed.
- The completed recording is reviewed by a physician, usually a neurologist, and a report is sent to the doctor who requested the test.

RECOVERY

If a sedative is used to help foster sleep during the test, the patient may be slightly drowsy following the test.

COMPLICATIONS AND RISKS

None.

ENDOSCOPY

Using a tube to look inside the body has been done for years. However, the wide variety of areas that can now be seen and the equipment used to visualize them have changed rapidly over the past two decades, making endoscopy one of the most versatile diagnostic tools.

Endoscopy is the use of a lighted tube inserted into the body to see internal structures. The tube may be rigid—for direct vision—or flexible with fiber-optic equipment—for transmitting images and even videotaping.

The type of physician who performs the endoscopy varies depending on which part of the body is to be inspected. Most procedures are done on an outpatient basis.

Examples of endoscopy that use the available openings in the body include

- Gastroscopy (stomach)
- Colonoscopy and sigmoidoscopy (colon)
- Bronchoscopy (lungs)
- Cystoscopy (bladder)
- Hysteroscopy (uterus)

In other cases, the skin may be opened to allow a scope to penetrate into an area. Among these procedures are

- Arthroscopy to look into a joint
- Laparoscopy to look in the abdomen

Besides helping to make a diagnosis, endoscopy can be used to treat certain conditions. RECTAL OR COLON POLYP REMOVAL, transurethral resection of the prostate (see PROSTATE GLAND REMOVAL), joint surgery, and a rapidly expanding area of endoscopic surgery for GALLBLADDER REMOVAL are just a few of the surgical applications for endoscopy.

PREOPERATIVE PREPARATION

- In most cases, some degree of fasting is best. This may be several hours or even overnight.
- For patients with HEART VALVE DISEASE, prophylactic antibiotics, such as ampicillin and gentamicin, may be needed.

ANESTHESIA

The kind of anesthesia used depends on the body part being viewed.

- No anesthesia may be necessary for sigmoidoscopy of the rectum and lower colon.
- Local anesthesia, using topical sprays to numb an area, may be used for bronchoscopy of the lungs.
- General or spinal anesthetic may be appropriate for laparoscopy of the abdomen or pelvis.

PROCEDURE

- The patient may be sedated with an intravenous injection before the procedure.
- The scope is passed carefully into the opening.
- All the areas passed are inspected and possibly photographed or even videotaped if necessary.
- BIOPSY may be performed, repairs made, and diseased parts may even be removed.
- The scope is removed.
- If an incision was necessary, it is closed and dressed.

HOSPITAL RECOVERY

Most endoscopy only requires a brief (less than an hour) observation period after the procedure. If sedation is used, the patient may be kept longer (up to one or two hours). For laparoscopic surgery, overnight stays may be necessary.

Mild analgesics like an acetaminophen and codeine combination may be needed for more involved procedures.

AT-HOME RECOVERY

When an incision in the skin was needed, keeping the wound clean and limiting activity for a few days may be required.

COMPLICATIONS AND RISKS

- Perforation of a body part, such as the colon, esophagus, or lung, with the scope is rare. The problem would be apparent within minutes to hours of the procedure. If perforation does occur, however, it can be a serious complication and may require surgery to repair.
- Local bleeding can usually be controlled without difficulty, but in rare circumstances, it can be excessive or life threatening.
- Infection is rare and can develop only if the skin is cut for the procedure or if the patient has other unusual risks such as HEART VALVE DISEASE.

FIBROID TUMOR REMOVAL

In the majority of women who undergo myomectomy, fibroids grow back and become problematic again.

The removal of FIBROID TUMORS of the uterus without removing the uterus itself is called *myomectomy*. It is performed when fibroids are large, cause pain, or cause abnormal bleeding *and* when the woman wants to bear children in the future. The operation can give a woman sufficient time to have children before fibroids necessitate a HYSTERECTOMY.

ALTERNATIVE TREATMENTS

Small fibroids or fibroids that cause no symptoms may be observed rather than removed. Nonsteroidal anti-inflammatory drugs such as ibuprofen may decrease pain and bleeding from fibroids.

Women who have problems with fibroids and do not desire children may elect to undergo HYSTERECTOMY. There is no permanent cure for symptomatic fibroids other than removal.

PREOPERATIVE PREPARATION

An ULTRASOUND is the most common test performed during the preparation for surgery.

Leuprolide (a synthetic form of the gonadotropin-releasing hormone) given in monthly injections for three to six months may decrease the size of fibroids, thereby allowing for easier surgery with less blood loss.

Prior to scheduled surgery, a woman will undergo preoperative BLOOD TESTS to assess her BLOOD COUNT, kidney function, and liver functions. Chest X ray (RADIOGRAPHY) and ELECTRO-CARDIOGRAPHY may be performed depending on a woman's age and hospital center.

The night before surgery, the woman usually has some sort of bowel cleansing, such as an enema, and must refrain from eating for 8 to 12 hours before surgery.

ANESTHESIA

General anesthesia or regional anesthesia, such as epidural or spinal block, may be used. With regional anesthesia, a sedative may be administered so that the patient is awake but not anxious.

PROCEDURE

- A six- to eight-inch incision is made in the abdomen.
- The uterus is raised out of the abdomen and a superficial incision is made over an accessible fibroid.
- The fibroid is shelled out and removed in one piece.
- If possible, all of the fibroids are removed through the same incision.
- The holes left by the fibroids in the uterus are then sewn tightly with thread that disappears over time.
- The abdomen is sewn closed in many layers.

Myomectomy is most commonly done as described; however, in certain cases, the procedure may be done vaginally or through hysteroscopy (a form of ENDOSCOPY).

HOSPITAL RECOVERY

Immediately after surgery, a woman has a catheter inserted in her bladder to remove urine and an intravenous tube inserted to deliver fluids and pain medicines. On the first postoperative day, she can and should be encouraged to walk. She is also allowed to drink fluids. Usually she can eat regular food once she has passed gas through her rectum. The length of the hospital stay is three to four days.

AT-HOME RECOVERY

The main instructions for recovery are rest and plenty of fluids. Pain medication, such as an acetaminophen and codeine combination, may be needed. The patient should refrain from using tampons or douches and from having sexual intercourse for the first month after surgery. Stairs must be taken slowly and activity gradually increased as tolerated. Most women can return to work in six weeks.

Women who desire immediate pregnancy are advised to wait three months before attempting conception. If the inside of the uterine cavity was entered, the uterine wall may be weak and cesarean section may be the only delivery option.

COMPLICATIONS AND RISKS

Infection, although rare, is a risk in any surgery.

GALLBLADDER REMOVAL

> The gallbladder is not absolutely necessary, and most patients have no problems after their gallbladders are removed.

The gallbladder can be removed in a procedure called *cholecystectomy* for any of three reasons:
- Gallstones that cause symptoms
- Complications of gallstones (see CHOLECYSTITIS AND CHOLANGITIS)
- Benign or malignant tumors (occasionally)

ALTERNATIVE TREATMENTS

The orally administered bile salts, ursodeoxycholate or chenodeoxycholate, dissolve cholesterol GALLSTONES in selected patients. Unfortunately, most patients have stones that are not amenable to this treatment. Dissolution requires from 12 to 24 months, the treatments are expensive, and stones recur in the majority of patients.

GALLSTONES have also been fragmented with sound waves (ULTRASONIC LITHOTRIPSY). The fragments are passed from the gallbladder and dissolved with bile salts. Again, this has only been effective in a select minority of patients, and recurrence rates are high.

PREOPERATIVE PREPARATION

Diagnostic tests to confirm the presence of stones include ULTRASOUND and sometimes X rays (RADIOGRAPHY) enhanced with different contrast agents depending on the nature of the problem suspected.

BLOOD TESTS and ELECTROCARDIOGRAPHY are standard before almost any surgery.

Overnight fasting is required with general anesthesia.

ANESTHESIA

General anesthesia.

PROCEDURE

For open cholecystectomy
- A standard incision is made in the upper middle of the abdomen or just below the ribs.
- The duct emptying the gallbladder into the common bile duct (the main duct connecting the liver to the

intestines) is identified, tied off with sutures or clips, and divided.

- The artery to the gallbladder is likewise identified, tied off, and divided.
- The gallbladder is then dissected from the liver and minor bleeding is controlled by electrocoagulation of small blood vessels.
- The surgeon may then perform an X ray (RADIOGRA-PHY) called an *intraoperative cholangiogram* before removing the gallbladder. (In this procedure, radiologic dye is injected into the gallbladder duct while the X ray is taken. The X ray shows the entire bile duct system, and any stones that have passed into the common bile duct can be seen. It also excludes injury to major bile ducts.)
- The abdominal wound is closed in layers with sutures, and the skin is closed with sutures or clips.

For laparoscopic cholecystectomy (Laparoscopy is a form of ENDOSCOPY.)

- A puncture wound is made near the navel.
- A camera is placed into the abdomen. (The surgeon and assistants can then watch the operation on a video monitor.)
- Three additional puncture wounds are made in the abdomen along the rib cage for other instruments to be inserted.
- The gallbladder is removed through one of the puncture wounds.
- Puncture wounds are closed with sutures or clips.

Laparoscopic cholecystectomy is possible in 95 percent of patients.

HOSPITAL RECOVERY

Patients requiring open cholecystectomy need three to five days to regain normal bowel function. Intravenous fluids and medications are necessary until liquid is tolerated orally. Activity is encouraged despite pain.

Patients undergoing laparoscopic cholecystectomy have less pain and take liquids within hours of the operation. They usually spend only one day in the hospital.

At-home recovery

Recovery from open cholecystectomy takes two to four weeks. Patients require pain medications such as an acetaminophen and codeine combination for one or two weeks, but are usually able to resume daily activities after one week. Strenuous activity and lifting of weight greater than about 20 pounds should be avoided for six to eight weeks.

Recovery time is markedly reduced with laparoscopic cholecystectomy. Most patients require pain medications for only several days and return to full activity after one or two weeks.

Patients may drive a car when they no longer have pain and when they are no longer taking pain medications that cause drowsiness.

Complications and risks

- Leakage of bile from the gallbladder bed can cause a collection of bile beneath the liver. This prolongs upper right ABDOMINAL PAIN and delays recovery from the operation. The collection of bile may have to be drained.
- Bile duct injury causes a leak of a large amount of bile. This causes the patient to develop jaundice and abscesses in the abdomen, especially near the liver. Bile may leak through the wound. This complication will require another operation for correction and can be quite serious.
- PNEUMONIA may result because postoperative incision pain may make deep breathing and coughing difficult.
- Wound infection is a possibility, but can be treated with antibiotics and by draining pus from the wound.

HEART VALVE REPLACEMENT

When a heart valve malfunctions enough to severely impair heart function (see HEART VALVE DISEASE), it may need to be replaced or repaired. During open heart surgery, cardiothoracic surgeons often decide to repair some heart valves, but sometimes only replacement with an artificial valve will suffice. Replacement valves are either categorized as mechanical valves, which are metallic or made of related alloys, or tissue valves, which are made from cow or pig tissue that has been specially processed.

The implantation of new valves is performed to relieve symptoms of congestive heart failure, fainting, or angina caused by a damaged valve.

ALTERNATIVE TREATMENTS

Special catheter treatments using balloons (valvuloplasty—a cousin of ANGIOPLASTY) can be useful in certain situations to delay the need for open heart surgery and valve replacement.

PREOPERATIVE PREPARATION

Echocardiograms (ULTRASOUND), CARDIAC CATHETERIZATION, and special exercise tests (CARDIAC STRESS TESTS) may be used to help decide the proper timing of valve replacement. This is often a difficult and unclear area. The physician does not want to put in an artificial valve too soon if the damaged one can be tolerated for additional months or years. Yet if one waits too long, sudden death or irreversible heart damage may occur.

ANESTHESIA

General anesthesia and a heart-lung machine are required for open heart surgery.

PROCEDURE

- The chest is opened and the ribs spread to allow access to the heart.
- The appropriate heart chamber is opened and the valve is inspected.
- If the valve can be repaired, it is (this option is often preferable).
- If the valve cannot be repaired, it is removed. Newer techniques attempt to preserve as much of the tissue supporting the old valve as possible.

- The appropriate artificial valve is sewn into place and the incisions are closed.

A heart-lung machine circulates and oxygenates enough blood to sustain life during the main parts of the operation.

HOSPITAL RECOVERY

Open heart surgery usually requires a five- to ten-day hospital stay. Anticoagulants such as heparin and warfarin may be needed to discourage clot formations. Chest tubes and continuous ELECTROCARDIOGRAPHY will be in place for the first few days, which are spent in a surgical intensive care unit.

AT-HOME RECOVERY

- Working and other activities are gradually increased.
- Driving can usually be resumed after six weeks.
- Wound care to avoid infections is necessary until healing occurs.
- Prophylactic administration of antibiotics such as ampicillin or gentamicin is helpful in preventing serious infections in patients with heart valve replacements. These drugs are given before certain procedures like dental work, bowel surgery, or vaginal surgery.

COMPLICATIONS AND RISKS

Valve replacement surgery can have mortality rates as high as five to ten percent, so it is done only when the risk of leaving the original valve in place is significantly greater than that of replacement.

Infection of the wound or valve and valve malfunction can occur at any time.

Clots may form on artificial valves and cause malfunction or even travel to the brain or limbs causing STROKE or gangrene. This occurs rarely and can be minimized with anticoagulants such as heparin or warfarin.

HEMORRHOID BANDING

Hemorrhoid banding is a method of destroying and thus eliminating internal HEMORRHOIDS. The rubber band that is applied causes the tissue to die and slough off while controlling the vein so that it doesn't bleed. The procedure is most often performed by a general or a colorectal surgeon in an outpatient setting.

ALTERNATIVE TREATMENTS

Patients may obtain temporary relief with warm baths (sitz baths), which soothe and cleanse the perianal area. Anal suppositories with or without cortisone may also ameliorate symptoms.

Other surgical treatments include HEMORRHOID REMOVAL and infrared or electrocoagulation of HEMORRHOIDS.

The development and progression of HEMORRHOIDS can be avoided or impeded by avoiding CONSTIPATION and straining with bowel movements. A high-fiber diet is best for long-term control of bowel habits, but many patients require fiber supplements such as psyllium or methylcellulose to control the consistency of bowel movements. Regular exercise may also be beneficial in the prevention of HEMORRHOIDS.

PREOPERATIVE PREPARATION

Patients should evacuate their rectum before the procedure. This usually requires an enema on the day of the procedure.

ANESTHESIA

None.

PROCEDURE

- Anoscopy (see ENDOSCOPY) is performed to locate the hemorrhoid to be banded.
- The area at the base of the hemorrhoid is grasped and tested to be sure that it is in an area where there are no pain fibers.

> Banding is particularly useful for patients with large or prolapsed internal hemorrhoids, but it is not effective with external hemorrhoids because application of a rubber band in this area is too painful.

- The hemorrhoid is grasped and pulled into a special instrument, and an elastic band is then released to contract around the base of the hemorrhoid.
- The band is left in place, and the instruments are withdrawn.

HOSPITAL RECOVERY

The procedure is usually performed in the office and requires no specific monitoring. Patients may feel pressure or mild discomfort in the rectum and are usually observed until that feeling subsides.

AT-HOME RECOVERY

Very little, if any, pain medication, such as an acetaminophen and codeine combination, is required. Diet should be altered and fiber supplements or stool softeners given to control bowel movements.

The patient may note minor RECTAL BLEEDING with bowel movements, especially as hemorrhoidal tissue sloughs.

COMPLICATIONS AND RISKS

- Excessive pain may result if the skin in the anal canal is included in the rubber band. It should be treated by removing the rubber band.
- Significant RECTAL BLEEDING can occur infrequently when the hemorrhoidal tissue sloughs, usually one to three days after treatment, and the patient should see his or her doctor at that time.
- Patients, especially elderly men, may have difficulty passing urine due to a reflex caused by the discomfort.
- Infection at the site of the treatment may occur but is rare.

HEMORRHOID REMOVAL

HEMORRHOIDS that cause persistent symptoms, especially bleeding, despite medical treatment, and that are not amenable to less invasive treatments require formal surgery to remove them. This operation is performed by a general or colorectal surgeon in a hospital setting.

ALTERNATIVE TREATMENTS

Patients can sometimes obtain relief from symptoms with warm baths (sitz baths), which soothe and cleanse the perianal area, thus avoiding all medical treatment. However, this is not a cure for HEMORRHOIDS, and severe cases need more aggressive therapy.

Dietary changes and fiber supplements can be instituted to control bowel habits. Anal suppositories with or without cortisone may ameliorate symptoms.

HEMORRHOID BANDING is a possible treatment in select patients with internal HEMORRHOIDS. Infrared or electrocoagulation of HEMORRHOIDS may also be an option.

PREOPERATIVE PREPARATION

It is helpful to control CONSTIPATION and bowel habits preoperatively with a high-fiber diet, fiber supplements, and stool softeners. The rectum should be evacuated with enemas on the night before and morning of surgery. Overnight fasting is required for general anesthesia.

ANESTHESIA

Local anesthesia with sedation, regional anesthesia (spinal block), or general anesthesia may be used for this surgery.

PROCEDURE

- The patient is placed in either a prone position with the buttocks taped apart or supine with the legs in stirrups.
- The anus is examined and the groups of hemorrhoids to be removed are identified.
- The hemorrhoid is tied off with a suture.
- The hemorrhoid is cut from the anal muscles and removed.

> Hemorrhoid removal is the most thorough method of removing symptomatic hemorrhoids, but recurrence is not uncommon.

- The wound in the rectum is closed with a running suture, but the external skin wound is left open. (If the anal skin is closed, there may be increased postoperative pain and a higher incidence of infection and stricture of the anus.)

HOSPITAL RECOVERY

Many patients can be discharged the same day of the operation. Those with pain that is not well controlled with oral pain medications, difficulty passing urine, and with concomitant medical problems may require observation in the hospital for one to two days.

AT-HOME RECOVERY

Patients require pain medication such as an acetaminophen and codeine combination for several days until pain subsides. Pain may be worse after bowel movements and medication may be required intermittently for one to two weeks. Bowel movements should be controlled with a high-fiber diet, fiber supplements, and stool softeners.

Sitz baths (soaking the anal area in warm water) are begun the day after surgery and are performed two to three times per day to soothe and cleanse the surgical sites. Activity is encouraged but limited by pain. Patients normally have a small amount of bleeding that ceases immediately after bowel movements.

COMPLICATIONS AND RISKS

- Infection is rare, but can be serious, causing FEVER and severe, worsening pain.
- In rare cases, significant postoperative RECTAL BLEEDING can occur; this complication requires prompt attention.
- Stricture, or stenosis, of the anal canal can occur as wounds heal, but is rare. In this complication, the patient has difficulty and pain passing bowel movements, and stool caliber is decreased.

HERNIA REPAIR

HERNIA is a common condition, and hernia repair is a commonly performed operation for general surgeons. A HERNIA in the groin or abdominal wall is repaired to ameliorate symptoms and to avoid future enlargement and any subsequent complications.

Patients should be able to return to full activity after recovery from the repair, but the HERNIA can recur in as many as ten percent of patients over their lifetime.

ALTERNATIVE TREATMENTS

There is no medical treatment for a HERNIA. In very ill patients, for whom surgery would be risky, a HERNIA may be observed and the operation reserved for complications, should they develop.

PREOPERATIVE PREPARATION

There are no specific tests required for hernia repair. Patients should be evaluated and prepared as appropriate for their medical problems and for the type of anesthesia they will require. BLOOD TESTS and ELECTROCARDIOGRAPHY are not uncommon; overnight fasting is required for general anesthesia.

A bowel preparation involving the removal of fecal contents and the administration of antibiotics (see SMALL BOWEL RESECTION) may be performed before repair of a complex incisional HERNIA.

ANESTHESIA

Simple hernia repairs can be performed under local anesthetic with intravenous sedation. A more complex operation will require a general anesthesia. Laparoscopic repair (see below) always requires a general anesthetic.

PROCEDURE

For open repair
- An incision is made directly over the area.
- The incision is carried through the skin, subcuta-

Hernia repair is usually a low-risk operation, but a large, complex hernia, especially one arising in abdominal scars, may require a more involved, riskier procedure.

neous tissues, and the strong connective tissue that gives the abdominal wall its strength (called the superficial fascia).

- The hernia is located and the sac of herniated tissue is opened.
- Abdominal contents are reinserted.
- The base of the sac is closed with sutures and the excess sac is removed.
- One of several repairs is then performed: 1) A section of deep fascia is sutured over the defect; or 2) if the fascia is weak, as it often is with a recurrent hernia, a piece of woven mesh material is used to close the defect or reinforce the repair.
- The incision is sutured closed in successive layers.

For laparoscopic repair

- The abdominal cavity or the space between the abdominal cavity and the hernia is filled with carbon dioxide gas through a puncture wound near the navel to give the surgeons room to work.
- A laparoscope is inserted through a small incision and placed into the space, allowing the surgeon and surgical assistants to watch the procedure on a video monitor.
- Instruments are placed through two other puncture wounds.
- The hernia is reduced from the inside, and the edges of the defect and fascia important for its repair are cut free.
- A piece of mesh material is put over the defect and stapled in placed.
- The puncture wounds are closed with sutures.

An incisional HERNIA is repaired by reopening the abdominal wound. The edges of the defect are defined and cut back to normal muscle and fascia. The wound is reclosed using sutures. If the defect is large, a piece of mesh may be required to bridge the defect or to reinforce the repair.

HOSPITAL RECOVERY

Patients most often undergo hernia repair as an outpatient; that is, they leave the hospital as soon as they recover from the anesthetic and are able to walk. Some patients may require admission to the hospital to observe and treat coexisting medical problems.

Patients who require incisional hernia repair are hospitalized for several days, since they essentially undergo abdominal surgery when their wound is reopened and reclosed. They may develop decreased bowel motility and may not be able to eat. Therefore, they often require intravenous fluids until they can tolerate food.

AT-HOME RECOVERY

- Normal activity is encouraged, but patients will require pain medication such as an acetaminophen and codeine combination.
- Strenuous activity, including lifting of weight greater than 10 to 20 pounds, is restricted for six to eight weeks.
- Patients may drive a car when they no longer have pain and when they are not taking pain medications that make them drowsy.

Many surgeons are more liberal after laparoscopic repair and allow patients to return to full unrestricted activity as soon as their pain subsides.

COMPLICATIONS AND RISKS

Wound infection causes redness and swelling, FEVER, increasing pain, and, possibly, drainage from the incision. It is treated with antibiotics and with drainage of pus from the wound.

Ecchymosis refers to a small amount of bleeding under the skin causing a large amount of black and blue in the area around the wound. In the groin, ecchymosis can extend into the scrotum and penis. This can be quite alarming to the patient, but has no significance. Ecchymosis disappears spontaneously over 10 to 14 days.

Hematoma is a collection of blood below the wound, manifested by a firm swelling. It may be associated with ecchymosis. If large, a hematoma may cause discomfort and should be evaluated by the surgeon.

Recurrent HERNIA is not uncommon and requires repair, usually with prosthetic mesh material.

HIP ARTHROPLASTY

Total hip replacement is usually a very successful operation; it has a satisfaction rate greater than 90 percent.

The goal of a hip arthroplasty (total hip replacement) is to replace the hip joint surfaces that are painful and degenerated from OSTEOARTHRITIS or RHEUMATOID ARTHRITIS with an artificial ball and socket joint made of advanced metal, plastic, and ceramic materials. The operation, performed by an orthopedic surgeon, promises improved function and decreased pain.

ALTERNATIVE TREATMENTS

The decision to have a hip arthroplasty is based on how the symptoms of the hip arthritis interfere with everyday life activities. No medications or noninvasive techniques for improving the quality of worn or damaged hip joint surfaces are currently available.

PREOPERATIVE PREPARATION

General laboratory BLOOD TESTS and other diagnostic tests such as ELECTROCARDIOGRAPHY are usually done to evaluate general health status. RADIOGRAPHY may be used to help plan the operation.

ANESTHESIA

General anesthesia or regional anesthesia (spinal or epidural block) is used. A sedative may be given with regional anesthesia so that the patient is awake but not anxious.

PROCEDURE

- A variety of surgical incisions are made on the side of the upper thigh.
- The muscles are moved to the side to expose the hip (ball and socket) joint area.
- Using power instruments, the upper end of the femur (the ball) and the acetabulum (the socket) are cut and reamed to remove worn cartilage.
- Implants sized to fit the patient are then either press fitted or cemented onto the femur and into the acetabulum to create a new, low-friction ball and socket joint.
- Muscles involved in movements of the hip are then reattached to their normal positions.

HOSPITAL RECOVERY

Most patients will be in the hospital for about five to ten days after the operation. Intravenous or intramuscular pain medicine is generally used for the first several days after surgery; patients can usually be changed to oral pain medicine such as an acetaminophen and codeine combination after that time.

Physical therapy is initiated in the hospital to educate patients about restrictions and to start exercises for range of motion and strengthening. Depending on the type of hip arthroplasty, patients will start with limited weight bearing with an assistive device (crutches or a walker).

AT-HOME RECOVERY

Patients continue the rehabilitation process at home with an emphasis on improving range of motion and hip muscle strength. Restrictions on weight bearing decrease as the hip heals and muscle strength returns. There may be some restrictions on certain sitting positions and on stooping and bending until soft tissues around the hip are healed.

Therapists provide some assistive devices to aid in everyday activities that stress the hip (special aids for the bath and shower, and grabbers for picking up objects from the floor, for example).

Oral pain medications such as an acetaminophen and codeine combination may be required for two to four weeks after the patient comes home.

COMPLICATIONS AND RISKS

- As with any surgical procedure, there is a small risk of surgical wound infection.
- Dislocation of the hip joint before the soft tissues heal may occur if patients are not careful about positioning restrictions.
- Deep vein THROMBOSIS is a serious but rare occurrence.

HYSTERECTOMY

A *total* hysterectomy is the operation to remove the uterus and cervix (which is the bottom part of the uterus). A *partial* hysterectomy, removal of the uterus without the cervix, is performed very rarely. Hysterectomy does not include removal of the fallopian tubes and ovaries, although this is often done at the same time.

Hysterectomies may be performed by one of two routes, depending upon the indication. Abdominal hysterectomy—removal of the uterus through an incision in the abdomen—is used when there are very large FIBROID TUMORS, UTERINE CANCER, OVARIAN CANCER, or scarring from previous abdominal surgery or infection such as PELVIC INFLAMMATORY DISEASE.

In *vaginal* hysterectomy, the uterus is removed through an incision in the vagina. Although recuperation is much easier from this type of surgery, it is only practical when the uterus is not greatly enlarged. Indications for vaginal hysterectomy include symptomatic small to moderate FIBROID TUMORS, persistent abnormal VAGINAL BLEEDING, certain precancerous conditions of the uterus, and when the uterus is falling (prolapsing) into the vagina. A vaginal hysterectomy can also be performed with the aid of laparoscopy (a form of ENDOSCOPY), which makes the procedure more versatile.

ALTERNATIVE TREATMENTS

Alternative treatments depend on the indication for the surgery. Small or asymptomatic fibroids may be observed rather than removed. Abnormal uterine bleeding may be controlled by hormones—estrogen, progesterone, or a combination of the two. In certain cases abnormal uterine bleeding may be prevented by ablation, or charring, of the interior lining.

PREOPERATIVE PREPARATION

During the workup before a hysterectomy, women most frequently have a pelvic ULTRASOUND to assess the uterus and ovaries. In cases of abnormal bleeding, a BIOPSY of the inside lining of the uterus (endometrium) may be performed to rule out cancer, such as UTERINE CANCER.

Preoperative BLOOD TESTS may include BLOOD COUNTS, liver and kidney assessments, and a sampling of blood to be kept in the blood bank in case the need for transfusion arises. A chest X ray (RADIOGRAPHY) and ELECTROCARDIOGRAPHY may be performed depending on the woman's age and the hospital center.

The night before surgery the woman usually has some kind of bowel cleansing such as an enema and does not eat for eight to twelve hours prior to surgery.

ANESTHESIA

General anesthesia and regional anesthesia (spinal or epidural block) are both options. A sedative may be given with regional anesthesia so that the patient is awake but not anxious.

PROCEDURE

For abdominal hysterectomy
*   An incision is made in the abdomen.
*   The blood vessels to the uterus and the surrounding tissue are cut and tied off.
*   The uterus is removed through the abdominal incision.
*   The abdomen is then sewn closed in many layers with thread that disappears over time.
*   The skin is closed with thread or staples.

For vaginal hysterectomy
*   An incision is made at the top of the vagina.
*   The blood vessels and surrounding tissue are cut and tied off.
*   The organs are removed through the vaginal incision.

To perform a laparoscopically assisted vaginal hysterectomy, small incisions are made near the navel and at two other sites in the lower abdomen to allow a laparoscope (see ENDOSCOPY) to pass into the abdominal cavity. The surgery is performed with the aid of images obtained through the scope.

Hospital recovery

Immediately after surgery, a catheter is placed in the bladder for urination and an intravenous catheter is inserted to deliver fluids and pain medications. On the first postoperative day, the patient should be encouraged to walk as much as possible. Depending on the type of surgery, she may be able to drink fluids and consume a general diet on the first day. After an abdominal hysterectomy, a patient drinks clear fluids and consumes regular food only after having passed gas through her rectum. Diet may be advanced more quickly after vaginal surgery.

The hospital stay is usually three to four days for an abdominal hysterectomy and two to three days for a vaginal hysterectomy.

At-home recovery

The main instructions for recovery are rest and plenty of fluids. Pain medication, such as an acetaminophen and codeine combination, may be needed. The patient should refrain from using tampons or douches and from having sexual intercourse for the first month after surgery. Stairs must be taken slowly and activity gradually increased as tolerated. Most women are healthy and feel capable of returning to a normal routine in six weeks.

Complications and risks

All types of hysterectomy, like all other surgery, carry risks of infection. Blood loss, anesthesia problems, and injury to other organs, such as the intestines and bladder, are remote possibilities.

ILEOSTOMY

An ileostomy is an opening created between the abdominal wall and the portion of the small intestine called the *ileum*. The patient has bowel movements through the opening, called a *stoma*, and must wear an appliance that holds an impermeable plastic bag in place to collect the wastes. Ileostomy is required for patients who have their large intestine removed because of disease such as COLORECTAL CANCER or who need to have the fecal stream diverted from the large intestine as in some cases of ULCERATIVE COLITIS.

ALTERNATIVE TREATMENTS

None.

PREOPERATIVE PREPARATION

An ileostomy is performed during another procedure, usually removal of part or all of the colon. If the procedure is scheduled in advance, the patient is taught about the ileostomy and a point on the abdominal wall suitable for the ileostomy is marked before the operation so that it will be located in the optimal position.

BLOOD TESTS, ELECTROCARDIOGRAPHY, and other tests to evaluate general health status are standard before almost any surgery.

Overnight fasting is required with general anesthesia.

ANESTHESIA

General anesthesia.

PROCEDURE

Ileostomy is usually performed in conjunction with another operation, which means an abdominal incision has already been made.

- After the other procedure, such as SIGMOID COLON REMOVAL, an opening is made in the abdominal wall, usually in the right lower abdomen.

An ileostomy can be temporary if the bowels are to be reattached at some point, or it can be permanent when the large intestine has been removed.

- The end, or sometimes a loop, of small intestine is brought out through the opening and sewn to the skin edges to create an opening in the bowel for bowel movements.
- The opening is covered with an ileostomy appliance and a bag.

Hospital recovery

It depends on the primary operation, but ileostomy generally requires a hospital stay of three to seven days. Liquids and soft foods are introduced after a few days.

At-home recovery

It depends on the primary operation, but activity should generally be restricted for three to six weeks. Pain medication, such as an acetaminophen and codeine combination, may be prescribed if necessary.

Complications and risks

- The end of the bowel may retract into the abdominal wall, causing difficulty with fitting the appliance.
- Infections can occur alongside the stoma.
- If the appliance does not fit properly, leakage of fecal material can damage the skin around the ileostomy.
- DIARRHEA may occur since absorption of water by the colon is no longer possible, and patients are more susceptible to DIARRHEA during gastrointestinal illnesses.

KIDNEY REMOVAL

Kidney removal, also called *nephrectomy*, is necessary in several circumstances. Severely infected or cancerous kidneys are candidates for removal. A nonfunctioning kidney (KIDNEY FAILURE) may need to be removed to make room for a KIDNEY TRANSPLANT. A functioning kidney from a living donor is also removed in this manner.

PREOPERATIVE PREPARATIONS

Intravenous pyelogram (RADIOGRAPHY) and COMPUTED TOMOGRAPHY are usually necessary. BLOOD TESTS and ELECTRO-CARDIOGRAPHY are also standard before almost any surgery. Overnight fasting is required with general anesthesia.

ANESTHESIA

General anesthesia.

PROCEDURE

- A generous incision is made along the flank.
- The renal vein, renal artery, and the ureter are tied off and cut, and the organ is removed.
- The kidney's attachments to the surrounding structures are cut, and the organ is removed.
- Internal muscles are repaired and vessels tied off.
- The external incision is closed with sutures.

HOSPITAL RECOVERY

Hospital stay is usually five to seven days. Fluids are administered intravenously for several days until the patient can eat.

AT-HOME RECOVERY

Activity should be limited for approximately six weeks.

COMPLICATIONS AND RISKS

- Excessive bleeding (hemorrhage) is a danger with this procedure and may require transfusion.
- Because the incision in the flank is so large and so near the bottom of the lung, pneumothorax (collapsed lung) is a possible complication.

Because the body is equipped with two kidneys, one can be removed without severely compromising the body's ability to eliminate wastes through the urine.

KIDNEY TRANSPLANT

With current methods to control rejection, kidney transplantation is likely to be successful if a suitable donor can be found.

In this procedure, a kidney from a living related donor or from a compatible organ donor is transplanted into a person with KIDNEY FAILURE. The operation is performed in the hospital setting by either a transplant specialist or a urologist.

ALTERNATIVE TREATMENTS

Although dialysis can offset many of the problems associated with failing kidneys, quality of life may often be better with transplantation.

PREOPERATIVE PREPARATION

The donated organ and the recipient patient must be precisely cross-matched to minimize the risk of rejection. Cross-matching usually entails BLOOD TESTS.

As with other major sugery, overnight fasting and preoperative tests, such as BLOOD TESTS and ELECTROCARDIOGRAPHY, are usually required.

ANESTHESIA

General anesthesia.

PROCEDURE

The diseased kidney can be removed from the transplant recipient (KIDNEY REMOVAL) well before the transplant operation—up to several weeks in advance—with kidney functions being performed through dialysis. The donor kidney, however, cannot be removed any sooner than about 12 hours before transplantation. Once the donor kidney is available, the procedure can begin:

- An incision is made along the flank.
- The vein and artery that will be connected to the graft kidney are identified.
- The graft kidney is placed in the selected site.
- The graft kidney's artery and vein are attached to the patient's own vessels.
- The graft kidney's ureter is connected to the patient's bladder.
- The surgical incision is closed with sutures.

HOSPITAL RECOVERY

The length of time the patient must stay at the hospital is extremely variable and depends on the occurrence of complications. Three weeks is common. Occasionally, part of the postoperative stay is in the intensive care unit, and some dialysis treatments may still be required. Part of the treatment immediately after transplantation includes immunosuppressive medication, such as cyclosporine, azathioprine, and prednisone, which can cause significant side effects.

Sutures stay in place for about one week, and the intravenous line remains for a few days.

AT-HOME RECOVERY

Recovery at home takes a minimum of six weeks—often longer, depending on any complications. Recovery entails significant restrictions on activities and close monitoring of health status.

COMPLICATIONS AND RISKS

- Poor graft function can be a temporary or long-term problem. Poor urine output can signal diminished function.
- Graft rejection is the most feared of the complications. In rejection, the host's body treats the new kidney as an invader and the immune system attacks it (hence the use of immunosuppressant medication after surgery). Pain in the area of the transplant and FEVER are warning signs of rejection.
- Opportunistic infections are a danger because the artificially weakened immune system makes the recipient unable to fight off otherwise simple bacterial and viral invaders.

KNEE ARTHROPLASTY

> More than 90 percent of patients with advanced knee arthritis have decreased pain and improved function after knee arthroplasty.

The goal of knee arthroplasty is to replace worn and arthritic knee cartilage with metal, plastic, or ceramic surfaces to improve function and decrease pain. This operation is done by an orthopedic surgeon.

ALTERNATIVE TREATMENTS

Degenerative conditions of the knee such as OSTEOARTHRITIS and RHEUMATOID ARTHRITIS are treated initially with anti-inflammatory or pain medicines, such as ibuprofen and acetaminophen, and with decreased activity. Physical therapy may be helpful.

No medications or noninvasive techniques for improving or restoring degenerative knee cartilage surfaces are currently available.

PREOPERATIVE PREPARATION

Laboratory tests, such as BLOOD COUNT and other BLOOD TESTS, and other diagnostic tests, such as ELECTROCARDIOGRAPHY and chest X ray (RADIOGRAPHY), are done to evaluate general health.

Overnight fasting is required for general anesthesia.

ANESTHESIA

General anesthesia and regional anesthesia (spinal or epidural block) are both options. A sedative may be given with regional anesthesia so that the patient is awake but not anxious.

PROCEDURE

- An incision is made on the front part of the knee.
- By moving the patella (knee cap) and its associated tendons out of the way, the worn surfaces of the knee joint (femur and tibia) are exposed.
- Using power instruments and special surgical guides to align the cut surfaces, the worn surfaces are removed.

- The removed material is replaced by metal and plastic implants that are sized to the individual patient and are then press fitted or cemented into place.
- The patella mechanism is then allowed to return to its normal position.
- The incision is closed with sutures.

HOSPITAL RECOVERY

Most patients undergoing knee arthroplasty will be in the hospital between five and ten days. Intravenous or intramuscular pain medications may be administered for the first several days; patients can usually switch to oral pain medicine, such as an acetaminophen and codeine combination, at that time.

Physical therapy to regain range of motion and improve strength is initiated in the hospital. Patients are generally limited to restricted weight bearing with an assistive device (crutches or walker).

AT-HOME RECOVERY

Patients continue the rehabilitation process at home—either with at-home physical therapy or as an outpatient. Exercises are continued to improve range of motion and strength. Restrictions on activity and weight bearing are progressively relaxed as the knee heals.

Patients may continue to use oral pain medicine, such as an acetaminophen and codeine combination, for two to four weeks after they come home.

COMPLICATIONS AND RISKS

- As with any operation, there is a small risk of surgical wound infection.
- On rare occasions, blood clots in the legs (deep vein THROMBOSIS) can be a dangerous complication.

LUMBAR DISK REMOVAL

Lumbar disk removal is helpful for about 80 percent of the patients who experience no improvement with conservative treatment.

The objective of a disk removal surgery, called *diskectomy*, is to decompress nerve roots that are irritated by a portion of the intervertebral disk (see HERNIATED DISK). Disk removal surgery is done by surgeons with specialized training in spine surgery, usually orthopedic surgeons or neurosurgeons.

Although most of the time the surgery is done in a hospital setting, some types of diskectomies may be done as outpatient surgery.

ALTERNATIVE TREATMENTS

Almost all patients with disk problems should initially undergo conservative treatment with rest, anti-inflammatory medication such as ibuprofen, and possibly physical therapy to allow for recovery without surgery.

PREOPERATIVE PREPARATION

An evaluation of the patient's general health can include routine BLOOD TESTS and more specialized tests such as ELECTROCARDIOGRAPHY and chest X rays (RADIOGRAPHY) as needed.

Overnight fasting is required for general anesthesia.

ANESTHESIA

Anesthesia is usually general, but occasionally regional anesthetic (anesthesia of the lower back and legs) or local anesthetic (anesthesia of the surgery site only) may be used with or without a sedative.

PROCEDURE

The goal of the diskectomy is to free affected nerve roots that are compressed or stretched by HERNIATED DISK material. This may be done through an open incision with the aid of magnifying glasses or a microscope, or by an endoscopic approach (see ENDOSCOPY).

For the microdiskectomy

- An incision is centered over the affected disk space.
- The overlying soft tissues are carefully cut to reveal the nerve root.
- The nerve is carefully moved to the side, and the offending disk material is removed.
- The wound is closed with sutures in layers.

In the endoscopic approach
- A small tube that allows passage of small instruments and an endoscope is passed through the muscle along the spine and placed in the center of the disk.
- Disk material is then removed in front of the bulging material to decompress the nerve root indirectly.

HOSPITAL RECOVERY

Depending on the setting of the procedure, some patients may be able to go home the same day or the day after the procedure. Patients can generally walk unassisted after the operation on that same day.

Oral pain medicine such as an acetaminophen and codeine combination is usually adequate to control discomfort; some patients may require some intravenous or intramuscular pain medicine right after the procedure, however.

AT-HOME RECOVERY

Most patients require a period of convalescence and reduced activity after surgery. Patients should avoid repeated stooping, bending, lifting, and prolonged sitting for several weeks. Some patients with less demanding jobs may be able to return to limited work as soon as two to three weeks after the operation.

Oral pain medicine (acetaminophen and codeine combination) is generally needed for several weeks after the operation.

COMPLICATIONS AND RISKS

As with any surgery, there is a small risk of surgical wound infection, but it is rare.

Surgery around the irritated nerve root may cause some additional pain, NUMBNESS, or tingling similar to the original symptoms of a HERNIATED DISK with nerve root entrapment, and should be evaluated by a physician.

LUMBAR PUNCTURE

A lumbar puncture is performed to test for such diseases as multiple sclerosis or meningitis and to inject drugs in the spinal cord area to treat some conditions.

During the lumbar puncture, or spinal tap, a small needle is put into the fluid-filled space that surrounds the brain and spinal cord to remove fluid for laboratory tests. The needle is inserted between the bones of the spine in the lower back below the end of the spinal cord. This test is performed to diagnose infections, such as meningitis, and bleeding into this space (subarachnoid hemorrhage), as well as to obtain fluid to test for other diseases such as MULTIPLE SCLEROSIS.

PREPARATION

There is no specific preparation for this test.

ANESTHESIA

A local anesthetic is used.

PROCEDURE

Usually the patient is asked to curl up on his or her side, although sometimes the patient is asked to sit and bend forward. Sometimes the test is done in an X-ray (RADIOGRAPHY) room where a fluoroscope can be used to aid the procedure.

- The skin is cleaned with an antiseptic and a local anesthetic is injected.
- A needle is inserted into the spinal canal.
- Once the needle is in the spinal fluid, the pressure may be measured and fluid collected.
- Once the spinal fluid has been collected, the needle is removed.

RECOVERY

The patient is usually kept flat in bed for about an hour following the test and then may resume normal activity but should avoid lifting or straining for 24 hours. There may be soreness in the lower back for a few days.

COMPLICATIONS AND RISKS

In extremely rare cases in which there is an unsuspected increase in the pressure in the brain, a lumbar puncture can cause a worsening of neurologic symptoms.

LUNG RESECTION

Lung resection can be used to remove suspicious nodules, or "spots," in the lung or, in a relatively new procedure, to reduce lung volume in patients with EMPHYSEMA.

Removal of suspicious lesions is often needed for diagnosis and attempted cure (see LUNG CANCER).

Volume reduction surgery removes lung tissue damaged by EMPHYSEMA, decreasing lung volume and allowing the rib cage and diaphragm to assume a more normal position. Removing damaged lung also allows the more normal lung tissue to function better.

Specific criteria must be met before patients are deemed candidates for this surgery. In general, patients must have severe EMPHYSEMA with significant lung overinflation. Patients are not candidates if they are active smokers, are extremely obese, or have another severe illness.

ALTERNATIVE TREATMENTS

For emphysema patients, optimal medical therapy should be attempted before surgery.

PREOPERATIVE PREPARATION

For lung resection of suspected LUNG CANCER, an evaluation for any possible spread of the cancer is performed. COMPUTED TOMOGRAPHY is often used for this purpose.

Other tests used before lung surgery may include
- BLOOD TESTS, including BLOOD COUNT
- ELECTROCARDIOGRAPHY
- PULMONARY FUNCTION TESTING
- Chest X ray (RADIOGRAPHY)

Overnight fasting is required for general anesthesia.

ANESTHESIA

General anesthesia.

PROCEDURE

There are two major approaches: open surgery or surgery using thoracoscopy (a form of ENDOSCOPY).

For open surgery
- An incision is made in the center of the chest.
- The sternum (breastbone) is separated.

Lung resection is
the surgical removal
of a portion of
the lung.

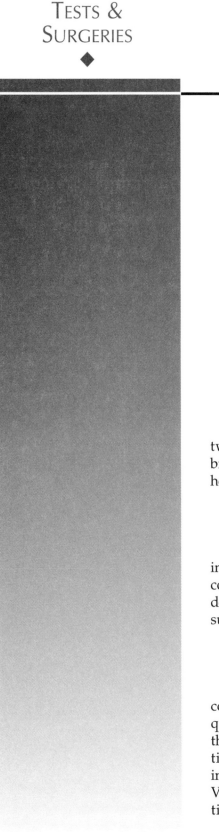

- The suspicious nodule or the portion of the emphysematous lung is removed with a stapling device that cuts and seals lung tissue with staples.
- A strip of bovine (cow) heart tissue may be used to strengthen the incision.
- The incision is closed in layers with sutures.

For the thorascopic approach

- Three small holes are made on one side of the chest.
- The thoracoscope and other instruments are inserted through the holes.
- Surgical removal is performed as above except through the thoracoscope.
- The instruments are removed and the puncture wounds closed.

HOSPITAL RECOVERY

Chest tubes and intravenous fluids are usually required for two to three days after the surgery. Mechanical ventilation (a breathing machine) may also be needed initially. The total hospital stay is usually between five to seven days.

AT-HOME RECOVERY

Over three to six weeks, activity may be gradually increased. Pain medication, such as an acetaminophen and codeine combination, may be prescribed. Driving is usually deferred for six weeks if the breast bone was cut during surgery. Some wound care is necessary.

COMPLICATIONS AND RISKS

Wound infection, excessive bleeding, PNEUMONIA, and other complications of major surgery are a possibility. Also, the quantity of remaining lung tissue has to be enough to sustain the patient. Preoperative tests are used to predict postoperative lung function, but patients are sometimes left with an inadequate amount of functional lung tissue after resection. Very rarely, patients require prolonged use of mechanical ventilation (a breathing machine).

MAGNETIC RESONANCE IMAGING

Magnetic resonance imaging (sometimes called MR or MRI) is a form of radiologic testing that allows physicians to distinguish fine details of internal structures. Unlike RADIOGRAPHY and COMPUTED TOMOGRAPHY, magnetic resonance imaging does not use X-ray radiation.

The technology used is very complex: Using an extremely powerful magnetic field, some portion of the body's atoms are lined up parallel to each other like rows of magnets. A pulse of radio waves transiently shifts the atom particles and they emit a detectable radio signal as they shift back into line. The signals are assembled with the help of a computer to build an image of the body area.

PREPARATION

Patients with heart pacemakers, hearing aids, or any other metal parts in the body may not be able to have the test and need to tell their doctors before an exam. Otherwise, no special preparation is necessary.

ANESTHESIA

None is needed, but in rare instances, patients who are claustrophobic may need sedation before the procedure.

PROCEDURE

- The patient lays down and is moved into the large cylinder that houses the magnets.
- Sometimes a special dye or contrast medium is used to enhance the images, and this is injected by vein into the body.
- The test may take 30 to 90 minutes, during which time the patient must remain very still.

RECOVERY

None.

COMPLICATIONS AND RISKS

There are no known risks associated with this procedure.

Although relatively new, magnetic resonance imaging is now a frequently used diagnostic technique that has a wide variety of applications.

MALIGNANT MELANOMA REMOVAL

A malignant melanoma is a pigmented form of SKIN CANCER. It begins as a result of an abnormal proliferation of the pigment-producing cells in the skin called *melanocytes*.

ALTERNATIVE TREATMENTS

Malignant melanoma requires surgical removal.

PREOPERATIVE PREPARATION

Overnight fasting is usually required for general anesthesia.

ANESTHESIA

General anesthesia or regional anesthesia may be used.

PROCEDURE

For superficial tumors
* The surgeon numbs the skin with a local anesthetic.
* The surgeon uses a scalpel to cut around the tumor.
* Adequate margins of normal skin are also removed.
* The two sides are then stitched together.
* The removed tissue is examined to make sure all of the tumor has been removed.

When the tumor is deeper and when the skin area of the tumor drains to a defined set of lymph nodes, the lymph nodes may also need to be surgically removed and examined for any melanoma cells that may have spread from the skin to the bundle of lymph nodes. If cells are found in the lymph nodes, medicines that kill cancer cells (chemotherapy) may be given to treat melanoma cells that may have spread to other sites besides the skin and lymph nodes. The patient will also undergo a variety of X-ray (RADIOGRAPHY) methods to search for signs of tumor in other sites.

RECOVERY

No hospital stay is usually required.

COMPLICATIONS AND RISKS

Infection and excessive bleeding are possible but rare.

MASTECTOMY, MODIFIED RADICAL

The modified radical mastectomy, or total mastectomy, is a time-honored treatment for BREAST CANCER. It involves the removal of the entire breast and contents of the armpit area. The operation is most commonly performed in the hospital by a general surgeon or a surgical oncologist.

ALTERNATIVE TREATMENTS

Lumpectomy (MASTECTOMY, PARTIAL) and radiation treatments may be appropriate for some tumors of the breast.

PREOPERATIVE PREPARATION

The patient undergoing modified radical mastectomy requires mammography (RADIOGRAPHY) to assess the health of the opposite breast. Patients should have a chest X ray (RADIOGRAPHY) and a battery of tests that include serum liver function tests to exclude tumor in the liver (see BLOOD TESTS).

Some patients with large cancers should have a bone scan (see NUCLEAR MEDICINE) and tests to examine the liver, such as COMPUTED TOMOGRAPHY or liver scan (see NUCLEAR MEDICINE), to exclude the possibility that the tumor has spread to the bones or to the liver.

Overnight fasting is required for general anesthesia.

ANESTHESIA

General anesthesia.

PROCEDURE

- The patient is placed on the operating room table on her back.
- An incision is made over the breast and skin flaps are created to close the wound by cutting between the skin and the breast tissue.
- The breast is then removed from the chest wall by removing the fascia (the lining of the chest wall muscles).
- The muscles of the chest wall are preserved. (Previously the operation—called the radical mastectomy—removed these muscles and caused significant chest wall deformity. This is no longer considered necessary.)

In most cases, radiation treatments are not required if a modified radical mastectomy is performed, but depending on the stage of disease, patients may require chemotherapy.

- The blood vessels and important nerves in the
  armpit area are identified through the same incision
  and preserved.
- The contents of the armpit, including the lymph
  nodes, are removed and sent for pathologic examination (see BIOPSY).
- The skin is closed with sutures or clips.

Some women choose to have breast reconstruction, either
immediately or later, after they have recovered from the operation and treatment. This is performed by a plastic surgeon.

HOSPITAL RECOVERY

Since lymph fluid may collect in the wound, a drainage
tube is sometimes placed in the armpit and under the skin
flaps. The surgery requires a short one- to three-day hospital
stay. Patients require oral pain medications such as an acetaminophen and codeine combination. They are encouraged to
resume normal activity, to perform exercises, and to use their
arms as soon as possible after the operation.

AT-HOME RECOVERY

Patients may continue to require pain medications such as
an acetaminophen and codeine combination at home. They
should increase their activity and their exercises. Many
patients go home with drains in their armpits and must care
for and empty the drains until they are ready to be removed.
Chemotherapy, if needed, is begun when the wounds are
healed and the drains are removed.

COMPLICATIONS AND RISKS

- Hematoma is a collection of blood in the wound. It
  usually resolves spontaneously, but if large, it may
  have to be evacuated surgically.
- Seroma is a collection of lymph fluid in the armpit.
  It can occur despite the use of drains. It may resolve
  on its own, but if uncomfortable, it may need to be
  aspirated with a needle.
- Wound infection is a possibility with all surgery, but
  it is rare.

MASTECTOMY, PARTIAL

A partial mastectomy is the removal of part of the breast to treat benign and malignant tumors of the breast (see BREAST CANCER). Removal of a cancer of the breast with an adequate margin of tissue is called *lumpectomy*. Sometimes an entire quadrant of the breast is required to remove a cancer. The operation is most commonly performed in a hospital by a general surgeon or a surgical oncologist.

ALTERNATIVE TREATMENTS

Modified radical mastectomy is another more involved operation to treat tumors of the breast (see MASTECTOMY, MODIFIED RADICAL).

PREOPERATIVE PREPARATION

The patient undergoing breast BIOPSY (removal of a lump for diagnosis) usually requires mammography (RADIOGRAPHY) to assess the characteristics of the lump and to be sure there are no other lesions in the same or opposite breast.

Patients with BREAST CANCER should have a chest X ray (RADIOGRAPHY) and a battery of tests including serum liver function tests (see BLOOD TESTS) to exclude tumor in the liver. Some patients with large cancers should have a bone scan (see NUCLEAR MEDICINE) and tests to examine the liver, such as COMPUTED TOMOGRAPHY or a liver scan (see NUCLEAR MEDICINE), to exclude spread of the cancer.

Overnight fasting is required for general anesthesia.

ANESTHESIA

Breast BIOPSY and lumpectomy may be performed under local anesthesia. Many patients require general anesthesia when BIOPSY of the armpit lymph nodes or a larger resection is required.

PROCEDURE

- The patient is placed on the operating room table on her back.
- An incision is made over the lump.
- The lump and an appropriate amount of surrounding tissue are removed.

For most types of breast cancer, lumpectomy is followed by sampling of lymph nodes from the armpit area, radiation treatments, and depending on the stage of the disease, chemotherapy.

- The lump is sent for pathologic examination (BIOPSY).
- If the contents of the armpit need to be removed or sampled, another incision is made in the armpit.
- Wounds are closed with sutures or clips.

HOSPITAL RECOVERY

Breast BIOPSY is usually performed as an outpatient, but more extensive operations, such as lumpectomy or quadrantectomy, require a short one- to two-day hospital stay. Since lymph fluid may collect in the wound, a drainage tube is sometimes placed in the armpit area and left in place to collect fluid until drainage ceases. Patients require oral pain medications such as an acetaminophen and codeine combination. Patients are encouraged to resume normal activity, perform exercises, and use their arms as soon as possible after the operation.

AT-HOME RECOVERY

Patients may continue to require pain medications at home. They should increase their activity and their exercises gradually. Many patients go home with wound drains in place and must care for and empty the drains until they are ready to be removed.

Radiation and chemotherapy can begin when wounds are healed and drains are removed.

COMPLICATIONS AND RISKS

- Hematoma is a collection of blood in the wound. It usually resolves spontaneously, but if large, it may have to be evacuated surgically.
- Seroma is a collection of lymph fluid in the armpit. It can occur despite the use of drains. It may resolve on its own, but if uncomfortable may need to be aspirated with a needle.
- Wound infection is a possibility with all surgery, but it is rare.
- Recurrence of tumor may occur in some patients. Total mastectomy (MASTECTOMY, MODIFIED RADICAL) may be required at that time to eliminate the disease.

MEDICAL HISTORY

PHYSICAL EXAMINATION and diagnostic tests contribute only a small portion of the information required to make a diagnosis. A medical history involves the communication of information about a patient's symptoms, past illnesses, health habits, family history, and other pertinent topics.

PREPARATION

To get the most from a medical history, it helps to organize and even write down information to give to the doctor or to refer to during the history. For example, dates of prior hospitalizations, immunizations, and surgeries are important pieces of information. It's also helpful to record any adverse or allergic reactions one had to a specific medication.

Some aspects of the family history are very helpful and worth asking a relative about. For example, the patient should know about any family history of

- Unexpected deaths at a young age
- BREAST CANCER
- COLORECTAL CANCER
- Thyroid cancer
- Premature heart disease such as a HEART ATTACK
- DIABETES

If the visit to the doctor is to evaluate a specific symptom, read the appropriate section in this book, note what symptoms make the problem more or less suspicious, the timing and duration of the symptom, and any other clues.

PROCEDURE

The key aspects of a medical history are

- The chief complaint—the main reason a patient is seeking medical advice
- History of the present illness
- Past medical history
- Family medical history
- Social history including occupation, hobbies, smoking and alcohol use, sexual orientation
- General review of body systems

Depending on the setting, a doctor may focus on a limited number of topics or cover most of this list.

It is very important to be as open as possible about answers, even if they are embarrassing; a physician is in a better position to help if he or she knows the whole story.

> In approximately 70 percent of cases, all a physician really needs to make a diagnosis and address a problem is the information a patient can provide.

NUCLEAR MEDICINE

Nuclear medicine
encompasses a wide
variety of tests and
therapies. It can be
used to obtain
images useful in
diagnosis, and it
can actually treat
certain disorders.

Nuclear medicine is the use of radioactive chemicals for a medical purpose. Some type of scan or imaging of the body is the most common use. The radioactive substance is injected into the body and its radio signal is then detectable from the outside. Common scans using nuclear techniques include bone scans, heart muscle scans, thyroid scans, and lung scans.

Radioactive iodine to treat HYPERTHYROIDISM is an example of the therapeutic use of nuclear medicine. A radiopharmacist may prepare the material, but a radiologist or cardiologist certified in nuclear medicine usually performs the test or treatment.

PREPARATION

This varies widely with the specific test. Preparation mainly consists of communicating the appropriate information to the physician conducting the test. The physician must know about

- Any medications the patient is taking, because they may need to be avoided for a day or so before the test (Theophylline, for example, must be discontinued before certain heart scans.)
- Any chance that the patient is pregnant (Nuclear medicine can adversely affect a developing fetus.)

PROCEDURE

Almost all nuclear scans require injecting a radioactive material into the bloodstream. Then special cameras record the radiation coming from the organ being studied.

Scans commonly take 20 to 60 minutes, and patience is required because of the time it takes to get a useful picture.

RECOVERY

For hyperthyroidism treatment with radioactive iodine, patients may be kept in a hospital room for a day or so.

COMPLICATIONS AND RISKS

The radiation dose is generally quite small, and for the average patient, the cumulative exposure is insignificant.

OCCULT BLOOD TESTING

Occult blood testing of stool is an attempt to detect the small amounts of blood emitted by COLORECTAL CANCER that are not otherwise visible. The test also detects blood from sources other than cancers—from meat or benign gastrointestinal problems—leading to false alarms. Despite the frequent false-positive results, the test is useful. One recent study documented the benefit, albeit modest, of a yearly occult blood test: The mortality from colon cancer over a 13-year period in people aged 50 to 80 dropped from 8 deaths per 1000 people to 5 deaths per 1000 people in those who had an occult blood screening yearly. The use of flexible sigmoidoscopy (a form of ENDOSCOPY) may be an alternative to occult blood screening.

PREPARATION

One should follow the directions included with each testing kit, but in general, to minimize the chances of a false-positive result, one should avoid red meat and aspirin or other anti-inflammatory drugs such as ibuprofen for a few days before the test.

PROCEDURE

The test is performed by the subject at home with a special kit. Because different kit manufacturers have slightly different procedures, it is important to follow the directions on the particular package. Generally, stool is sampled over a period of three days.

COMPLICATIONS AND RISKS

There is nothing dangerous about this test, but false positive results do generate additional tests and costs (for example, ENDOSCOPY and RADIOGRAPHY).

Approximately half of all colorectal cancers bleed at some time, and this bleeding is not always enough to be noticed. A laboratory test for this occult (hidden) blood is often necessary.

OVARIAN CYST REMOVAL

Persistent ovarian cysts may need to be removed. Ruptured or twisted cysts may need emergency surgery. There are several techniques available for the procedure including traditional open surgery and removal with laparoscopy (a form of ENDOSCOPY).

PREOPERATIVE PREPARATION

BLOOD TESTS and possibly an ULTRASOUND may be necessary. Overnight fasting is required with general anesthesia.

ANESTHESIA

General or spinal anesthesia is the norm, but local anesthesia with sedation may be possible with laparoscopy.

PROCEDURE

For open surgery
- An incision is made in the abdomen.
- The blood vessel to the ovary is clamped.
- If the cyst is malignant, the ovary is removed.
- The incision is sewn shut in layers with sutures.

For surgery using laparoscopy (ENDOSCOPY), the procedure is performed through small puncture wounds in the abdomen.

HOSPITAL RECOVERY

An abdominal incision may require three to seven days in the hospital, less with a laparoscopy.

AT-HOME RECOVERY

Patients should limit vigorous activity for about six weeks. Sexual activity may be resumed when the doctor feels the wounds have healed.

COMPLICATIONS AND RISKS

- Infection at the site of entry through the skin
- Persistent bleeding, but this occurs rarely

PACEMAKER INSERTION

A pacemaker is an electronic device that helps regulate the heart rhythm and correct ARRHYTHMIAS. There are many types of pacemakers today. They all have a battery, one or more electrode wires that go to the heart, and a control center. Standard pacemakers keep the heart from going too slow in order to avoid FAINTING OR FAINTNESS or cardiac arrest. Newer types of pacemakers have features that can speed up the heart during exercise.

Related devices, such as implantable defibrillators and anti-tachycardia pacemakers, can deliver electrical shocks to automatically abort abnormal rhythms.

A cardiologist or cardiothoracic surgeon usually performs the procedure.

ALTERNATIVE TREATMENTS

For abnormally slow heart rhythms causing symptoms of FAINTING OR FAINTNESS, a pacemaker is the most appropriate treatment. There are some drug therapies for certain ARRHYTHMIAS, however. Some abnormally fast rhythms (called *tachycardias*) may respond to the selective use of medications such as

- Procainamide
- Quinidine
- Sotalol
- Amiodarone

PREOPERATIVE PREPARATION

ELECTROCARDIOGRAPHY and special pacing studies of the heart may be required. BLOOD TESTS to assess general health may also be performed.

ANESTHESIA

Local anesthesia is used under the collarbone near the vein where the electrode wire is passed.

PROCEDURE

- The pacemaker battery and control center are placed under the skin.

A pacemaker is inserted to help regulate the heart rhythm and especially to keep the heart from going too slow and causing faintness.

- The electrode wire is passed via one of the large veins nearby into the heart's inside wall.
- X rays (RADIOGRAPHY) are used to confirm or adjust the location of the electrode.
- The pacemaker's performance is tested and adjusted, and the incision is closed.

HOSPITAL RECOVERY

Pacemaker insertions are now done as outpatient surgery or with very brief hospital stays of one to two days. The heart is monitored with ELECTROCARDIOGRAPHY and the arm on the side of the incision is restricted in its motion for a short time.

AT-HOME RECOVERY

Vigorous activity with the arm should be avoided for a few weeks so that the electrode gets a chance to settle into the heart muscle and continues to make good electrical contact with the tissue.

Especially in the early weeks after a pacemaker insertion, antibiotics may be recommended to avoid infection in patients undergoing procedures, such as dental work, in which bacteria could be released into the blood stream.

COMPLICATIONS AND RISKS

A wound infection, purulent drainage, or FEVER can occur early after the surgery, as can excessive bleeding.

The pacemaker signal wire can dislodge or even, rarely, perforate the heart wall, although this can be adjusted again in most cases.

Pacemaker electrodes or batteries can malfunction, leading to loss of function and causing FAINTING OR FAINTNESS.

A pacemaker can be a lifesaving procedure and is well worth the risks when inserted in appropriately selected patients.

PAP SMEAR

The Pap smear tests for cancer or precancerous changes in the uterine cervix (see CERVICAL CANCER). The Pap smear is performed in the office by a primary care physician or an obstetrician-gynecologist. This is a painless, though possibly uncomfortable, part of a routine pelvic examination.

Women who are sexually active or who have reached 18 years of age should have routine pelvic examinations and Pap smears.

PREPARATION

None.

PROCEDURE

- A speculum is inserted to open the vagina.
- Cells shed from the cervix are collected by means of scraping the inside of the cervix with a small wooden spatula.
- The cells collected are spread on a slide and sent to the laboratory to be examined (see CYTOLOGY).

If an abnormality is detected, further testing may be required, including

- A procedure called colposcopy (a form of ENDOSCOPY and BIOPSY)
- Another pelvic examination with insertion of a speculum to visualize the cervix
- BIOPSY of the cervix

RECOVERY

This is an outpatient procedure and is usually performed in a doctor's office.

COMPLICATIONS

Occasionally, there may be troublesome VAGINAL BLEEDING, requiring sutures to be placed. This rarely happens with the new office procedures. Other possible complications include local or systemic infections requiring antibiotic therapy. Patients should call the doctor if there is any bleeding that is heavier than a normal menstrual period (MENSTRUAL IRREGU-LARITIES), DIZZINESS, FEVER, or increasing pain unresponsive to mild pain medication, such as ibuprofen or naproxen.

Pap smear is short for the *Papanicolaou* smear, named for the Greek physician who developed the test.

PERIODONTAL SURGERY

A component of preventive dental care, periodontal surgery manipulates soft (gingiva) and hard (bone) tissues supporting the teeth to correct various problems that could result in tooth loss if left uncorrected.

ALTERNATIVE TREATMENTS

Treatment alternatives may include more frequent dental hygiene visits for nonsurgical periodontal procedures such as scaling and root planing.

PREOPERATIVE PREPARATION

Diagnostic casts to examine the occlusion as well as X rays (RADIOGRAPHY) and measurements of gingival pocket depths are used to determine the need for surgical treatment.

ANESTHESIA

Local anesthetic.

PROCEDURE

Periodontal surgery aims at reducing or eliminating gum pockets around the teeth by removing infected gingival tissue, encouraging reattachment of healthy gingival tissue, or grafting of gum tissue and bone.

Synthetic membrane barriers are used to help guide regeneration of bone. These fibers are placed into the gum lining, and synthetic bone grafts may be used.

RECOVERY

Postoperative management is performed routinely one week after treatment to see if the graft has taken. Consistent dental hygiene visits are necessary to maintain the health of the gum tissues.

COMPLICATIONS AND RISKS

On occasion, exposure of the root surface and sensitivity may initially be present after surgical treatment. Additional complications may arise if the grafted material does not function properly.

> Nearly all periodontal surgery is preventable with good oral hygiene.

PHYSICAL EXAMINATION

The physical examination consists of careful looking (inspection), tapping with the fingers (percussion), feeling with the fingers (palpation), and listening with a stethoscope (auscultation). Depending on the body part examined, a doctor may use all of these methods (as during an examination of the heart, lungs, or abdomen) or just one or two (as during an examination of the skin). Occasionally, even smell is useful; for example, ketoacidosis—a condition in DIABETES—produces a characteristic odor to the breath, and wounds that are infected can smell.

A primary care physician has a broader repertoire of physical examination techniques to choose from. A specialist may examine a patient in greater depth, but the examination is usually limited to one organ system.

PREPARATION

None.

ANESTHESIA

None.

PROCEDURE

An examination may focus on one or two body parts or be more general, depending on the patient's need, the problem, and the available time.

An almost endless number of individual steps can be performed during a physical examination. For example, hundreds of techniques can be used to test the nervous system alone.

Although it's not possible to perform a truly "complete" physical examination, a general physical exam usually includes

- Vital signs, including body temperature, blood pressure (see BLOOD PRESSURE TEST), pulse, respiratory rate, and general characteristics such as weight and height
- Head, eyes, ears, nose, and throat (often using special scopes)
- Neck, including the glands, the arteries that carry blood to the head, and thyroid
- Chest, including heart and lungs

Along with the medical history, the physical examination is the most basic and the oldest of diagnostic explorations.

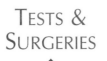

- Abdomen
- Pelvic examination in women
- Scrotal examination in men
- Rectal exam in both women and men
- Legs, arms, spine, and other joints
- Skin
- Nervous system, including reflexes, muscle strength, coordination, and mental function

In recent years, the belief has become more accepted that certain parts of a general screening examination are much more important than others. For example, depending on the patient's age, sex, and individual risk factors, a doctor may be much more effective spending more time on a skin or breast examination than a nervous system or joint examination.

HOSPITAL RECOVERY

None.

AT-HOME RECOVERY

None.

COMPLICATIONS AND RISKS

None. A physical examination is extremely safe.

PROSTATE GLAND REMOVAL

Removal of the prostate is an operation performed for PROSTATE CANCER that is confined to the prostate. The procedure is also used to treat advanced cases of enlarged prostate that cannot be managed by other means (see PROSTATE, ENLARGED).

The surgery is performed in the hospital, usually by a urologist. There is more than one technique used for this surgery: the *retropubic* approach and the *perineal* approach.

ALTERNATIVE TREATMENTS

Radiation therapy and hormonal (palliative) therapy are alternatives for select patients.

PREOPERATIVE PREPARATION

- A needle BIOPSY is usually needed to confirm the diagnosis.
- A bone scan is performed to look for evidence that the cancer has spread. (see NUCLEAR MEDICINE).
- The patient should have no food or drink after midnight the night before surgery.

ANESTHESIA

General anesthesia.

PROCEDURE

- In the retropubic approach, the incision is made in the lower abdomen. In the perineal approach, the incision is made in the area between the scrotum and the anus.
- The lymph nodes in the area are removed (retropubic approach only).
- The prostate gland is cut away from the urethra and the bladder.
- The gland is removed.
- The bladder and the urethra are connected to each other again.
- The external incision is closed with sutures.

For patients with cancer confined to the prostate, prostate gland removal offers an excellent chance of cure.

HOSPITAL RECOVERY

- The patient usually has to spend another three to five days in the hospital.
- Pain medication such as acetaminophen and codeine combination is prescribed as needed.
- An intravenous line is usually left in place for two days.
- Solid food is resumed after one to two days.

AT-HOME RECOVERY

- A Foley catheter that runs from the bladder down the urethra and out the penis is left in place for two to three weeks to drain urine.
- Activity must be restricted for approximately six weeks.

COMPLICATIONS AND RISKS

The two biggest complications associated with prostate gland removal are

- INCONTINENCE—Most patients leak urine after the catheter is removed. This condition generally improves with time; after about six months, approximately 90 percent of men have no leakage problems or leak only a small amount when they are straining or lifting.
- IMPOTENCE—Despite techniques to spare the nerves responsible for achieving erection, IMPOTENCE is still common after prostatectomy.

PULMONARY FUNCTION TESTS

A number of physiologic tests can be performed in a pulmonary function laboratory for the purpose of establishing lung function. These measurements often include

- The total lung volume
- The ability to exhale forcefully
- The total amount of air exhaled in a full breath
- The diffusing capacity of the lung (how quickly and evenly a gas distributes in the lung)

These tests are often used in the diagnosis of diseases such as ASTHMA, EMPHYSEMA, and chronic bronchitis (BRONCHITIS, CHRONIC).

PREPARATION

None.

PROCEDURE

To test lung volume, either the helium-dilution technique or body plethysmography are used. The helium-dilution technique involves inhaling a known volume and concentration of helium for several minutes. The concentration of helium decreases as it enters the lung. By measuring the decrease in helium concentrations caused by its larger volume of distribution, lung volume can be estimated. Body plethysmography requires patients to sit inside an air-tight box and breathe through a mouthpiece. Lung volume is determined by measuring the change in box volume and pressure.

To test the ability to exhale, patients are asked to take in a full breath and then forcefully exhale as long and hard as they can. The volume of the air exhaled in the first second of trying, called the FEV_1, can help demonstrate when airflow obstruction is present. The total amount of air exhaled from a full exhalation (called the *forced vital capacity*, or *FVC*) is also helpful in diagnosis.

Another commonly performed pulmonary function test is the diffusing capacity for carbon monoxide. In this test, patients are asked to inhale minute quantities of carbon monoxide to test the diffusion of this gas into pulmonary blood vessels.

COMPLICATIONS AND RISKS

None.

> Pulmonary function tests measure lung size or volume and the ability to exhale air forcefully, which helps to identify lung disease.

RADIOGRAPHY

When diseases or abnormalities are suspected, radiography is used to view internal parts of the body.

Using X rays to take pictures of parts of the body not easily seen is called *radiography*. X rays can identify broken or diseased bones, chest abnormalities, or signs of perforated organs in the abdomen. Special X-ray techniques can detect foreign bodies such as glass under the skin; they can also be used to detect signs of BREAST CANCER (a test called *mammography*).

Primary care physicians, emergency medicine physicians, surgeons, and other specialists all use X rays for various reasons.

Some X rays require injection of special dye, or contrast material, to make certain structures more visible on the X-ray film. The contrast material may be injected into a vein in the arm or via a catheter directly into blood vessels near the body part being studied; for example, in an angiogram, the dye is injected into the blood vessels that are under examination. Other X rays require drinking a liquid with barium in it (the upper gastrointestinal, or GI, series) or running barium into the colon (the lower GI series) to enhance X-ray images of the esophagus, stomach, and intestines.

PREPARATION

Individuals who are allergic to the contrast material used for some X rays may need special preparation with antihistamines or other drugs to suppress adverse reactions. Such drugs include prednisone and diphenhydramine.

If there is any chance of pregnancy, the patient should discuss it with her doctor, because X rays may cause abnormalities in the early development of a fetus.

Some examinations require fasting.

ANESTHESIA

None.

PROCEDURE

- Contrast material, if any is needed, is administered, orally or by injection.
- The patient is positioned in front of the source of the X rays.
- A special film is placed behind the patient to receive the X-ray image.

- A lead apron can be placed over areas not in the picture.
- The technician usually steps out of the room, and the picture is taken.

RECOVERY

None, except that angiograms or delayed films (if needed) may require a few hours.

COMPLICATIONS AND RISKS

- The risk of X rays is generally insignificant except to a fetus early in development. However, some X rays involve more radiation than others, and excessive repeat examinations over a period of years could increase a person's risk for certain cancers or LEUKEMIA. Therefore, doctors try to order X rays only when necessary.
- The radiation from a chest X ray is said to be comparable to the amount one would get from a day on the beach.
- Allergic reactions to contrast materials can range from mild flushing to wheezing, low blood pressure, or even death. Serious reactions are extremely rare and can be treated promptly with diphenhydramine, fluids, and epinephrine.
- There is an extremely small risk of perforation of the colon with a lower GI series.

RECTAL OR COLON POLYP REMOVAL

A COLON POLYP or rectal polyp is an abnormal growth in the colon or rectum. It may be benign, but many benign polyps have the potential to become malignant (to become COLORECTAL CANCER) and should be removed. Many polyps contain cancer already and have to be removed. Polyps may be removed without surgery using colonoscopy (a form of ENDOSCOPY). Other polyps are too large or too broad based for colonoscopy and require more traditional surgical removal in a hospital setting.

ALTERNATIVE TREATMENTS

A polyp that is small (less than four millimeters in diameter) can be observed with regular ENDOSCOPY, but usually it is easier to remove it.

PREOPERATIVE PREPARATION

Patients who are to undergo polyp removal receive a mechanical bowel preparation. This consists of the removal of fecal contents by beginning a liquid diet one to two days before the operation. Later, a large volume of nonabsorbable liquid is ingested or laxatives are given to clear the intestine of feces. Some patients also require enemas.

Patients undergoing surgical removal are also given oral nonabsorbable antibiotics to kill bacteria in the bowel and, therefore, lessen any chance of postoperative infection. The patient is not allowed any food or water after midnight on the night preceding polyp removal.

ANESTHESIA

Endoscopic polypectomy can be performed with sedation alone. Surgical removal of polyps requires a general anesthetic.

PROCEDURE

Endoscopic polypectomy:
- A flexible scope is passed through the rectum and colon.

- The polyp is located and the feasibility of resection is assessed.
- A wire snare is passed through the scope and looped around the base of the polyp.
- The loop is tightened and electrocautery is used to cut the base of the polyp and coagulate any blood.
- When free, the polyp is grasped, taken out through the anus, and sent to the laboratory for pathologic examination.

Surgical removal of a polyp:

- An abdominal incision is made.
- Although the growth can be removed by opening the colon and removing the polyp, it is more often removed with a whole segment of colon in case cancer is later found in the polyp (see SIGMOID COLON REMOVAL).

HOSPITAL RECOVERY

Endoscopic polyp removal can be performed as an outpatient procedure or with a short hospital stay. Surgical removal requires more extensive recovery (see SIGMOID COLON REMOVAL).

AT-HOME RECOVERY

Endoscopic polyp removal requires no special at-home recovery. Recovery from open surgical removal may require several weeks (see SIGMOID COLON REMOVAL).

COMPLICATIONS AND RISKS

- Perforation of the bowel may occur with endoscopic polyp removal.
- RECTAL BLEEDING may occur after endoscopic polyp removal.
- See SIGMOID COLON REMOVAL for complications of surgical polyp removal.

SIGMOID COLON REMOVAL

The sigmoid colon is removed most frequently for benign and malignant tumors (COLORECTAL CANCER) and for diverticulitis (DIVERTICULAR DISEASE). It is occasionally removed if the colon twists on itself (a condition called *volvulus*), for inflammatory disease of the colon such as CROHN DISEASE, and for ENDOMETRIOSIS. The operation is performed by general or colorectal surgeons.

ALTERNATIVE TREATMENTS

Endoscopic polyp removal (see RECTAL OR COLON POLYP REMOVAL) may be an option for smaller tumors.

PREOPERATIVE PREPARATION

Patients receive a mechanical and antibiotic bowel preparation. This consists of the removal of fecal contents by beginning a liquid diet one to two days before surgery. Later, a large volume of nonabsorbable liquid is ingested or laxatives are given by mouth to clear the intestine of feces. Some patients also require enemas. Finally, oral nonabsorbable antibiotics are given to kill bacteria in the bowel. Overnight fasting is required for general anesthesia.

ANESTHESIA

General anesthesia.

PROCEDURE

- An abdominal incision is usually made vertically down the middle.
- The blood supply to the sigmoid colon and the fatty tissue in which it runs (mesocolon) is divided between clamps and tied with sutures.
- The bowel is clamped and divided above and below the diseased area.
- The affected segment is removed.
- Colonic continuity is restored either by suturing the ends together or by stapling them with a specially designed colonic stapling device.
- If a COLOSTOMY is required, the colon is brought out through the abdominal wall.
- The abdominal wall is closed in layers with sutures.

HOSPITAL RECOVERY

Intestinal motility decreases after the operation, and patients do not tolerate oral nutrition or fluid until bowel function returns. Bowel function, manifest by return of bowel sounds and passing of flatus and feces, returns in about three to five days. Intravenous fluids and pain medications such as morphine and meperidine are required until that time. Once bowel function resumes, a liquid diet is begun and patients are advanced to a regular diet as tolerated. Intravenous fluids are stopped, and oral medications such as an acetaminophen and codeine combination are begun.

The patient is encouraged to get out of bed and walk as soon as possible and to cough and take deep breaths to avoid respiratory complications.

Patients are discharged from the hospital as soon as they are on a regular diet. This usually takes seven to ten days.

AT-HOME RECOVERY

Recovery at home requires another several weeks. Patients gradually increase their activity as pain subsides. Bowel habits usually return to normal as the patient resumes normal dietary habits and daily routines.

Patients may drive a car when their pain has subsided, and they are not taking pain medications that cause drowsiness.

COMPLICATIONS AND RISKS

- Postoperative ileus is prolonged loss of motility after abdominal surgery. Eating causes ABDOMINAL SWELLING and VOMITING. The patient may require parenteral nutrition (nutrition not delivered orally). Prolonged ileus usually resolves spontaneously, but it does prolong hospitalization.
- Postoperative INTESTINAL OBSTRUCTION can be caused by scars from the operation or problems at the area where the bowel was sewn together.
- Anastomotic leak is a failure of the intestine to heal, causing leaking of intestinal contents, an abscess, or soiling of the abdominal cavity.
- PNEUMONIA may result because postoperative pain may make deep breathing and coughing difficult.
- Wound infection is an unlikely possibility.

SPLEEN REMOVAL

Spleen removal is performed to remove and evaluate the extent of tumors, to treat abscesses, and to remove the organ when it is trapping and sequestering blood cells or platelets.

The spleen is an organ in the upper left abdomen, which is part of the immune system. It also clears old and damaged blood components from the circulation. The spleen can be involved with malignant tumors (especially LYMPHOMA, NON-HODGKIN), can develop abscesses, and may enlarge considerably in response to other systemic illnesses. Spleen removal (splenectomy) may be necessary to remove and evaluate the extent of tumors, to treat abscesses, or to remove the organ when it is trapping and sequestering blood cells. Finally, the spleen is susceptible to injury during trauma to the chest, flank, and abdomen. Removal of the spleen may be necessary to stop bleeding.

Splenectomy is performed by a trauma or general surgeon.

ALTERNATIVE TREATMENTS

Most disorders of the spleen are treated initially with medications such as prednisone for autoimmune diseases. Removal of the spleen is performed when medical treatment is not effective.

Techniques have been developed to remove the spleen using laparoscopy (a form of ENDOSCOPY), which decreases postoperative pain and recovery time.

PREOPERATIVE PREPARATION

Patients undergoing elective removal of the spleen receive pneumococcal vaccine several weeks before the operation. BLOOD TESTS and ELECTROCARDIOGRAPHY are sometimes performed to assess general health before the operation. Overnight fasting is required with general anesthesia.

ANESTHESIA

General anesthesia.

PROCEDURE

For surgical removal
- An incision is made in the middle of the upper abdomen or below the left rib cage.
- The spleen's attachments to other organs are cut.
- The splenic artery and vein (the main blood supply) are then tied with sutures and divided.

- The spleen is removed.
- The abdominal wound is closed in layers with sutures and the skin is closed with sutures or clips.

For laparoscopic removal

- Five or six puncture wounds are made.
- A video camera is inserted through one of these wounds and instruments through the others.
- The surgeon and assistants remove the spleen while watching the surgery on a video monitor.
- The surgery is similar to the open procedure described above.
- The spleen is divided into smaller pieces and is removed through one of the puncture wounds.
- The puncture wounds are closed with sutures.

HOSPITAL RECOVERY

Patients undergoing open splenectomy remain in the hospital for three to ten days, depending on the reason for removal of their spleen. They are not able to take liquids or foods early after the surgery and need intravenous fluids and medications such as morphine and meperidine.

Patients who undergo laparoscopic removal of the spleen remain in the hospital for one to five days.

AT-HOME RECOVERY

Postoperative convalescence at home is variable and ranges from two to eight weeks for open operation and from one to three weeks for laparoscopic surgery. Patients may require oral pain medication such as an acetaminophen and codeine combination.

Patients may drive a car when their pain has subsided, and they are not taking pain medications that cause drowsiness.

COMPLICATIONS AND RISKS

- Postoperative bleeding may occur.
- An intra-abdominal abscess can cause FEVER, ABDOMINAL PAIN, and prolonged recovery.
- PNEUMONIA may result, because postoperative incisional pain may make deep breathing and coughing difficult.
- Wound infection is an unlikely possibility.

THYROIDECTOMY

The thyroid gland is located in the neck. Its hormone is vital to proper metabolic functioning. A number of conditions related to the thyroid gland may require surgical treatment.

A surgeon treats three groups of patients with thyroid disease: those with an overactive gland (HYPERTHYROIDISM), those with an underactive gland (HYPOTHYROIDISM), and those with suspicious masses (tumors, cysts, or nodules) in the gland. Removal of all or part of the thyroid may be required in each of these situations. The operation is performed by a general surgeon, an endocrine surgeon, or an otolaryngologist (an ear, nose, and throat specialist).

Surgery is also performed for goiter—a benign enlargement of the gland—when the goiter causes symptoms.

ALTERNATIVE TREATMENTS

HYPERTHYROIDISM may be treated with antithyroid drugs and radioactive iodine. The type of treatment is based on many factors, including the patient's age, other medical conditions, and the severity and progression of the disease.

HYPOTHYROIDISM can be treated with replacement of thyroid hormone.

Nodules in the thyroid gland consist of masses that function and those that do not (cysts and solid growths). Cysts may be treated with thyroid hormone if they show no signs of cancer on aspiration. Functioning nodules may be observed if the patient does not have HYPERTHYROIDISM.

PREOPERATIVE PREPARATION

Patients should have thyroid function tests (see BLOOD TESTS) and a thyroid scan (see NUCLEAR MEDICINE). Patients with nodules should also undergo BIOPSY to distinguish among cysts, benign nodules, and cancer.

Patients with HYPERTHYROIDISM who are candidates for surgery require suppression of the gland with iodine alone or with a combination of iodine and propylthiouracil. Some patients are also given propranolol to block the effects of thyroid hormone on other organs.

BLOOD TESTS and ELECTROCARDIOGRAPHY, among other tests of general health, are standard before almost any surgery. Overnight fasting is required with general anesthesia.

ANESTHESIA

General anesthesia.

PROCEDURE

- An incision is made across the lower neck, and skin flaps are made above and below the incision.
- The muscles covering the thyroid gland are retracted or divided, and the gland is exposed. The vein to the middle of the gland and the arteries to the top and the bottom are identified, tied off, and cut.
- The lobe is removed from the windpipe with the isthmus (the portion that connects the two lobes).
- If the entire gland is to be removed, the opposite lobe is removed in a similar manner.
- The wounds are closed with sutures or clips.

HOSPITAL RECOVERY

Hospital stay is usually one to two days. Patients usually experience postoperative pain and require pain medications such as acetaminophen and codeine combination.

Sutures may be removed in three to five days.

AT-HOME RECOVERY

Patients who have had a total thyroidectomy require life-time replacement of thyroid hormone.

COMPLICATIONS

- Thyroid storm refers to a severe case of HYPERTHY-ROIDISM that may occur in patients who have not been adequately prepared preoperatively with antithyroid medications.
- A hematoma is a collection of blood beneath the wound. If large, it can press on the windpipe and interfere with breathing.
- Injury to the recurrent laryngeal nerve causes paralysis of the vocal cord and a hoarse voice.
- HYPOTHYROIDISM will occur when all or most of the thyroid gland is removed. It is treated by giving thyroid hormone replacement.

TRACHEOSTOMY

A tracheostomy is a procedure that establishes an alternative pathway for the passage of air while breathing. An opening is made in the neck into the trachea (the windpipe) to allow passage of air if the upper airway is obstructed or if long-term ventilation of the lungs is required.

Indications for tracheostomy fall into three major categories, including

- Upper airway obstruction resulting from tumors such as LARYNGEAL CANCER, trauma, infection, neuromuscular disorders, or malformations
- Diseases of the lungs such as EMPHYSEMA or severe PNEUMONIA that require prolonged ventilator support
- The inability of the patient to manage secretions from either the mouth or the lungs

Surgeons and emergency medicine physicians are trained in this procedure.

ALTERNATIVE TREATMENTS

When an emergency airway is required, there are several options. Often, ventilation can be achieved using an oxygen mask over the nose and mouth. An endotracheal tube can be passed through the mouth and larynx and into the trachea if this is medically safe and possible.

PREOPERATIVE PREPARATION

In an emergency setting, there is often little time for preoperative preparation.

When the tracheostomy is elective, routine preoperative tests such as BLOOD COUNT and other BLOOD TESTS are performed.

Overnight fasting is required with general anesthesia.

ANESTHESIA

Anesthesia may be either general or local. Local anesthesia is often combined with sedation.

PROCEDURE

- An incision is made in the front of the neck over the trachea.

> Tracheostomy is often performed as an emergency procedure when airway obstruction is acute.

- The midline of the muscles of the trachea is identified, and the muscles are gently separated.
- Retraction is used to hold the muscles to the sides, exposing the area of the trachea and the thyroid.
- An opening is made in the front wall of the trachea and secretions are immediately suctioned out.
- A tube is placed through the opening into the trachea, sutured to the skin, and secured around the neck with a cloth band.

HOSPITAL RECOVERY

Recovery usually includes a one night stay in the intensive care unit followed by one week in the hospital. During this time, the patient and caregivers learn proper care and cleaning of the tracheostomy tube.

AT-HOME RECOVERY

Recovery at home is centered on proper care of the tracheostomy tube. Since the normal airflow is diverted from the nose, the functions of air humidification and clearance of secretions are altered. Initially the patient will require humidified air. Suctioning of secretions from the lungs with a catheter is necessary.

A tracheostomy can be temporary. When the tube is removed, the opening will slowing close by contracture of scarring. A few patients will need an operation to completely close the opening.

COMPLICATIONS AND RISKS

A blockage of the tube may occur if the tube is not cleaned frequently enough to keep it clear. Mucus or dried secretions may plug the trachea or deeper bronchi in the lungs if proper humidification and suctioning are not observed.

The tracheostomy tube may become dislodged from the trachea if the cloth ties securing it around the neck are not kept snug.

Finally, in rare cases, there may be bleeding from the tube. Bleeding from the trachea is potentially a very serious sign of erosion of the tracheostomy tube into an artery.

TUBAL LIGATION

Tubal ligation is a permanent form of contraception. This procedure should be considered only by women who have completed childbearing or by women who do not desire to bear children. Tubal ligation is highly effective: Less than 0.5 percent of patients undergoing the procedure become pregnant. However, if the procedure fails, approximately 50 percent of pregnancies will be ectopic. Therefore, if a woman misses a period following tubal ligation, a pregnancy test is mandatory. Should the test be positive, the woman must seek immediate medical care.

ALTERNATIVE TREATMENTS

Alternatives to tubal ligation include VASECTOMY for the woman's partner and injectable or implantable hormonal contraceptives. These methods are as effective as tubal ligation. However, the latter two are reversible. Other birth control methods such as intrauterine devices (IUDs) and barrier methods are available, but they are not as consistently effective as surgical sterilization.

PREOPERATIVE PREPARATION

Tubal ligation should be performed within the first ten days of the menstrual cycle to ensure that the patient is not pregnant. A BLOOD COUNT and pregnancy test are done upon admission. Overnight fasting is required for general anesthesia.

ANESTHESIA

The majority of tubal ligations are performed under general anesthesia, although spinal anesthesia is an alternative.

PROCEDURE

For tubal ligation performed by laparoscopy (a form of ENDOSCOPY)

- Two incisions, a half inch in size, are made at the belly button and pubic area.
- A laparoscope is inserted through the lower incision.
- Gas is used to distend the abdomen.

> Tubal ligation is a highly effective, permanent contraceptive procedure that only women who do not desire any more children should undergo.

- The pelvis is examined.
- A segment of the fallopian tube is destroyed, which prohibits the passage of the egg and sperm so that fertilization of the egg does not occur.
- The laparoscope is then removed, the gas allowed to escape, and the incisions at the belly button and pubic area are closed with sutures.

Vaginal and postpartum tubal ligations entail a different approach, but most tubal ligations are performed laparoscopically.

HOSPITAL RECOVERY

A tubal ligation is an outpatient procedure. After the surgery, a nurse monitors vital signs and observes the patient for surgical or anesthetic complications. Pain medicine such as an acetaminophen and codeine combination may be administered, and most patients will get drowsy.

If no problems arise, the patient will be given liquids, and when able, will be assisted to the rest room. Most patients remain in the recovery room for approximately two hours after the procedure. Rarely, patients will experience nausea and VOMITING severe enough to require an overnight stay.

AT-HOME RECOVERY

Upon arrival home, the patient should rest. Fluids and a bland diet are best the day of surgery. Ibuprofen is effective for relief of cramping. Driving is not recommended for 24 hours following surgery, but within three days of surgery, the patient should be able to resume normal activities. Intercourse and use of tampons are restricted for two weeks after tubal ligation.

COMPLICATIONS AND RISKS

Major complications of tubal ligation are rare (less than one percent). They include internal bleeding and intra-abdominal infection. A laparotomy (incision of the abdomen) may be needed to correct these complications. Death occurs in 1 in 30,000 procedures.

ULTRASONIC LITHOTRIPSY

Ultrasonic lithotripsy is a procedure in which kidney stones or gallstones are broken into fragments using shock waves.

An ultrasonic lithotripter is a device designed to fragment KIDNEY STONES and GALLSTONES without surgery. After fragmentation, the pieces of the stone either pass spontaneously in urine or bile, are dissolved, or must be removed using ENDOSCOPY or surgical techniques.

ALTERNATIVE TREATMENTS

See KIDNEY STONES and GALLSTONES.

PREOPERATIVE PREPARATION

Stones must be identified before the procedure with X rays (RADIOGRAPHY) for KIDNEY STONES, and ULTRASOUND for GALL-STONES. Overnight fasting is required for general anesthesia.

ANESTHESIA

Intravenous sedation or general anesthesia is used.

PROCEDURE

- The patient is placed into a water bath or in contact with a gel-filled flexible membrane.
- Shock waves are sent through the water or gel.
- X rays (RADIOGRAPHY) for KIDNEY STONES, or ULTRA-SOUND for GALLSTONES are used to locate the stones.
- Shock waves are generated by the lithotripter and focused precisely on the stone.
- Fragmentation requires multiple shock waves.

HOSPITAL RECOVERY

Patients are discharged the same or the next day.

AT-HOME RECOVERY

Patients may require pain medication such as an acetaminophen and codeine combination after treatment.

COMPLICATIONS AND RISKS

- Shock waves can damage tissues near the stone.
- Patients can experience bleeding in the urine or bile.

ULTRASOUND

Ultrasound uses sound waves, like sonar, to bounce off a body part under the skin. The reflection can be used to give a picture of the shape and consistency of the internal organs. Ultrasound has a wide variety of uses, including looking for GALLSTONES, clots in blood vessels, or ATHEROSCLEROSIS. When used for studying the heart valves and heart muscle, it is called *echocardiography*.

PREPARATION

There may be minor preparation, such as drinking lots of fluids to fill the bladder, before certain pelvic ultrasounds.

PROCEDURE

- When the test is to be performed entirely externally, a special gel is put on the skin to help the ultrasound probe make optimal contact with the skin.
- The transducer—the device that generates and collects the sound waves—is placed in direct contact with the skin and passed over the area to be viewed.
- The pictures can be seen in real time on a video monitor or as still images.

There are also special ultrasound probes that are passed into the body. Examples of these include a rectal probe to look at the prostate, a vaginal probe to look at the pelvic organs, a probe on an endoscope (see ENDOSCOPY) to go down the esophagus to look at the heart and aorta (transesophageal echocardiography), and even special ultrasound probes that can pass through the skin into an artery.

RECOVERY

Usually, no observation is required for an ultrasound. In the case of passing an ultrasound catheter into an artery, an overnight stay may be necessary. If a sedative is used, then observation for an hour or so may be needed.

COMPLICATIONS AND RISKS

Routine ultrasound tests are without any significant side effects. If an artery is penetrated to study it from the inside, there is a small chance of bleeding and other risks.

Unlike other radiologic imaging techniques, ultrasound uses no radiation and no iodinated contrast materials or dyes.

URINALYSIS

A urinalysis helps in the diagnosis of many conditions affecting the kidneys, urinary tract, liver, and other metabolic functions.

Urine is the liquid produced by the continuous filtration of blood by the kidneys. The kidneys are very efficient, so urine should not contain any blood sugar or blood cells, and only minimal amounts of protein.

Urine is a "window" to the kidneys and can serve as an important clue to kidney function, urinary tract infections, and even liver and other metabolic diagnoses. Urine can also be analyzed for additional chemicals and special proteins. In some cases, a 24-hour collection is needed.

PREPARATION

When looking for infection, caution must be used in the collecting of a urine specimen to minimize contamination with skin near the urethra, the passageway and body opening where urine comes out. Prolonged standing can affect the amount of protein lost in the urine in some individuals, so specific instructions may be given if this is suspected.

PROCEDURE

- The opening of the urethra to the outside of the body is cleansed with a sterile pad.
- The middle portion of the urine stream (after the first few seconds) is the portion that is caught in a sterile cup.
- The sample is sent to the lab for analysis.

RECOVERY

None.

COMPLICATIONS AND RISKS

None.

VARICOSE VEIN REMOVAL

VARICOSE VEINS, found usually in the legs, result when the valves of the veins break and are unable to keep blood from backing up. Blood has a tendency to stagnate in the dilated veins. Because the pressure inside VARICOSE VEINS is greater than that of normal veins, the veins are engorged and visible on the surface of the skin.

A tendency to develop VARICOSE VEINS seems to run in families. Other predisposing factors include previous clots or inflammations of the leg veins, called thrombophlebitis, or any condition that obstructs the normal outflow of the venous blood from the legs, such as pregnancy, tight garments, or obesity.

ALTERNATIVE TREATMENTS

The first approach to VARICOSE VEINS should be the use of support stockings with pressure capacities between 30 and 50 mm Hg. Elevating the legs, avoiding prolonged standing, and removing any potential outlet obstruction of the legs are important first steps. However, once the valves in the veins are broken, or collapsed, there is no way to repair them. In rare severe cases, deep vein replacement surgery can be attempted.

There are no strictly medical therapies that eliminate VARICOSE VEINS.

For very small, thin VARICOSE VEINS, or small dilated surface blood vessels, another technique is available. The surgeon can introduce a small needle into the vessel and inject salty water or a chemical that causes the vessel to contract and become occluded (closed off). This procedure is called *sclerotherapy*. After the procedure, the patient usually wears a compression bandage or garment to keep the treated, sclerosed veins occluded and allow scar formation to make the occlusion permanent.

Newer technology consists of machines that emit laser light. One wavelength of laser light is very well absorbed by the pigment inside the blood vessels but not by skin tissues. Therefore, the laser light can obliterate vessels containing red blood cells and not injure the other skin tissues. This technology is starting to be used to treat small superficial vessels in the skin of the legs when patients desire varicose vein removal for cosmetic reasons.

> Because there is no evidence that proves the removal of superficial leg veins will truly alter the course of disease due to varicose veins, removal of the superficial veins is considered a cosmetic procedure.

Preoperative preparation

None.

Anesthesia

Usually none is needed for sclerotherapy. For vein removal, a local anesthetic is used.

Procedure

- The surgeon makes an incision in the skin above the vein.
- The varicose vein is then cut through and tied off at both ends of the cut with a suture.
- The surgeon performs the same procedure at another part of the same vein some distance away.
- The surgeon can then remove the tied-off vein through the skin. (The patient is left with two small scars at each end of the site where the vein was removed.)

Again, whether this procedure prevents the occurrence of conditions resulting from VARICOSE VEINS is controversial, but it definitely removes the unsightly vein.

Hospital recovery

The procedure is usually performed on an outpatient basis and requires no hospital stay.

At-home recovery

Wound care is necessary for the first few weeks.

Complications and risks

Excessive bleeding and local wound infection are possibilities but are rare.

VASECTOMY

Vasectomy is a minor surgical procedure to cut the tubes that carry sperm from the testes to the urethra. This elective procedure is done for sterilization only. Usually performed by a urologist, vasectomy takes place in an outpatient setting.

ALTERNATIVE TREATMENTS

There are no other options as far as male sterilization is concerned. Other methods of birth control are available, of course.

PREOPERATIVE PREPARATION

The scrotum is usually shaved in the areas of the incision. Otherwise, there are no special preparations.

ANESTHESIA

Local anesthesia.

PROCEDURE

- A small incision is made in the skin of the scrotum.
- The vas deferens (the duct that runs from each testicle) is identified and cut; the ends are then tied off.
- The incision is sewn up.
- The procedure is then repeated on the opposite side.

A postoperative semen analysis is sometimes performed to ensure the absence of sperm. Other birth control is necessary until the laboratory studies confirm the sterility.

RECOVERY

Activity should be restricted for one or two days. Oral pain medication such as an acetaminophen and codeine combination may be prescribed if necessary. It can be helpful to wear underwear with good scrotal support (briefs, for example) for a few weeks after surgery.

COMPLICATIONS

Complications are very uncommon. The only dangers are excessive bleeding and the remote possibility of infection at the wound site.

> Vasectomy is probably the most effective form of birth control. The procedure is simple and very safe.

INDEX

Retropubic prostate gland removal, 363
Reye syndrome, 193
Rheumatic heart disease, 97, 128, 168
Rheumatoid arthritis
  anemia and, 80
  backache and, 12
  causes, 253
  complications, 254
  diagnosis, 254
  ear ringing or buzzing and, 27
  eye pain and, 31
  loss of appetite and, 11
  lupus erythematosus and, 209
  neck pain and, 47
  numbness and, 49
  psoriasis and, 248
  symptoms, 253
  treatment, 255
Ringworm, 51
Rocky Mountain spotted fever, 18, 51
Rotavirus, 23
Rubella, 51

S
Salmonella, 23, 158
Salt (sodium) intake
  atrial fibrillation and, 97
  congestive heart failure and, 127
  fainting or faintness and, 34
  hypertension and, 183
  weight gain and, 72
Scabies, 51
Scaling and root planing, 241, 360
Sciatica, 49
Sclerosing cholangitis, defined, 132, 272
Sclerotherapy, 278, 383
Scrotum, 38, 58. *See also* Testicular cancer.
Scurvy, defined, 18
Seizures, 313
Senile tremor, defined, 60
Sepsis, 102. See also Infection
Septicemia, 102. See also Blood poisoning.
Septoplasty, 48
Seroma, defined, 352
Sexual intercourse
  bladder infection and, 98, 99
  cervical cancer and, 117, 118
  endometriosis and, 150
  impotence and, 188–189
  ovarian cysts and, 229
  post-hysterectomy, 334
Sexually transmitted diseases
  AIDS and, 75, 77

Sexually transmitted diseases *(continued)*
  hepatitis and, 171, 173
  painful urination and, 63
  pelvic inflammatory disease and, 238, 239
  vaginitis and, 66, 275, 276
Sezary syndrome, 139
Shigella, 23, 158
Shingles
  AIDS and, 75
  causes, 256
  complications, 257
  diagnosis, 256
  earache and, 29, 30
  prevention, 257
  rash and, 51
  symptoms, 256
  treatment, 257
Sigmoid colon removal, 125, 370–371
Sigmoidoscope/sigmoidoscopy, 14. *See also* Endoscopy.
Sinus rhythm, defined, 97
Sinusitis, 37
Sitz baths, hemorrhoids and, 52, 170, 323, 325, 326
Sjögren syndrome, 254
Skin cancer
  causes, 258
  diagnosis, 259
  prevention, 259
  rash and, 51
  skin changes and, 53, 54
  symptoms, 258
  treatment, 259, 348
Skin changes
  as a symptom, 53–54
  varicose veins and, 277, 278
Skin conditions, 138, 139. *See also* Boils; Dermatitis; Psoriasis; Shingles.
Skin tests, allergy, 280–281
Sleep apnea, defined, 35.
Sleep problems, 35–36, 62
Slipped disk. *See* Herniated disk.
Smoking
  asthma and, 90
  chronic bronchitis and, 108, 109
  cough and, 21
  emphysema and, 147, 149
  gingivitis and, 160
  heart attack and, 164, 166
  laryngeal cancer and, 202, 203
  lung cancer and, 207, 208
  oral cancer and, 221, 222
  pancreatic cancer and, 231, 232
  periodontitis and, 240, 241
  stroke and, 262, 263

Sodium. *See* Salt (sodium) intake.
Spastic colon, defined, 196
Spinal tap, defined, 344
Spleen removal (splenectomy), 179, 205, 372–373
Sprue, 23
Squamous cell skin cancer, 258, 259
Staphylococcus aureus, 104, 105, 139
Status *asthmaticus*, defined, 91
Stenotic heart valve, defined, 167
Stents, defined, 84, 282
Sterilization, 378–379, 385
Steroids. *See* Corticosteroids.
Stoma, defined, 287, 288, 303, 335
Stomach cancer
  appetite, loss of, 11
  causes, 260
  complications, 261
  diagnosis, 260–261
  prevention, 261
  symptoms, 260
  treatment, 261
  weight loss and, 73
Stones. *See* Bladder stones; Gallstones; Kidney stones.
Stool, abnormal appearance
  colorectal cancer and, 124
  pancreatic cancer and, 231
  as a symptom, 55
  ulcerative colitis and, 271
  ulcers and, 269
Stool impaction, 13–14
Stool softeners, 130, 146
Strangulated hernia, 174, 175
Strep throat infections, heart valve disease and, 97, 128, 168
Streptococcus pneumoniae (pneumococcal pneumonia), 242, 243
Streptokinase, 165, 251, 267
Stress incontinence, defined, 190
Stress reduction. *See also* Anxiety.
  arrhythmia and, 88
  Crohn disease and, 132
  dizziness and, 26
  headaches and, 41
  hypertension, 183
Stroke
  anemia and, 81
  arrhythmia and, 88
  atherosclerosis and, 93, 94
  atrial fibrillation and, 96
  cardiomyopathy and, 113
  carotid endartectomy, 296–297
  causes, 262
  complications, 263
  congestive heart failure and, 127
  diagnosis, 263